ALIMENTARY SPHINCTERS
AND THEIR DISORDERS

ALIMENTARY SPHINCTERS AND THEIR DISORDERS

Edited by

Paul A. Thomas

Senior Lecturer and Consultant Surgeon, The London Hospital, London, E1 1BB

and

Charles V. Mann

Consultant Surgeon, The London and St Mark's Hospitals, London

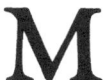

First published 1981 by
Scientific and Medical Division
MACMILLAN PUBLISHERS LTD
London and Basingstoke
Companies and representatives throughout the world

Filmset by Reproduction Drawings Ltd., Sutton, Surrey

ISBN 978-1-349-03942-5   ISBN 978-1-349-03940-1 (eBook)
DOI 10.1007/978-1-349-03940-1

Contents

The Contributors

W. N. W. Baker, MS, FRCS
Dept of Surgery
Ashford Hospital
Middlesex

T. W. Balfour, MB, ChB, FRCS
Dept of Surgery
Nottingham Medical School

A. Bennett, BPh, DSc, PhD
Dept of Surgery
King's College Hospital Medical
School
London, SE5

A. D'Mello, MSc, PhD
Dept of Pharmacology
The London Hospital Medical
College
London, E1 2AD

E. P. DiMagno, MD
Gastroenterology Unit
Mayo Clinic
Rochester, Minnesota 55901,
USA

H. L. Duthie, MD, ChM, FRCS
Welsh National School of
Medicine
Cardiff, South Glamorgan

C. E. Gabriel, MB, ChB, DLO
Dept of Otorhinolaryngology
ENT Hospital
Greenock, Scotland

A. G. Johnson, MCh, FRCS
University Surgical Unit
Hallamshire Hospital
Sheffield, South Yorkshire

F. B. Keane, MB, FRCS
Dept of Surgery
St James Hospital
Dublin, Irish Republic

P. McKelvie, MD, ChM, FRCS
Dept of Otorhinolaryngology
The London Hospital
London, E1 1BB

C. V. Mann, MCh, FRCS
Dept of Surgery
The London Hospital
London, E1 1BB

A. G. L. Peel, MA, MChir,
FRCS
North Tees General Hospital
Stockton-on-Tees
Cleveland

D. R. E. Reeve, PhD, MD,
FRCS
Dept of Anatomy
The London Hospital Medical
College
London, E1 2AD

P. A. Thomas, BSc, MS, FRCS
Dept of Surgery
The London Hospital
London, E1 1BB

H. H. Thompson, BSc, FRCS
Dept of Surgery
The London Hospital
London, E1 1BB

Preface

What is a sphincter? It used to be thought that the function of the specialised areas defined as 'sphincters' was to delay the onward passage of the fluids and solids from the organs which 'emptied' through them. It is now realised that this concept was too facile, and that these zones act in a very complex regulatory fashion and that they are able to change their functions to suit the requirements of the whole gastrointestinal tract. Nor is the organisation of each sphincter an exact replica of the rest: some are 'closed' and some are 'open'; some have a well-defined anatomical structure, others are not defined at all; some act as 'brakes' but others can possess an acceleratory characteristic.

With the increasing power of modern pharmaceutical ingredients, many of which (e.g. ganglion-blocking agents and prostaglandins) act directly on the smooth muscle of the alimentary canal, as well as the much increased safety and numbers of major surgical interventions, we considered it appropriate to draw together the current knowledge and ideas concerning the sphincters of the gastrointestinal tract. As these sphincteric regions are perhaps the most widely investigated areas of alimentary motor function, they provide well-defined examples of the correlation between gastrointestinal motor dysfunction and recognised clinical disorders. It is hoped that showing how they perform their functions will stimulate further research as well as increasing the respect that they deserve from all those physicians and surgeons who interfere with them.

The book would not have been possible without the full co-operation of the contributors. Each has brought to his work a high level of expertise, thoughtfulness and clarity of expression. It is especially relevant that most of the contributors are actively involved in the practice of clinical gastroenterology, which has enabled them to provide a relevant correlation between basic scientific data and the clinical disorders of sphincteric

ix

function. We are extremely grateful to them all for their contributions.

On a sad note, we have to report the untimely death of Mr David Reeve, whose surgically orientated chapter on the anatomy of alimentary sphincters provides the introduction to this book.

We are indebted to Ms Linda Bray for helping with the editing and typing of the manuscripts, together with Ms Lynda Randall, Diane Tolfree and Jenny Bignold.

Finally, our publishers have been helpful throughout, and we are grateful to Mr R. M. Powell of Macmillan Publishers for his succinct advice on the practicalities of producing a book such as this one.

London, 1981   PAT
                                                                                 CVM

1
Anatomy of the Sphincters of the Alimentary Canal

D. R. E. Reeve

INTRODUCTION

The word 'sphincter' is derived from the Greek *sphingein* (to bind tight), and means a ring-like muscle which controls the opening of a body orifice or constricts the lumen of a natural body passage.

Sphincters are found in the respiratory, genito-urinary and alimentary tracts, but particularly in the latter. This is only to be expected, considering the complex changes of physical and chemical form which take place in ingested materials during their delayed passage from mouth to anus. It is this delay which is one of the essential functions of the alimentary sphincters. Food is delayed in the stomach while it is mixed with acid and enzymes; this mixture is then delayed in the small intestine during digestion and absorption; and finally the faeces are delayed in the colon and rectum for water and ion exchanges and for storage prior to expulsion when the opportunity arises. Looking overall at sphincters, this is an oversimplification. There are many other functions which may be attributed to sphincters and there are many functional aspects which are, as yet, imperfectly understood. Of the more obvious specialised functions, for example, the larynx presents a primary method of defence against the inhalation of ingested food, the cardiac sphincter prevents the reflux of gastric contents into the oesophagus, and the anal sphincters maintain faecal continence.

An anatomical study of the well-recognised sphincters runs into difficulties if the traditional definition of a sphincter is adhered to—i.e. the demonstration of a ring-like muscle controlling a body opening or natural passage. In some instances (the gastro-oesophageal sphincter, for example) no ring-like muscle can be demonstrated in man, and yet clearly a functional sphincter exists. In such cases the anatomical horizons have to be widened beyond the accepted conventions of the subject in order to relate the physiological aspects of the subject to the architectural structure, which may fail to concur with the expected traditional anatomical arrangement. It is unfortunate that we have burdened ourselves with terminological distinctions such as 'anatomical sphincter' and 'physiological sphincter' when the functional result is the same, rather than to correlate the anatomical facts with the functional mechanisms as they become known. This is especially true of the alimentary tract, which is becoming more and more physiologically complex and where structural dogmatism can add little to the advancement of function understanding.

PHARYNX

There are three well-recognised sphincter mechanisms to be considered in the pharyngeal part of the gastrointestinal tract. First, the palatopharyngeal sphincter, which prevents the bolus from passing upwards into the nasopharynx during swallowing; second, the larynx, which prevents the inhalation of swallowed liquids and solids; and third, the cricopharyngeus, which acts as an upper oesophageal sphincter which relaxes to allow the bolus to pass into the oesophagus.

Palatopharyngeal Sphincter

This is formed by a constant band of muscle which is considered to be part of the palatopharyngeus muscle and is often termed the palatopharyngeal constrictor muscle. It arises from the lateral and anterior aspects of the superior surface of the palatine aponeurosis, and passes backwards lateral to levator veli palatini to unite with the muscle of the opposite side on the anterior surface of the superior constrictor muscle with which it blends. This band produces a ridge on the pharyngeal wall when the soft palate is elevated during swallowing, known as the ridge of Passavant. The soft palate, duly tensed and elevated, meets the protruding fold, forming an effective seal to protect the nasopharynx. As swallowing proceeds, the palate and fold move downwards, carrying the bolus with them. It has been suggested by Ramsay *et al.* (1955), using cinefluorography, that Passavant's ridge is produced, at least in part, by the localised activity of the superior constrictor muscle, because Passavant's ridge, as it descends during swallowing, is often succeeded by a second and lower fold in the posterior pharyngeal wall. This may be true, but that a major role during swallowing is played by the palatopharyngeal constrictor muscle is strongly suggested by the considerable hypertrophy of the muscle that occurs in cases of complete cleft palate.

The Larynx

The primary function of the larynx is to act as a sphincter to protect the respiratory passages during the act of swallowing; phonation should be considered to be a secondary function. The detailed anatomy of the larynx is not pertinent here, but the relevant structures which are held to be responsible for this function may be briefly listed.

The Epiglottis

It has been said by Ramsay *et al.* (1955) that as the larynx rises during swallowing the epiglottis folds backwards over the larynx. This protective function has been affirmed and denied, both before and after this report, and the exact mechanism and purpose of this proposed movement, passive or active, remains a mystery. However, it seems clear that the epiglottis, in any case, functions as a diverter of the bolus away from the midline through the piriform fossae into the hypopharynx. It appears unlikely that it is the major laryngeal sphincter mechanism, because patients who have the epiglottis removed for carcinoma, or those in whom it has been destroyed by disease, have no difficulty in swallowing.

The Sphincter of the Inlet

The free upper edge of the quadrate membrane contains a muscle, the aryepiglottic muscle, which connects the sides of the epiglottis to the opposite arytenoid cartilage. This muscle has been conceived of as being a complete sphincter of the laryngeal inlet which, on contraction, opposes the arytenoids to each other and to the posterior surface of the epiglottis in the region of its cushion. This muscle is not always well developed around the free edge of the quadrate membrane, in which case its function is ascribed to the thyro-epiglottic muscle, which lies outside the quadrate membrane.

The Vestibular and Vocal Folds

It seems unlikely that these folds act as the primary laryngeal sphincters, but rather as secondary mechanisms of defence. However, Ramsay *et al.* (1955) considered that the vestibular fold and sometimes the vocal folds are responsible for the protection, particularly in the case of liquids, of the laryngeal inlet.

In cases where the aryepiglottic and thyro-epiglottic muscles are paralysed (e.g. by damage to the recurrent laryngeal nerves), the inlet of the larynx is not closed during swallowing, and the lax aryepiglottic folds collapse medially and allow fluids to overflow into the larynx. Even so, in these patients inhalation is comparatively rare, and the isthmus must be protected in these cases by the vestibular and vocal folds in the absence of any alternative sphincter mechanism.

Cricopharyngeal Sphincter

Around the upper end of the oesophagus there is a collection of almost circular muscle fibres belonging to the inferior constrictor muscle, which normally keeps the oesophagus closed off from the hypopharynx. This muscle relaxes in advance of the propulsive contractions of the constrictor muscles of the pharynx during the act of swallowing.

The inferior constrictor is the thickest of the constrictor muscles and consists of two parts, named after the origins of the particular muscle fibres—the thyropharyngeus and the cricopharyngeus. The muscle arises from the oblique line of the thyroid cartilage, from an area of the surface of the lamina behind this line and from a tendinous band which passes from the inferior thyroid tubercle to the cricoid cartilage. In addition, a small slip of muscle arises from the inferior cornu of the thyroid cartilage; the whole of this muscular origin constitutes the thyropharyngeus.

Muscle fibres which arise from the cricoid cartilage in the interval between the origin of cricothyroid anteriorly and the articular facet for the inferior cornu of the thyroid cartilage posteriorly constitute the cricopharyngeal part of the inferior constrictor. The fibres of thyropharyngeus pass backwards, medially and upwards as far as the pharyngeal ligament and insert with the muscle of the opposite side into the pharyngeal raphe, which lies in the posteromedian plane of the pharyngeal wall. Some of the fibres of cricopharyngeus insert in a similar fashion into the pharyngeal raphe, but the inferior fibres are circular and continuous with the circular muscle layer of the oesophagus. The ascending fibres of thyropharyngeus surround the middle constrictor muscle where the lumen of the pharynx is widest; descending from this point, the lumen decreases in size and is at its narrowest at the level of the circular fibres of the cricopharyngeus muscle. During the act of swallowing, the middle constrictor muscle and the thyropharyngeal part of the inferior constrictor act as propulsive muscles for the bolus, while cricopharyngeus acts as the sphincteric part of the muscle, which relaxes to allow of the passage of the bolus into the oesophagus.

Pharyngeal Diverticula

These occur in the lower part of the pharynx in most instances, close to the junction of the pharynx and oesophagus. Various causes have been ascribed to the formation of these pouches, the most common being that they are pulsion diverticula which herniate through an area of congenital weakness in the muscle coat of the pharyngeal wall. This appears to be most unlikely, at least as regards a congenital weakness, as most occur in later life and are rare before the age of 20 years.

Pharyngeal diverticula have been noted in cases of oesophageal obstruction, and it is easy to visualise that the increased muscular power produced by the pharynx in an effort to overcome the oesophageal obstruction could cause a mucosal hernia through an area of weakened muscle. In most cases of pharyngeal diverticula, however, there is no obvious oesophageal obstruction. Killian (1908) suggested that a mechanical obstruction could be produced by the cricopharyngeus going into spasm during the act of swallowing, which could eventually result in the formation of a pulsion diverticulum. As yet, there is no conclusive evidence to support or disprove this hypothesis, although it is difficult to imagine what could produce spasm in the cricopharyngeus without causing noticeable dysphagia to the patient, a symptom rarely complained of prior to the formation of the diverticulum. Killian suggested that with increased tone in the cricopharyngeus a raised hypopharyngeal pressure could be produced on swallowing by a failure of this muscle to relax. He considered that the main supportive argument for this concept lay in the nerve supply to the inferior constrictor muscle. The thyropharyngeal part of the inferior constrictor is supplied by the pharyngeal plexus; the motor component arises from the nucleus ambiguus in the medulla, which sends efferent fibres via the cranial part of the XI (accessory) nerve to join the X (vagus) nerve at the base of the skull which distributes a pharyngeal branch to the pharyngeal plexus. The cricopharyngeal part of the inferior constrictor, however, is supplied to the recurrent laryngeal nerve, a branch of the X (vagus) nerve which loops around the ligamentum arteriosum on the left and the subclavian artery on the right side, and by the external laryngeal branch of the vagus. Killian suggested that asynergia between the two nerve components of the inferior constrictor muscle, motor via the pharyngeal branch to thyropharyngeus and inhibitory via the recurrent laryngeal branch to cricopharyngeus, might be a precipitating cause for pharyngeal herniations.

As regards the site of pharyngeal diverticulae, accounts vary as to whether herniation occurs through, above or below cricopharyngeus. Laimer described a triangular area (figure 1.1) situated just below the cricopharyngeus where the posterior oesophageal wall is particularly thin, as the longitudinal fibres of this organ are sweeping laterally, upwards and forwards to reach their attachment to the midline ridge on the cricoid lamina. Consequently, only circular muscle is found in this triangular area and would appear to be a potential site of weakness, although Moynihan (1927) denies this. Killian (1908) went further in his description of

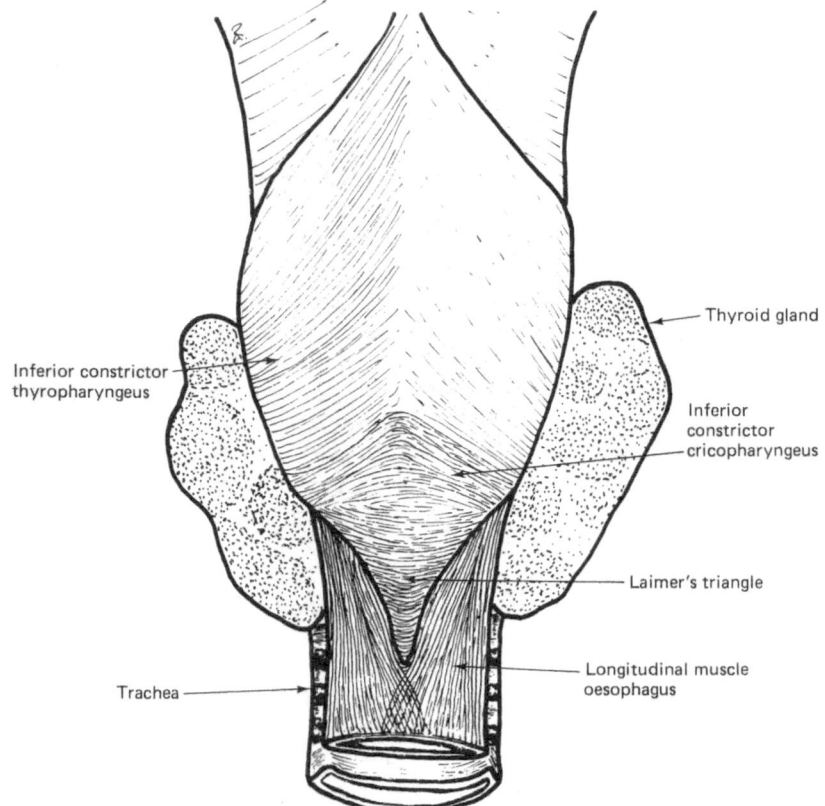

Figure 1.1 Diagram of the posterior wall of the hypopharynx, showing Laimer's triangle.

cricopharyngeus by demarcating two components of this muscle: the ascending constrictor fibres, which he considered to be supplied by the pharyngeal plexus, and the lower purely sphincteric part, which he considered to be the only portion of cricopharyngeus supplied by the recurrent laryngeal nerves. He stated that the effects of muscular asynergia of the two components would be felt maximally at this area of muscular dehiscence (figure 1.2).

Moersch and Judd (1934) thought that the herniating mucous membrane pierced the muscle between the cricopharyngeus and thyropharyngeus. There is, however, very little difference between this spot and that described by Killian, the difference depending purely on which muscular fibres are designated to belong to the cricopharyngeus or the thyropharyngeus. To all practical purposes, these arguments are not important in the clinical situation, as the symptoms, signs and approach to treatment are quite

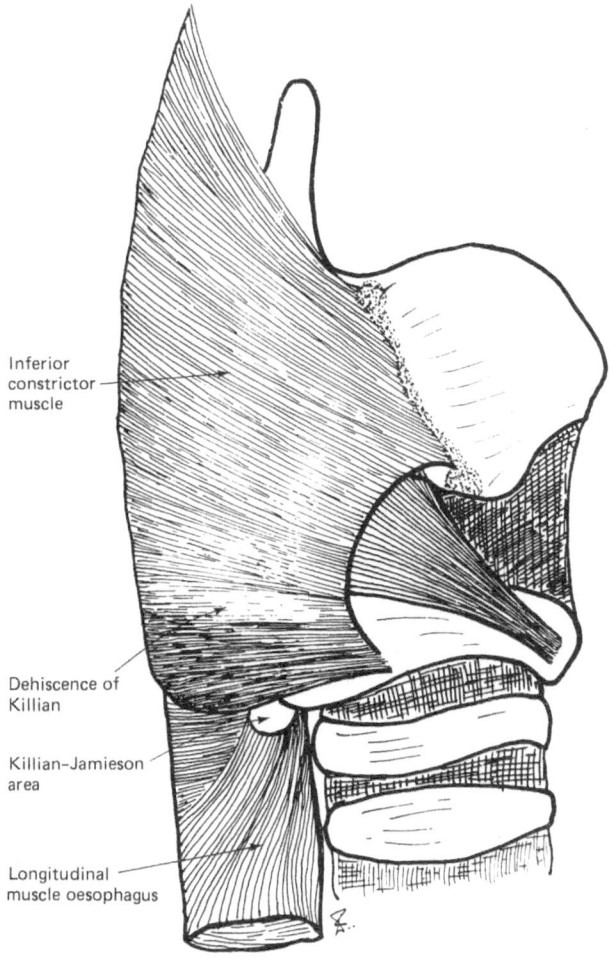

Figure 1.2 Diagram to show the dehiscence of Killian and the Killian–Jamieson area, through which the inferior laryngeal neurovascular bundle enters the larynx.

independent of the exact site of the diverticulum. Although the symptoms of a pharyngeal diverticulum can be distressing for the patient, many diverticula are large when first seen, and at operation are found to lie between the prevertebral and pretracheal fasciae to produce pressure on the surrounding structures of the neck. The fact that they are large makes it difficult for the surgeon to define the exact origin of the hernia; the neck of the sac is often correspondingly large and wide, and the anatomy so distorted that even the correct plane of origin (posterior or lateral), let alone the precise definition of the muscular component, is impossible to discover.

There have been alternative suggestions as to the site of origin of pharyngeal diverticula. Shallow (1936) believed that most occurred in the area between the cricopharyngeus and the rest of the muscle, but originated along the branch of the inferior thyroid artery which enters the pharynx at this point. This would suggest that pharyngeal diverticulae should be equally distributed on both sides, but in fact they are far more commonly found on the left side than on the right. There is no apparent explanation for this clinical fact. It is common for a constant artery to be larger on one side than on the other; perhaps this is true of the left inferior thyroid artery, although this has not been confirmed.

Shallow considered that the next most common area for herniation in the pharynx was through the Killian–Jamieson area (figure 1.2), the gap between cricopharyngeus and the upper circular fibres of the oesophagus. The least common area was higher in the pharynx through the inferior constrictor muscle, where the inferior thyroid artery penetrates the pharyngeal wall.

It is interesting to compare the aetiology of pharyngeal diverticulae with that of colonic diverticulae where arteries piercing the muscle walls of the gut are considered to produce areas of weakness through which mucosa can herniate when initiated by a raised intracolonic pressure. However, it is difficult to relate completely this hypothesis with the sex incidence in pharyngeal diverticula, as they are three times as common in males as in females. Perhaps the mature male larynx is responsible, constantly rubbing against the bony cervical vertebrae and, remembering the large variation in its size among individuals, perhaps producing an area of muscular weakness in the pharyngeal wall due to the resulting trauma.

GASTRO-OESOPHAGEAL (CARDIAC) SPHINCTER

It has long been known, from radiological studies, that swallowed food is held up at the lower end of the oesophagus before entering the stomach. Obviously some mechanism must exist in the region of the junction of oesophagus and stomach that produces this delay in the passage of swallowed material into the stomach and also prevents the regurgitation of gastric contents. It is certain in man that the mechanism involved is not a true sphincter as defined by conventional anatomical nomenclature, as no thickening of the circular muscle has been satisfactorily demonstrated at the cardiac orifice (Lendrum, 1937). Lendrum examined 150 cardio-oesophageal junctions from bodies of all ages and could not find, in any case, a thickening of circular muscle or other evidence of an anatomical sphincter. Also, he failed to demonstrate any thickening of the elastic tissue present in the oesophagus which may have influenced the sphincteric function of the cardiac orifice.

A wide variety of alternative factors have been implicated in the sphincteric effects at the lower oesophagus, and it is probable that there are several factors involved at this site. The following have been recorded as being important mechanisms in the prevention of gastro-oesophageal reflux.

(1) The acute angle lying between oesophagus and the fundus of the stomach. Loss of this angle may occur particularly if the diaphragmatic hiatus is widened, allowing herniation of the lower oesophagus and stomach into the chest.

(2) The phreno-oesophageal ligament. This extends from the abdominal aspect of the diaphragm through the oesophageal hiatus, to join and blend with the submucosa and the intermuscular fibrous septa of the muscle of the terminal part of the thoracic oesophagus. It contains a variable amount of fibrous tissue and may be disrupted or stretched by hiatal hernias.

(3) The rosette of mucosal folds around the cardiac orifice, which allows of opposition of the gastric mucosa.

(4) The diaphragmatic hiatus, which may become unduly widened owing to muscular weakness or obesity.

(5) There is no doubt that there are circularly running fibres in both the oesophagus and stomach on either side of the cardiac hiatus. It has been considered that this muscle, aided by the encircling muscular fibres from the right crus of the diaphragm, constitutes the cardiac sphincter, although the latter is in dispute (Atkinson *et al.*, 1957). In addition, the oblique layer of muscle of the stomach makes U-shaped loops at the cardiac incisura and may aid the sphincter by functioning as a 'pinchcock' in closing the cardiac orifice.

Little detail is known about the nerve supply of the cardiac sphincter area of the oesophagus. Vagal stimulation produces an increase in tone and motility of the lower oesophagus and relaxes the muscle in the sphincter area. In contrast, the sympathetic nerve supply via the coeliac axis decreases the tone in the oesophagus but increases the tone of the muscle in the supposed area of the cardiac sphincter.

It is possible that the muscular arrangement at the cardiac end of the oesophagus with the nerve supply described above is sufficient in itself to prevent gastro-oesophageal reflux. More recently, workers in this field have regarded the physiological lower oesophageal sphincter as the main determinant of gastro-oesophageal competence. This will be discussed elsewhere.

PYLORUS

The muscularis externa of the stomach contains a middle uniform layer of circular fibres over the whole of the stomach, between the external longitudinal fibres and the inner oblique fibres. At the terminal aspect of the stomach they are most abundant and thickened, and are aggregated into a ring of muscle called the pyloric sphincter, which is not independent of the preceding portion of the stomach muscle. In contrast to the oesophagus, where the circular muscle is in continuity with the muscle of the stomach, the pyloric sphincter muscle is demarcated from the duodenum by a layer of connective tissue. Horton (1928) described a complete separation by connective tissue between the circular muscle of the pylorus and the duodenum. He also described about 50 bundles of longitudinal muscle fibres of the pylorus dipping into the pyloric ring, to which he ascribed the function of a dilator of the pylorus. Torgersen (1942) agreed essentially with the description of Horton, except that he considered the connective tissue separation of the pylorus and duodenum to be only partial, as he felt that the muscular fibres along the lesser curve of the stomach were continuous with those of the duodenum but that those along the greater curvature of the stomach were not. He also described the sphincter as consisting of two parts, a pyloric and duodenal portion, being separated by the fibrous connective tissue septum already described. The exact mechanism of control of the transfer of chyme from the stomach to the duodenum through the pylorus is still not fully understood. The peristaltic contractions of the pyloric antrum mix the stomach contents in this region, squirting some into the duodenum and returning some into the body of the stomach for further mixing. The pyloric sphincter undergoes intermittent contraction during the contractions of the pyloric antrum. In addition, the pylorus has been seen to contract when the stomach is empty and no free acid or food is present (Shay and Gershon-Cohen, 1934). Normally when the stomach is at rest, however, the pylorus is relaxed, leaving the gastroduodenal aperture open (Spira, 1957).

SPHINCTER OF ODDI

The intestinal part of the common bile duct (CBD) and ampulla of Vater is surrounded by a sheath of smooth muscle called the sphincter of Oddi. This muscle is regarded as being continuous with the circular layer of muscle of the duodenal wall (Kirk, 1944). In fact, the narrowest part of the opening is through the duodenal wall, where a gallstone commonly lodges and produces obstructive symptoms.

Various distinct parts have been ascribed to this sphincter (figure 1.3):

(1) a circular sheath of muscle which surrounds the preampullary part of the CBD, which is known as the sphincter of the CBD or sphincter choledochus;

(2) a number of longitudinal muscular fasciculi between the CBD and the pancreatic duct;

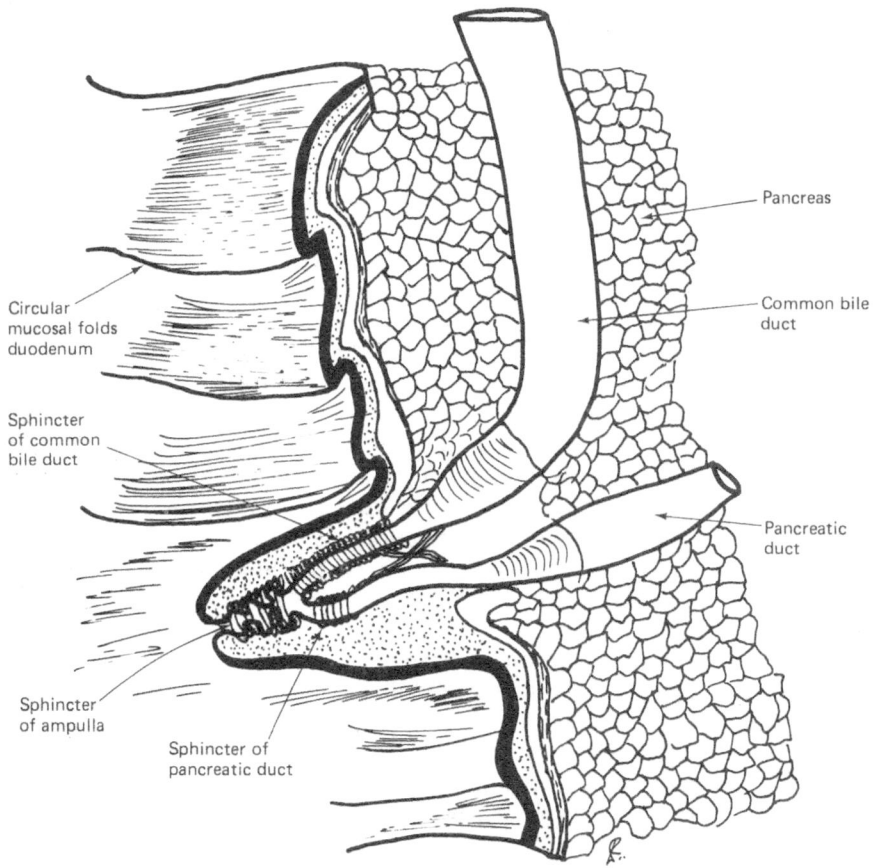

Figure 1.3 Diagram of the sphincter of Oddi. The main part of this sphincter surrounds the common bile duct.

(3) a circular muscle sphincter of the ampulla;

(4) a number of variable collections of sphincteric fibres around the main pancreatic duct to form a sphincter pancreaticus.

It is difficult to be precise in ascribing a function to the various descriptive parts of this complex sphincter. The sphincter choledochus could constrict the CBD and so impede the flow of bile. The longitudinal muscle fasciculi could shorten the intestinal CBD, produce an effective dilation and facilitate the flow of bile. On the other hand, the ampullary sphincter on contraction could impede the flow of bile and pancreatic juice.

Boyden (1937) considers that the sphincter choledochus is the most important part of the sphincter of Oddi and that the muscle of the ampulla is often weak. Also, there is considerable variation in the pancreatic and ampullary parts of the sphincter, which may even be absent; this could be a factor in the causation of pancreatic reflux of bile (Kreilkamp and Boyden, 1940).

It has been found that the sphincter can contract independently of the duodenal wall muscle. This suggests an independent nerve supply and, certainly in the human, the myenteric (Auerbach's) plexus is well developed at the site of termination of the ducts.

Following cholecystectomy there is often a loss of tone in the sphincter of Oddi, which produces a low ductal pressure (Puestow, 1938). However, the ducts often appear dilated, which does not appear to comply with a low intraductal pressure. Colp et al. (1936) noted in the dog that hypotonicity in the duct system did not always occur after a cholecystectomy and that when the ampullary region was stimulated the muscle could still become tonic with an associated increase in the intraductal pressure.

Histology shows that the terminal aspect of the united bile and pancreatic ducts is packed with villous folds of the mucous membrane which contain cores of connective tissue and muscle bundles derived from the outer muscle coats. It would appear that contraction of the muscle fibres results in retraction and erection of the mucosal folds, a mechanism which could prevent the reflux of duodenal contents into the duct and which could control the exit of bile into the duodenum.

As stated above, the sphincter of Oddi has a rich nerve supply and in the cat stimulation of the vagus nerves results in relaxation of the sphincter choledochus and an outpouring of bile into the duodenum. On the other hand, the mechanism for emptying the gall bladder appears to be mainly hormonal rather than nervous, and occurs when fat or acid in the duodenum causes the liberation of cholecystokinin which stimulates contraction of the gall bladder.

ILEOCAECAL VALVE

This structure is found where the lower end of the ileum opens into the posteromedial aspect of the large intestine at the junction between ascending colon and caecum. As the ileum penetrates the wall of the large intestine (figure 1.4), its orifice is provided with two transverse folds of the lining mucosa known as the ileocaecal valve. The protrusions of the mucous membrane also contain the submucous layer and the circular muscle of the terminal ileum which pouts into the lumen of the caecum. The two folds, or labia, which serve the valve are orientated so that they lie horizontally—superior and inferior to the ileal orifice. The superior labium is large, protrudes into the caecum for some 1.5 cm and is attached to the line of junction of the ileum with the colon. The inferior labium is smaller,

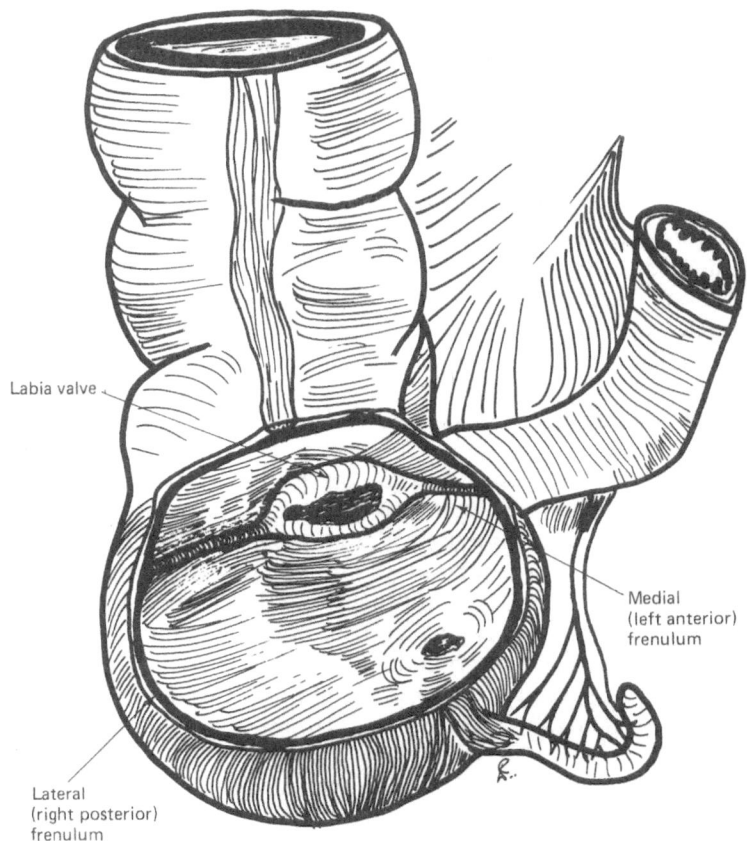

Labia valve

Medial
(left anterior)
frenulum

Lateral
(right posterior)
frenulum

Figure 1.4 The ileocaecal valve.

protrudes into the lumen by about 0.5 cm and is attached to the line of junction of the ileum with the caecum. Although generally smaller than the superior labium, it is often larger and more concave. The labia fuse with each other at the ends, to form the frenulae of the valve. In the fresh state or in specimens fixed *in situ* the medial (or left anterior) aspect of the valve is rounded, while the lateral (or right posterior) aspect is narrower and pointed; both are contiguous with two transverse folds of the mucosa which project into the lumen of the large bowel as they continue around the circumference of the caecocolic junction. Histological examination of the ileocaecal valve shows that the mucous membrane of the ileal aspect of the valve is typical of the small intestine with villi, while the caecal aspect of the valve is covered with mucosa typical of the large intestine with crypts and mucous glands.

The circular and longitudinal muscle coats of the terminal part of the ileum are continued into the valve to form a sphincter which Rutherford (1926) described as a caecocolic sphincter which could close the caecal lumen to prevent the accumulation of faeces in the caput caeci.

The precise way in which this valve functions is still not clear. Apart from its passive valvular action, Beattie (1924) thought that it acted as a muscular sphincter, a view also supported by Bargen *et al.* (1940). However, no tonic contractions of the valve are apparent which are typical of a true sphincter, although stretching the valve does apparently produce a contraction. Moreover, direct observations of the valve through a caecostomy (Rosenberg and Didio, 1969) even failed to confirm the normal descriptive form of the valve, as it appeared papillary in shape. Also, radiological observations during barium follow-through examinations fail to demonstrate any effective valvular mechanism at this site.

Apart from regulating the flow of small intestinal contents into the caecum, the valve is considered to prevent the reflux of contents from the caecum into the terminal ileum, by maintaining a state of tonic contraction by sympathetic nerve impulses. These impulses are reduced or abolished when food passes from the stomach into the small intestine accompanied by the passage of ileal contents through the relaxed ileocaecal valve into the large intestine. However, if the large intestine is distended, the contractions of the valve and, hence, its function are inhibited (Fleischner and Bernstein, 1950). The latter workers state that reflux of intestinal contents from the colon to ileum readily occurs if the caecum and colon are distended and palpable.

In the case of the cardiac sphincter there is no anatomical evidence for the undoubted sphincteric mechanism which occurs at this site, while in the case of the valve and, hence, its function are inhibited (Fleischner and Bernstein, limited evidence that it acts as such. Unfortunately, most methods of examining this sphincter involve serious interference with the normal anatomy of the area, which may affect its function. Perhaps the colonoscope may provide more satisfactory answers about these problems by providing a more 'natural' means of obtaining functional observations.

ANAL SPHINCTERS

The anal canal is surrounded by a complex arrangement of sphincters, which may be divided into an internal and an external group of muscles.

Internal Anal Sphincter

The smooth muscle of the rectum consists of an inner circular coat and an outer longitudinal coat derived from the muscular taeniae of the sigmoid colon. The circular muscle in the lower aspects of the rectal wall thickens and ends just above the level of the anal verge. This thickening is readily demonstrated but has no sharply defined upper margin. It surrounds the anal canal for some 30 mm (its upper three-quarters) and its lower margin is free and easily palpable on rectal examination; it constitutes the internal sphincter. This sphincter is separated from the upper portions of the external sphincter by the longitudinal muscle of the rectum, while a fascial septum derived from the inferior muscle fasciculi of the longitudinal coat separates the internal sphincter from the subcutaneous part of the external sphincter (figure 1.5). The above fascia separating the two sphincters is very fibrous around the anal canal, and the majority of its fibres run beneath the border of the internal sphincter to insert into the modified skin of the anal canal, which Milligan and Morgan (1934) called the anal intermuscular septum. The area of the anal canal into which the major proportion of its fibres insert is the area below the pectinate line known as the pecten band, which is now conceded to be synonymous with Hilton's white line. The gap at the lower border of the internal sphincter through which the intermuscular septum passes is called the intermuscular sulcus and is readily palpated in the living subject.

Regarding the exact relationships between the two anal sphincters, it is now generally accepted by anatomists and proctologists that the deep or

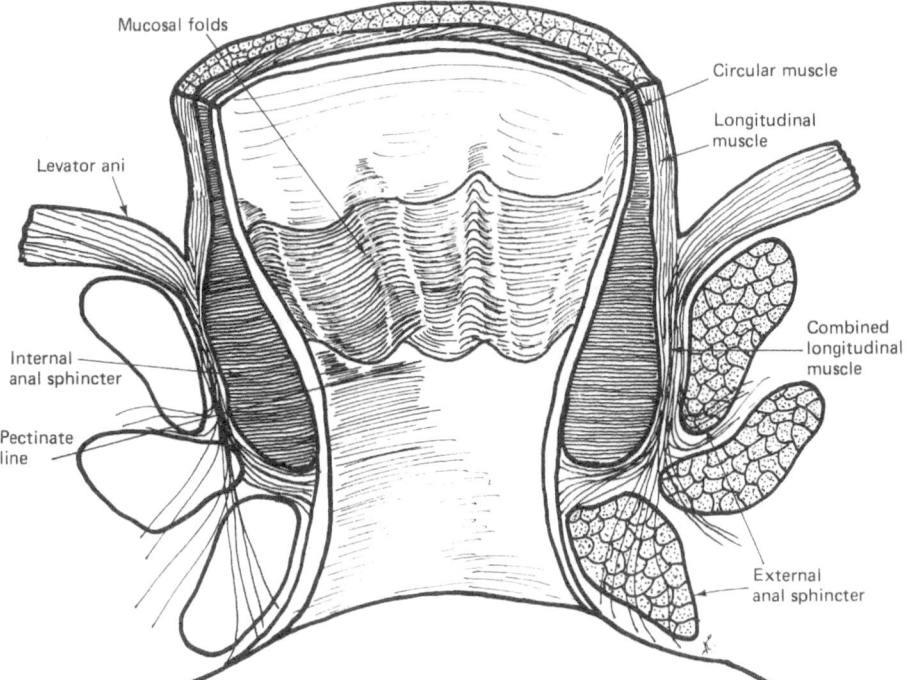

Figure 1.5 The musculature of the anal canal and lower rectum.

profundal part of the external sphincter surrounds the internal one and that, as noted above, the intermuscular septum separates the internal sphincter only from the upper border of the subcutaneous part of the external sphincter, and not the whole of it, as was thought long ago (Milligan and Morgan, 1934).

Fistulae

Into the anal sinuses or crypts open the terminal ducts of structures called the anal glands or anal ducts, which extend down through the longitudinal muscle of the anal canal and into parts of the external sphincter. Those anal glands which are posteriorly situated open into the space outside the subcutaneous external sphincter and between the posterior limbs of the superficial external sphincter known as the triangular space of Minor. It is now generally accepted that infections of the anal glands, ducts or sinuses may lead to the formation of a fistula which opens internally into the anal sinus and opens to the exterior somewhere in the perianal region. Because of the frequent course the posterior anal ducts take, fistulae in this region commonly take the path between the subcutaneous and superficial parts of the external anal sphincter, following the fibrous septae which radiate from the lower aspect of the intermuscular septum. In order to get a fistula to heal, it must be opened, which invariably means that the anal valve, pecten band and internal sphincter need to be sectioned if the primary and secondary openings are internal—i.e. all the structures internal to the course of the fistula tract. If, on the other hand, the fistula opens externally, at least the subcutaneous part of the external sphincter will need to be sectioned, as the fistula invariably follows the fibrous septae which radiate through this part of the external sphincter. It is generally agreed by proctologists that the internal sphincter and at least the subcutaneous part of the external sphincter may be sectioned without loss of continence, and most will agree that the superficial part of the sphincter may be sectioned, also with safety. It must not be forgotten that infected anal glands which extend into the ischiorectal fossa following fibrous septae from the intermuscular septum may produce an abscess in this region. In these cases it is obvious that a simple drainage procedure is inadequate to effect a permanent cure.

Nerve Supply of the Internal Sphincter

The sympathetic nerves to the upper part of the anal canal and the internal sphincter pass mainly along the inferior mesenteric and superior rectal arteries, and partly via the superior and inferior hypogastric plexuses. From the plexuses nerves join the pelvic plexuses from which, in turn, are derived the middle rectal plexuses which supply the anal canal and sphincter. In theory, the sympathetic nerve supply should be inhibitory to the rectum and motor to the internal sphincter, but whether it has any real marked effect on anything other than blood vessels still remains to be elucidated. The parasympathetic supply is from the pelvic splanchnic nerves which pass from the sacral nerves to join the inferior hypogastric plexuses and pelvic plexuses around the rectum, being motor to the rectal musculature and inhibitory to the internal sphincter.

Voluntary Anal Sphincters

Levator Ani

Puborectalis was originally described as being part of pubococcygeus, one of the main muscular constituents of levator ani, and was, therefore, considered to belong to levator ani. It is now regarded as being part of the deep aspect of the external anal sphincter (Thompson, 1923). Puborectalis consists of paired muscle slips that arise with pubococcygeus from the posterior surface of the pubis (the most inferior fibres of this origin) and from the superior layer of fascia which covers the urogenital diaphragm. The fibres pass posteriorly on either side of the rectum and vagina to form a sling behind the bowel and anatomically demarcate the rectum from the anal canal. It is not surprising that puborectalis has been considered to be part of the levator ani muscle, because it is not easily separated from pubococcygeus. Courtney (1950), however, described the fibres of puborectalis as being attached to the coccyx, some decussating anterior to the rectum and mingling with the fibres of the external sphincter and some decussating posterior to the rectum to form the sling-like fibres normally ascribed to this muscle. He also described these sling fibres as mingling with the deep part of the external sphincter, and considered that this sphincter was formed by puborectalis and was, therefore, part of levator ani. Levy (1936) also subscribed to this view, and indeed most observers working on the sphincters have noted that it is very difficult to distinguish between puborectalis and the deep part of the external sphincter. Puborectalis has long been regarded as the main structure maintaining the perineal or anorectal flexure of the bowel. However, this flexure is also supported by the attachment of the bowel to the upper surface of levator ani as it passes through the hiatus and by the attachment to the perineal body inferiorly. It is easy to feel the point where the gut passes through the levator hiatus on rectal examination and may serve as the junctional point between rectum and anal canal.

Puborectalis has been considered important in maintaining faecal continence, acting in this respect with the external sphincter. Milligan and Morgan (1934) described puborectalis combined with the upper borders of the internal and external anal sphincters at the perineal flexure and extending downwards to surround the anal canal as the anorectal ring. They considered that part of this ring, at least, must be intact to maintain faecal continence. This still holds true today.

External Anal Sphincter

This sphincter is classically divided into three parts—deep, superficial and subcutaneous (figure 1.5)—which, as already seen with the deep part, have substantial continuity with each other.

The deep portion of the external anal sphincter surrounds the musculature of the rectum and anal canal and the internal anal sphincter. The deep fibres are inseparable from puborectalis (figure 1.6), and in front many fibres of the deep external sphincter decussate with the fibres of the

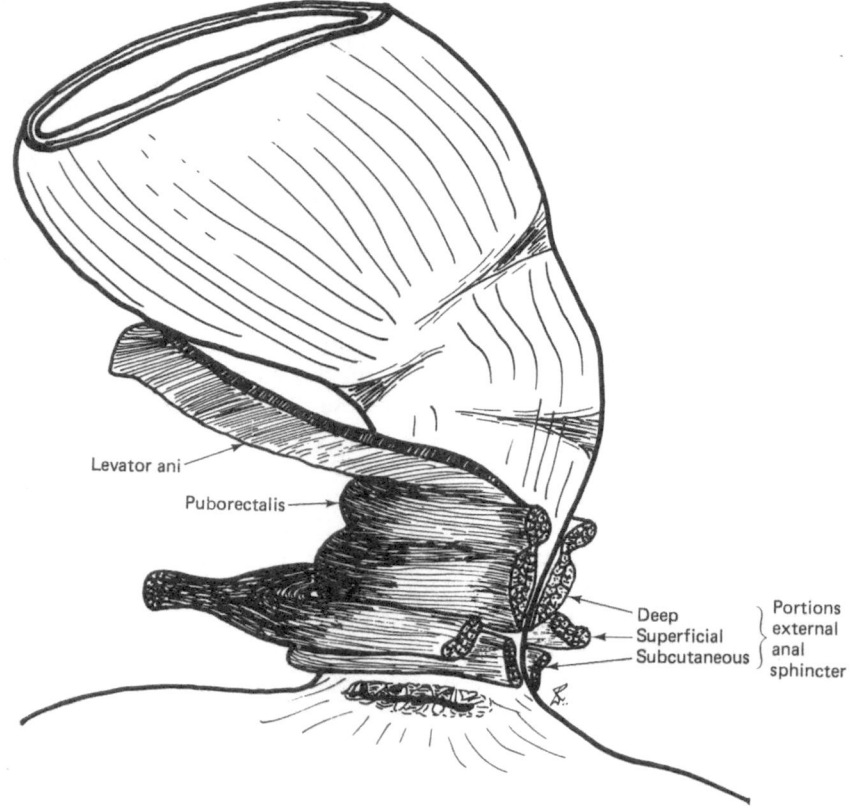

Figure 1.6 The external anal sphincter musculature. As noted in the text, many workers consider it impossible to distinguish clearly between these described portions of the external sphincter.

superficial transverse perineal muscles. Posteriorly some fibres of the deep part are attached to the anococcygeal ligament. Goligher *et al.* (1955) considered that it was not possible to clearly differentiate between puborectalis and the external sphincter or to distinguish the three parts of the sphincter from one another.

The subcutaneous part of the sphincter is usually described as a flat band of muscle about 15 mm broad which lies horizontally and surrounds the lower part of the anal canal. It lies below the internal sphincter and the termination of the longitudinal muscle of the anal canal, so that it bears the same relationship to the anal canal as the internal sphincter, although they are separated by the intersphincteric groove, which is occupied by the intersphincteric septum. It lies beneath the skin at the anal orifice and it is also subcutaneous at the white line of Hilton in the anal canal. Anteriorly some of its fibres attach to the perineal body, while posteriorly some fibres find attachment to the anococcygeal ligament or raphe.

It used to be thought that the intersphincteric groove completely separated the superiorly situated internal sphincter from the inferiorly situated external sphincter. In other words, the whole external sphincter lay below the intersphincteric sulcus. If this were true, then the internal sphincter would at least be at or above the level of the pelvic floor as demarcated by levator ani. There is no doubt that the deep part of the external sphincter in association with puborectalis and at least part of the superficial part of the sphincter is adjacent and closely associated to the whole of the internal anal sphincter.

The superficial part of the external sphincter is elliptical in shape and lies deep to the subcutaneous part. It is often described as being lateral to the subcutaneous part, on a level between the latter and the deep part of the sphincter (figure 1.6). Consequently, the superficial part is not quite so intimately related to the anal canal as the deep part, which clasps the tube-like anal canal, so that it is broader horizontally than the other parts, in the plane of the skin. It is the only part of the external sphincter that is attached to bone, arising posteriorly from the terminal segments of the coccyx by a fibrous aponeurosis and the anococcygeal raphe. It surrounds the anus and, hence, the lower aspect of the internal sphincter, and is inserted anteriorly into the perineum and the midline cutaneous raphe.

This arrangement of the three parts of the external sphincter gives rise to the anal spaces. The area behind the anus between the two limbs of the superficial part of the external sphincter is called the triangular space of Minor. Above it, but below the pelvic floor, is found the deep anal or post-anal space. Between the superficial part of the external sphincter and the skin posteriorly lies the superficial post-anal space. These latter post-anal spaces filled with connective tissue communicate via the space of Minor and also communicate laterally with the ischiorectal fossa of both sides.

This division of the external sphincter into three parts is the classical description most commonly met in most texts. This description has long been challenged by many individual workers in a number of minor ways, which do not, however, alter the functional anatomy of the area or the physiological understanding of their use. For example, Milligan and Morgan (1934) described the superficial and the deep parts of the external sphincter as being inseparable. Again, Courtney (1950) described the division of the sphincter into three separate parts as 'artificial'. However, these arguments, as already stated, do not alter the understanding of them or the surgical approach to fistulae or repairs for incontinence.

More recently the external sphincter has been the subject of intensive study and a new nomenclature has been suggested (Shafik, 1975a), although the essential topographical description remains unchanged from the more classical but contemporary views of proctologists. However, the concept does help to clarify the essential functions of levator ani and the anal sphincters, so that a brief review of the description by Shafik is relevant here.

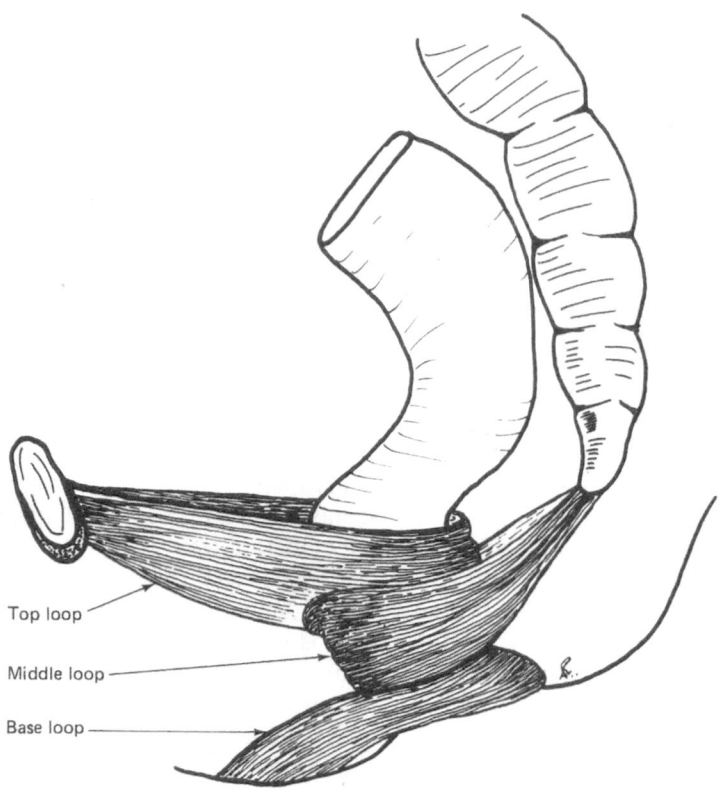

Top loop

Middle loop

Base loop

Figure 1.7 Diagram illustrating the triple-loop system of the external anal sphincter.

Shafik describes the external anal sphincter as a series of U-shaped loops (figure 1.7) which he names the top, middle and base loops, which essentially represent the deep, superficial and subcutaneous parts of the external sphincter.

The top loop consists of the deep portion of the sphincter as well as puborectalis. The top loop surrounds the back and sides of the upper part of the anal canal; puborectalis belongs to this loop, there being no morphological or histological distinction between the two. It passes forwards and medially upwards to attach to the lower part of symphysis pubis and the pubic bone. This concept concurs with those already noted above and the case can be argued on simple morphological grounds. First, the muscle bundles of puborectalis and the deep external sphincter have the same sort of arrangement, namely U-shaped loops around the sides and back of the upper anal canal. The fibres of both descriptive parts cannot be distinguished, as both are fused together. The fibres of puborectalis, on the other hand, are completely different from those found in the rest of levator ani, where they are almost horizontally orientated, as the levator diaphragm stretches across the pelvis. Second, puborectalis has the same action as the deep external sphincter, both being constrictors at the anorectal junction. Levator ani, however, dilates it. Third, both puborectalis and the deep external sphincter have the same nerve supply from the inferior haemorrhoidal nerve, and it is supplied from the perineal aspect of the muscle. Levator ani, however, is supplied by the perineal branch of S_4 from the pelvic aspect of the muscle.

The middle loop is separated from the top loop by fascia. The muscle arises from the tip of the coccyx and passes horizontally forwards, dividing into two halves, which run alongside the anal canal and meet in front of it. The muscle is a flat ribbon of fasciculi which overlap both the top and the base loops. It is supplied with nerves from the perineal branch of S_4.

The base loop is separated from the middle loop by fibrous prolongations which arise from the longitudinal muscle of the anal canal. It has no attachment to bone, arising from perianal skin anteriorly from, and close to, the midline. The muscle divides around the anal canal, passing posteriorly with an upward inclination to meet behind the anal canal. The lower and most medial bundles of fibres are circular, forming a complete ring. Fibrous septae from the inferior border of the longitudinal muscle of the gut fan out through the base loop to insert into the perianal skin. The base loop is supplied by the inferior haemorrhoidal nerve.

When the functions of this complex sphincter arrangement and the almost equally complex levator ani are considered, the two structures work in harmony to maintain faecal continence and to aid defaecation, while in other functions one or other of these structures is the more important—e.g. levator ani is the primary mechanism in preventing rectal and vaginal prolapse.

Continence

The anal canal is kept closed by the tonic contraction of the internal and external anal sphincters. The external sphincter is also a voluntary muscle, and this helps to maintain continence and to control the latter part of the defaecatory act. It appears that the internal sphincter by itself is of little importance in the maintenance of continence, which relies on the external sphincter with puborectalis. An 'air-tight' closure of the anal canal is achieved by the triple-loop system, with the middle loop acting as a fulcrum to fix the mid-anal part of the canal during the contraction of the top and base loops (figure 1.8). From a mechanical point of view, it seems that for striated muscle the triple-loop system allows for maximum efficiency in their performance of anal occlusion. This function is achieved by two main factors produced by the triple-loop system: first, direct compression by the external sphincter, and, second, a 'kinking' of the terminal bowel which

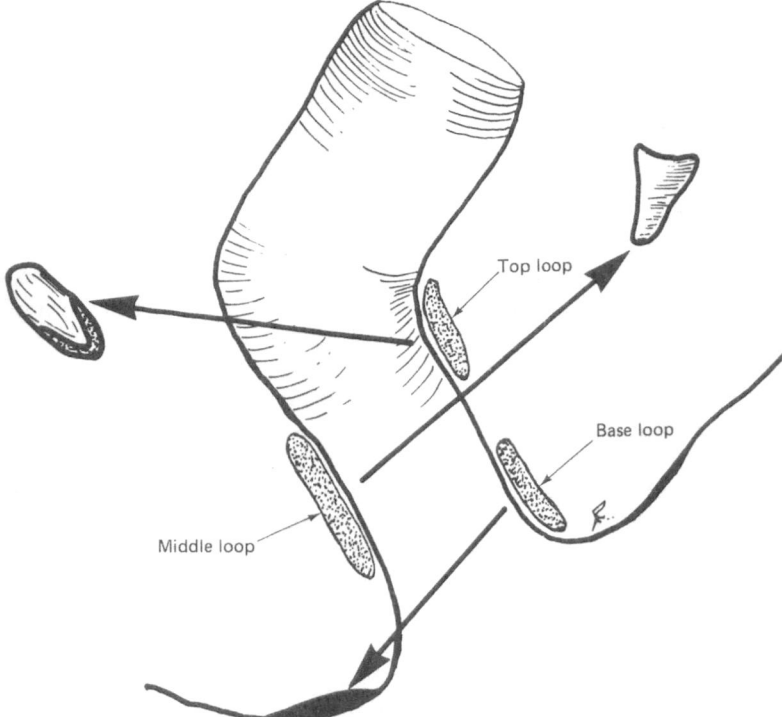

Figure 1.8 Diagram to show the mechanism of anal occlusion by the triple-loop system of the external anal sphincter. The arrows show the direction of contraction of external sphincter loops.

allows for a tight closure of the anal canal with the minimum of effort. Also, the triple loops possess propulsive powers to aid the latter part of defaecation.

There are other factors in the maintenance of faecal continence which are important adjuncts to the primary mechanisms. First, the obliquity of the anal canal helps; the presence of an almost 90° angle between rectum and anal canal is a physical factor aiding continence. Second, the longer post-anal canal wall compared with the anterior wall (about 1 cm longer) due to the right-angled bend in the terminal bowel noted above aids in the occlusion when the two walls collapse together. Both these factors must also facilitate closure of the anorectal junction by the top loop of the external anal sphincter.

Defaecation

Levator Ani

Before this function can be fully understood it is necessary to consider in more detail the anatomy of the levator ani muscle. The muscle consists of two parts, the pubococcygeus and the ileococcygeus, which are generally described as inserting into the midline anococcygeal raphe. Shafik (1975b), however, demonstrated a free passage, across the anococcygeal raphe, of the tendinous fibres of the two levators, indicating that the raphe is not the true line of insertion of the levator ani muscles. Rather it is the line along which the tendinous fibres from the two sides decussate with each other in their passage across the midline, to insert some way lateral to the anococcygeal raphe. This digastric pattern of insertion of the levators allows for the simultaneous contraction of the muscle on both sides, which contracts as a single sheet, being strengthened at its central and most vital part by the tendinous anococcygeal raphe. If the levators were directly continuous on both sides, their contraction would constrict the intrahiatal structures, but the presence of the decussating raphe prevents any such constriction. In fact, as the anococcygeal raphe changes the direction of pull of the muscle fibres, by its decussating arrangement, a dilator effect rather than a constrictor effect will occur. Such an arrangement would allow for appreciable changes in the length and breadth of the anococcygeal raphe, and, for reasons stated below, in the hiatal contents. In addition, this structure would be capable of considerable adaption as regards shape and the support it would give to the pelvic viscera, which is its main function in the upright position. All this is evidence, in addition, that the levator ani muscle is completely different in structure and function from puborectalis, which rightly belongs to the external anal sphincter.

The Levator Hiatus and Ligament

The levator hiatus is formed by the medial borders of pubococcygeus and not puborectalis, as is frequently mentioned in the literature (Morgan, 1949). Puborectalis lies outside a downward prolongation of the pubococcygeus muscle and therefore does not share in the structure of the hiatus. In the average adult this hiatus is about 2.5–3 cm across and 3.5–4.5 cm from pubis to the anorectal junction. The intrahiatal structures are attached to the edges of the levator hiatus by fibrous tissue derived from the pelvic fascia. At the level of the anorectal junction the fascia is more thickened; Shafik (1975b) has called this the 'hiatal ligament'. Obviously the presence of close-packed fibrous tissue at this site would ensure that contraction of levator ani would have an end result on the intrahiatal structures. It appears possible that if this ligament becomes unduly stretched by muscle weakness and obesity, with a raised intra-abdominal pressure, then a rectal or vaginal prolapse is more likely, particularly as this process will include weakening of the anococcygeal raphe which will allow of sagging of the levator diaphragm and further widening of the levator hiatus. With the decreased support which results from this process the pelvic viscera start to prolapse through the hiatus.

With the increase in intra-abdominal pressure which accompanies straining at stool, the pelvic diaphragm is raised and flattened as it contracts, which results in a shortening and widening of the levator hiatus (figure 1.9). These movements produce an expansion of the anal canal due

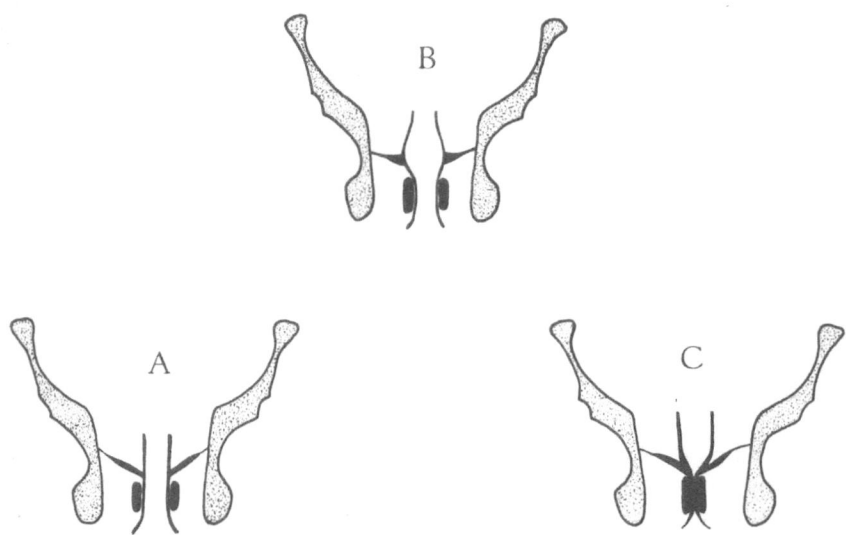

Figure 1.9 Diagram to show the mechanism of action of pubococcygeus and puborectalis. A, at rest; B, during defaecation pubococcygeus contracts and puborectalis relaxes; C, to oppose a call for stool puborectalis contracts and pubococcygeus relaxes.

to the pull of the hiatal ligament and an elevation of the levator hiatus above the descending faeces. The presence of faeces in the lower rectum and upper anal canal produces a reflex relaxation of the internal sphincter and then relaxation of the external sphincter in the absence of voluntary inhibition, so that the stool passes into the anal canal. The stool is evacuated by alternate relaxation and contraction of the levator muscles which 'milk' the stools down the gut aided by the alternate contractions of the triple-loop system. As the top loop contracts, the middle loop relaxes, and so on, in a manner similar to intestinal peristalsis. It is interesting to note that the differing nerve supplies of the parts of the triple-loop could aid this contraction and relaxation in a way similar to that discussed with the inferior constrictor muscle of the pharynx.

REFERENCES

Atkinson, M., Edwards, D. A. W., Honour, A. J. and Rowlands, E. N. (1957). The oesophagogastric sphincter in hiatus hernia. *Lancet, ii*, 1138

Bargen, J. A., Wesson, H. R. and Jackman, R. J. (1940). Studies on the ileocaecal junction (ileocecus). *Surg., Gynec. Obst.,* **71**, 33

Beattie, J. (1924). The early stages of the development of the ileocolic sphincter. *J. Anat.,* **59**, 56

Boyden, E. A. (1937). The sphincter of Oddi in man and certain representative mammals. *Surgery,* **1**, 25

Colp. R., Doubilet, H. and Gerber, I. E. (1936). Endocholedochal section of the sphincter of Oddi. *Arch. Surg.,* **33**, 696

Courtney, H. (1950). Anatomy of the pelvic diaphragm and anorectal musculature as related to sphincter preservation in anorectal surgery. *Am. J. Surg.,* **79**, 155

Fleischner, F. G. and Bernstein, C. (1950). Roentgen-anatomical studies of the normal ileocaecal valve. *Radiology,* **54**, 43

Goligher, J. C., Leacock, A. G. and Brossy, J. J. (1955). The surgical anatomy of the anal canal. *Br. J. Surg.,* **43**, 51

Horton, B. T. (1928). Pyloric musculature, with special reference to pyloric block. *Am. J. Anat.,* **41**, 197

Killian, G. (1908). Ueber den Mund der Speiseröchre. *Zeitschr. Ohrenh.,* **55**, 1

Kirk, J. (1944). Observations on the histology of the choledocho-duodenal junction and papilla duodeni, with particular reference to the ampulla of Vater and sphincter of Oddi. *J. Anat.,* **78**, 118

Kreilkamp, B. L. and Boyden, E. A. (1940). Variability in the composition of the sphincter of Oddi: a possible factor in the pathologic physiology of the biliary tract. *Anat. Rec.,* **76**, 485

Lendrum, F. C. (1937). Anatomic features of the cardiac orifice of the stomach: with special reference to cardiospasm. *Arch. Int. Med.,* **59**, 474

Levy, E. (1936). Anorectal musculature. *Am. J. Surg.,* **34**, 141

Milligan, E. T. C. and Morgan, C. N. (1934). Surgical anatomy of the anal canal, with special reference to anorectal fistulae. *Lancet, ii*, 1150, 1213

Moersch, H. J. and Judd, E. S. (1934). Diagnosis and treatment of pharyngo-oesophageal diverticulum. *Surg., Gynec. Obst.,* **58**, 781

Morgan, C. N. (1949). The surgical anatomy of the ischio-rectal space. *Proc. R. Soc. Med.,* **42**, 189

Moynihan, B. (1927). Diverticula of the alimentary canal. *Lancet, i*, 1061

Puestow, C. B. (1938). Changes in intra-choledochal pressure following cholecystectomy. *Surg., Gynec. Obst.,* **67**, 82

Ramsay, E. H., Watson, J. S., Gramiak, R. and Weinberg, S. A. (1955). Cinefluorographic analysis of the mechanism of swallowing. *Radiology,* **64**, 498

Rosenberg, J. C. and Didio, L. J. (1969). *In vivo* appearance and function of the ileum as observed directly through a cecostomy. *Am. J. Gastroenterol.*, **52**, 411

Rutherford, A. H. (1926). The frenula valvulae coli. *J. Anat.*, **60**, 564

Shafik, A. (1975a). A new concept of the anatomy of the anal sphincter mechanism and the physiology of defaecation. I. The external anal sphincter: a triple loop system. *Invest. Urol.*, **12**, 412

Shafik, A. (1975b). A new concept of the anatomy of the anal sphincter mechanism and the physiology of defaecation. II. Anatomy of the levator ani muscle with special reference to puborectalis. *Invest. Urol.*, **13**, 175

Shallow, T. A. (1936). Combined one stage closed method for the treatment of pharyngeal diverticula. *Surg., Gynec. Obst.*, **62**, 624

Shay, H. and Gershon-Cohen, J. (1934). Experimental studies in gastric physiology in man. II. A study of pyloric control; the roles of acid and alkali. *Surg., Gynec. Obst.*, **58**, 935

·Thompson, P. Quoted by Smith, W. C. (1923). The levator ani muscle: its structure in man, and its comparative relationships. *Anat. Rec.*, **26**, 175

Torgersen, J. (1942). The muscular build and movements of the stomach and duodenal bulb; especially with regard to the problem of the segmental divisions of the stomach in the light of comparative anatomy and embryology. *Acta Radiol. Suppl.*, **45**, 191

2
Pharmacology of Human Gastrointestinal Sphincters

A. D'Mello and A. Bennett

INTRODUCTION

Gastrointestinal sphincters have been defined on anatomical and functional criteria discussed fully elsewhere in this book. In this section it is adequate to reiterate that there should be anatomical evidence that the muscle arrangement differs from that of the adjacent muscle of the gut to permit of independent sphincteric activity. Functionally, it is thought that the sphincteric region is normally closed but relaxes in response to an advancing peristaltic wave, and can inhibit retrograde flow (or reflux) by its ability to contract and maintain an elevated pressure. It is likely, but not always essential, that the response of the sphincteric region to some endogenous or exogenous substances may differ from that of adjacent alimentary muscle. It is usually said that sphincters contract to noradrenaline, whereas the rest of the alimentary tract relaxes. The degrees to which the sphincters of the alimentary tract meet these requirements vary. Different groups of competent workers disagree even about the reliability of the methods used to locate sphincters and to measure the pressures which they can generate.

Since there are numerous and important species differences with respect to the mode of action of drugs on the alimentary tract, we have restricted our comments almost entirely to man.

The physiological and pathophysiological mechanisms modifying sphincter tone may include myogenic activity, neurally released transmitters, endocrine substances such as gastrin, or autacoids such as prostaglandins. Drugs may either mimic or alter the effects of the endogenous substances which affect sphincter activity.

The design of experiments to investigate the effects of drugs on physiological functions should be based on firm experimental procedures

27

such as those required for drug trials, including the use of controls, double-blind evaluation of effects and relevant statistical analysis of the results (Dunne, 1967). We draw attention to some cases where this design is faulty. A more detailed assessment of the value of various reports can be obtained by using a check list as described by Lionel and Herxheimer (1970); this may also indicate further areas of research.

RELATIVE ADVANTAGES OF *IN VIVO* AND *IN VITRO* TECHNIQUES FOR STUDYING SPHINCTERS

The relative advantages, disadvantages and relationships between *in vitro* experiments and motility studies *in vivo* with regard to the gastrointestinal tract in general have been discussed by Bennett (1968) and Sanger and Bennett (1981). In essence, it was pointed out that although a full understanding of the physiology and pharmacology of human gut muscle must involve studies in conscious subjects, such investigations are often limited on ethical and technical grounds. Furthermore, the gut *in vivo* may be influenced by numerous factors not effective in isolated tissues, including extrinsic nerves, reflexes from other regions of the gut, circulating hormones and changes in blood flow. These may be functionally important but difficult to control experimentally.

Studies on strips of gastrointestinal muscle from the specimens resected for surgical reasons measure only the direct effects of drugs on the muscle or its intrinsic nerves, and have the advantage and disadvantage that many of the variable factors *in vivo* are eliminated. The techniques are relatively easy and allow of analyses with drugs that could not ethically be given to human volunteers. It is difficult to obtain specimens of human tissue for perfusion through the blood vessels, and drugs administered to a tissue without a blood supply *in vitro* may diffuse in an abnormal manner compared with the *in vivo* situation. This diffusion might be better than that obtained by intravascular administration in mimicking the effects of substances released endogenously within the gut wall, but the added substance may also act on receptors which it does not normally reach. Another problem is that the existence of receptors for neurotransmitters in muscle strips does not necessarily indicate a physiological role for them; for example, blood vessels have muscarinic receptors without parasympathetic innervation. However, even with so many possible pitfalls, many substances induce responses of isolated muscle strips which correspond with motility changes *in vivo*.

The doses of hormones used to elicit responses of tissues *in vivo* and *in vitro* should be compared with the concentrations which occur *in vivo*, to differentiate between physiological, pathophysiological and pharmacological effects.

In vitro studies can be useful for investigating gastrointestinal disease. The responses of diseased and healthy tissue can be compared in an attempt to elucidate the disorder and to predict a remedy.

Investigating the Actions of Drugs *in vitro*

The way that tissues are studied *in vitro* can affect the response, and the conditions should always be stated. Comprehensive accounts of this topic have been published by Bennett (1973) and Sanger and Bennett (1980). Other practical details can be found in *Pharmacological Experiments on Isolated Preparations,* by the staff of the Department of Pharmacology, University of Edinburgh (1970). In brief, strips of human gastrointestinal muscle are obtained from surgical specimens. Since the resected specimen usually contains healthy gut, it is possible to examine both normal and diseased tissue from the same patient. Krebs' solution (table 2.1) at 37°C is usually used because its ionic composition and pH when bubbled with 5 per cent CO_2 (see Bennett, 1973) are similar to those of plasma.

Table 2.1   Composition of Krebs solution (Krebs and Henseleit, 1932), plus dextrose. Chemicals dissolved in glass-distilled or de-ionised water gassed with 5% CO_2 in O_2

Constituent	NaCl	KCl	MgSO$_4$.7H$_2$O	CaCl$_2$	KH$_2$PO$_4$	NaHCO$_3$	Dextrose
g/l	6.92	0.35	0.29	0.28	0.16	2.1	2.1
mM	118.5	4.7	1.2	2.5	1.2	25.0	11.7

Specimens of bowel should be placed in Krebs' solution immediately they are available, the mucosa and submucosa gently cut away, and strips (usually 2–4 mm thick and 2–4 cm long, often containing both muscle layers) cut in the direction of the longitudinal or circular muscle fibres. These are suspended in organ baths (e.g. figure 2.1), and responses are recorded usually under conditions of constant load or constant tissue length.

Although it is better to use fresh tissue, storage overnight at 4°C may be necessary and this does not usually produce qualitative changes in response to drugs (Bennett, 1973). However, there may be some degenerative changes—for example, of intramural nerves. Tetrodotoxin, which selectively blocks nerve transmission, is more effective on fresh than on stored (24–26 h) human anal sphincter strips (Burleigh *et al.,* 1979). It is generally reported that premedication and anaesthesia do not seem to affect the responses of human gut muscle strips to drugs (Fishlock and Parks, 1963; Bucknell, 1965; Bennett and Stockley, 1975; Burleigh *et al.,* 1979).

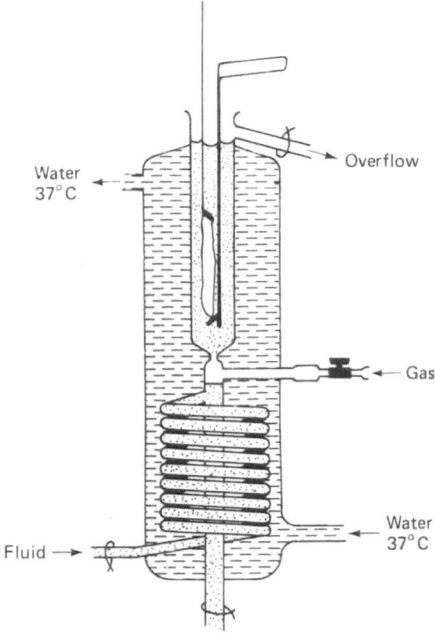

Figure 2.1   An isolated organ bath which maintains a constant environment around the tissue, which does not permit added drugs to diffuse out and which allows the fluid to be changed by upward displacement (from Bennett, 1964, by kind permission of the *Journal of Science Technology*).

A recommended procedure for electrical stimulation of intramural nerves is to use linked stimulators generating square-wave pulses of alternating polarity (e.g. Bennett and Stockley, 1975) to reduce artefacts induced by electrolysis. In the procedure described by Bucknell (1965) and Bennett and Stockley (1975) for human gut, platinum electrodes were placed at the top and bottom of the organ bath. However, the position of the electrodes affects the stimulation of intramural nerves in guinea-pig isolated ileum. Bennett and Stockley (1974) compared five electrode arrangements on responses of this tissue: longitudinal field stimulation (electrodes at the top and bottom of the bath); transverse stimulation using uninsulated platinum wires, one on each side of the ileum (Ambache and Freeman, 1968); wires each side of the tissue insulated where they enter the bath fluid (similar to Crema *et al.*, 1968); transmural stimulation with one electrode inside and another outside the lumen of the gut (Paton, 1955); ring electrodes 2 mm apart around one end of the segment (similar to Furness, 1970). Bennett and Stockley (1974) found that all electrode arrangements could produce tetrodotoxin-resistant contractions at higher frequencies, probably due to direct muscle stimulation, but this was most marked with longitudinal field stimulation (threshold 0.1 Hz).

As indicated above, the nature of responses to electrical stimulation can be tested with drugs such as tetrodotoxin which selectively block nerve conduction (Kao, 1966). Drugs such as hexamethonium which block ganglia can be used to determine whether pre- or postganglionic nerves are being stimulated.

Responses of tissues elicited by electrical stimulation in the absence of appropriate blocking drugs are the net effect of stimulating a mixture of excitatory and inhibitory nerves. Different responses may occur at different frequencies, probably due to variations in nerve sensitivity, but it is wise to use frequencies that occur in physiological or pathological conditions (Folkow, 1952; Douglas and Ritchie, 1957). Most studies have used square-wave pulses, although this is not the shape produced by natural stimuli.

Bennett and Stockley (1975) obtained results supporting the view that cholinergic nerves are stimulated at low frequencies, but frequencies above 8 Hz are required to stimulate adrenergic nerves in human taenia coli (Bucknell, 1965, 1966). Pulse width is also important, since pulses lasting more than 1 ms have a greater tendency to stimulate muscle directly. Stockley (1974) found that adrenergic and non-adrenergic inhibitory nerves mediated relaxation with 0.5 ms, but not with 1 ms pulses.

Relatively few experiments have been performed using human gastrointestinal sphincter tissue *in vitro,* partly because such material is not frequently available at surgery. However, the actions of drugs on other human gastrointestinal muscle have been extensively examined *in vitro,* and such experiments can provide a basis for planning investigations of the mode of action of drugs on human sphincter tissue. Selected examples will now be mentioned to illustrate the principles used in such investigations, but further details are given by Bennett (1973) and Daniel (1973).

In addition to electrical excitation, nerves in isolated tissues can also be stimulated by drugs. Nicotine or dimethylphenylpiperazinium (DMPP) activates nicotinic cholinergic receptors on the postsynaptic membrane in ganglia, leading to the release of neurotransmitter from the postganglionic nerve terminals. The ability of drugs to exert more than one action is showed by nicotine and DMPP, which can release noradrenaline directly from postganglionic sympathetic adrenergic nerves (evidence reviewed by Muscholl, 1970).

Other substances act directly on the muscle cells. Acetylcholine acts on muscarinic receptors on smooth muscle cells, as demonstrated by competitive antagonists such as atropine or hyoscine (figure 2.2). Noradrenaline, the transmitter at sympathetic nerve terminals, can stimulate both alpha- and beta-adrenoceptors, which may be present in varying proportions depending on the type of tissue, and may be blocked,

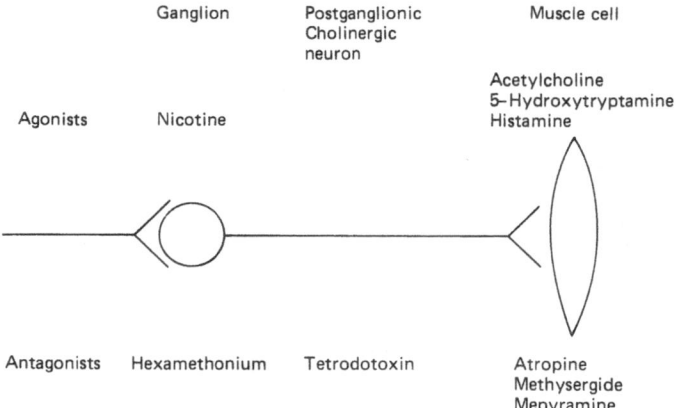

Figure 2.2   The sites at which some substances act on cholinergic nerves and on longitudinal muscle strip of human ileum.

respectively, by the competitive antagonists phentolamine and propranolol.

No drug interacts with only one type of receptor, although many have a sufficiently high degree of selectivity to permit of conclusions about the site of action. Nevertheless, it is advisable to substantiate the findings with one drug by several different procedures.

Although selective antagonists are known for many potent substances which occur in the body, such as acetylcholine, histamine, noradrenaline and 5-hydroxytryptamine, selective competitive antagonists are not available for others. With regard to prostaglandins, the antagonist SC-19220 (Sanner, 1969) and polyphloretin phosphate (Eakins *et al.,* 1970) cause selective blockade only in some tissues—for example, SC-19220 is not active against PGE_2 or $PGF_{2\alpha}$ on human gut muscle (Bennett and Posner, 1971). The lack of suitable antagonists is even greater with regard to most hormones. Failure to block responses to intrinsically released substances might, however, indicate only a difficulty of drug access to the receptor sites within the tissue.

The actions of drugs of potential or proven therapeutic value can be examined on isolated sphincter tissue to indicate the type of action and its mechanisms. However, care must be taken in extrapolating these findings to the *in vivo* situation, and even though receptor mechanisms can be demonstrated in a tissue, they are not necessarily important *in vivo*.

THE UPPER OESOPHAGEAL (CRICOPHARYNGEAL) SPHINCTER

The upper sphincter of the oesophagus is composed of the horizontal striated fibres of the cricopharyngeal muscle and is innervated by motor nerves which pass through the vagi without synapsing and terminate in motor endplates. At rest the sphincter is tonically contracted and relaxes on swallowing.

There is little information about the action of drugs on this sphincter in man. Up to 2 mg atropine intramuscularly did not affect sphincteric pressure, although below the sphincter there was a dose-related depression of peristaltic amplitude (Kantrowitz et al., 1966). Evidence from animal experiments supports the existence of nicotinic cholinergic neuromuscular transmission in this muscle, as in other striated muscles (Christensen, 1975).

THE LOWER OESOPHAGEAL SPHINCTER

The sphincter at the oesophagogastric junction is referred to as the lower oesophageal or cardiac sphincter. The muscle is thickened (Liebermann-Meffert et al., 1979) and develops a pressure, usually about 20 mmHg, which normally falls temporarily on swallowing, to allow of passage of oesophageal contents into the stomach. Many groups (for example, Fisher et al., 1977), have shown the importance of lower oesophageal sphincter pressure in preventing reflux of highly acid gastric contents into the lower oesophagus.

Studies of the Autonomic Nervous System in vitro

The effects of drugs on longitudinal and circular muscle strips from the lower oesophagus have been examined by several investigators (Ellis et al., 1960; Bennett et al., 1967; Misiewicz et al., 1969a; Bass et al., 1970; Stockley, 1974; Bennett and Stockley, 1975; Burleigh, 1979). Acetylcholine or its analogue bethanechol causes contraction which is blocked by atropine-like drugs, and is presumably due to an action on muscarinic receptors. α-Adrenoceptors also mediate contraction, but isoprenaline causes a relaxation which is antagonised by β-adrenoceptor antagonists.

However, various effects have been reported for the same sympathomimetic amine. Noradrenaline may cause relaxation (Misiewicz et al., 1969a) or contraction (Ellis et al., 1960); Burleigh (1979) found that noradrenaline consistently relaxed circular muscle strips by acting on β-adrenoceptors. Bass et al. (1970) found that adrenaline can cause contraction.

Nicotine has various effects on human gastrointestinal muscle, and is thought to cause contraction by stimulating enteric ganglia supplying cholinergic nerves, and relaxation by releasing catecholamines (Bennett and Whitney, 1966a). Ellis et al. (1960) found that circular muscle strips of lower oesophagus relaxed to nicotine, whereas the longitudinal muscle responded with contraction. However, Misiewicz et al. (1969a) and Stockley

(1974) found that nicotine usually relaxed both circular and longitudinal muscle strips. These relaxations were blocked by hexamethonium, by bretylium, which inhibits noradrenaline release, and by the β-adrenoceptor antagonist pronethalol (Misiewicz et al., 1969a).

The responses to electrical field stimulation also show inconsistency. Ellis et al. (1960) and Burleigh (1979) found that 1 ms pulses of 0.8–5 Hz caused relaxed circular muscle strips taken from the most distal sphincteric region of the oesophagus, but caused contractions or a biphasic response in the strips taken from a site well above this region. However, Bennett and Stockley (1975) found that the response of the circular muscle of the lower oesophagus to 1 ms pulses varied with the frequency of stimulation. For example, at low frequencies (0.5 Hz or less) most circular muscle strips contracted, but at 1–4 Hz almost half the strips relaxed. When the electrical stimulation ceased, the relaxation was followed by a rapid contraction. Even more complex patterns were seen at higher frequencies, some strips giving a triphasic response of contraction followed by relaxation and an after-contraction. Most of the longitudinal muscle strips responded with contraction. These effects were due mainly to stimulation of intrinsic nerves, since they were greatly reduced or prevented by tetrodotoxin and were the net result of stimulating excitatory and inhibitory nerves. Atropine frequently converted electrically induced contractions into relaxations, presumably by blocking cholinergic excitatory responses, but in about half of the circular or longitudinal muscle strips studied by Bennett and Stockley (1975) the contractions to low-frequency (<1 Hz) stimulation were unaltered or only slightly changed by drugs which potentiate or block cholinergic contractions. The excitatory transmitter therefore did not seem to be mainly acetylcholine, and experiments with the antagonist methysergide indicated that 5-HT was not involved. Although Ellis et al. (1960) did not use adrenergic blocking drugs, they assumed that electrical field stimulation of lower oesophageal muscle activated adrenergic nerves which relaxed the muscle by releasing a catecholamine.

In the experiments of Bennett and Stockley (1975) guanethidine or oxprenolol reduced, but did not prevent, the electrically induced relaxation of circular muscle strips, so that both adrenergic and non-adrenergic inhibitory nerves appear to be present. However, in Burleigh's (1979) experiments no adrenergic responses were demonstrated: the relaxation of the circular muscle was unaffected by propranolol, phentolamine, hyoscine or guanethidine, but was prevented by tetrodotoxin or lignocaine. Thus, at least some of the inhibitory nerves in human lower oesophageal sphincter appear to be mainly non-adrenergic. The weak motor effect of ATP on the tissue (Burleigh, 1979) does not necessarily mean that these nerves are not purinergic; other studies—for example, with stable ATP analogues—are necessary before a firm conclusion can be drawn.

Studies of the Autonomic Nervous System *in vivo*

Cholinergic Agonists and Antagonists

The conflicting reports prior to 1960 (reviewed by Bettarello *et al.*, 1960) on the effect of cholinergic muscarinic agonists and antagonists on the lower oesophageal sphincter appear to have been resolved. Bettarello *et al.* (1960) reported that bethanechol increased and atropine decreased intraluminal pressure in the distal portion of the oesophagus of patients. Subsequent work has confirmed these results. Thus, subcutaneous administration of the choline ester bethanechol, which acts mainly on muscarinic receptors, increased lower oesophageal sphincter pressure in patients with either a normal or incompetent sphincter (Roling *et al.*, 1972). Similarly, intravenous injection of the anticholinesterase edrophonium raised the pressure in incompetent sphincters (Farrell *et al.*, 1973). Cohen *et al.* (1972) reported that the pressure of normal and incompetent sphincters was increased by injected methacholine or edrophonium, whereas atropine reduced the response to methacholine without altering the baseline lower oesophageal pressure. Bethanechol, given orally, gave symptomatic relief in patients with gastro-oesophageal reflux (Farrell *et al.*, 1974).

Cholinergic agonists may induce many effects, including the release of hormones (Christensen, 1975). Since the lower oesophageal sphincter pressure might be increased indirectly by the release of gastrin, bethanechol and carbachol have been investigated for an effect on serum gastrin levels. Vatn *et al.* (1975) detected no significant change in plasma gastrin levels during an infusion of carbachol, and Boesby *et al.* (1976) made a similar observation with subcutaneously injected carbachol, although the gastro-oesophageal sphincter pressure rose. Bethanechol did not significantly affect blood gastrin levels in normal subjects or those with gastro-oesophageal reflux (Humphries *et al.*, 1974; McCallum *et al.*, 1975).

Cholinergic agonists therefore seem to stimulate lower oesophageal sphincter muscle *in vivo*, as *in vitro*, by acting on muscarinic receptors. A cholinergic mechanism seems involved in the control of the lower oesophageal pressure, since the resting sphincter closure tension in man is partly reduced by atropine (Lind *et al.*, 1968) or propantheline (Van Derstappen and Texter, 1964), and atropine can reduce the rise in sphincteric pressure caused by abdominal compression (Lind *et al.*, 1968). These effects of atropine might be expected to increase the incidence of gastro-oesophageal reflux, but Skinner and Camp (1968) found no correlation between the intraluminal pressure in the lower oesophagus and the incidence of reflux after atropine. Furthermore, Torgerson *et al.* (1979) have recently reported that in a controlled double-blind cross-over study, propantheline did not significantly alter lower oesophageal pressure in normal subjects.

Local chemoreceptors may reflexly alter sphincter closure. Acidification of the lower oesophageal mucosa raises the sphincter closure tension, with a peak effect at pH 3. Cholinergic nerves seem to be involved, since the effect is prevented by atropine (Giles *et al.*, 1969a).

Adrenoceptor Agonists and Antagonists

Zfass *et al.* (1970) found that isoprenaline reduced the resting closure tension of the lower oesophageal sphincter; the β-adrenoceptor antagonist alprenolol had little effect on resting closure tension but it increased the force and duration of sphincteric contraction that followed swallowing-induced relaxation. In the same study neither the α-adrenoceptor agonist phenylephrine nor the α-adrenoceptor antagonist phentolamine altered the sphincter pressure. Phentolamine had no cardiovascular effect, so that there is no evidence that α-adrenoceptor blockade was achieved, but phenylephrine raised the blood pressure. The results with alprenolol are consistent with, but not firm proof of, a β-adrenergic inhibitory modulation of the sphincter, and β-adrenoceptor blockers rarely produce symptoms of lower oesophageal sphincter dysfunction (Christensen, 1975).

Hormones

Gastrin in vitro

Bennett *et al.* (1967) found that gastrin heptadecapeptides I and II (and pentagastrin in the only strip studied) usually contracted the circular muscle of the lower oesophagus, and gastrin sometimes contracted the longitudinal muscle. Pharmacological analysis of the mode of action of gastrin on human stomach strips suggests that the hormone caused contractions directly without involving intrinsic nerves, since ganglion blockade, local anaesthetics, anticholinesterases or hyoscine did not alter the response of the muscle strips to gastrin. Burleigh (1979) also found that pentagastrin contracts strips of circular muscle from the sphincteric region and, as with human stomach (Bennett *et al.*, 1967), there was marked tachyphylaxis.

Gastrin in vivo

Bennett (1968) suggested that gastrin released by food may contribute to gastric motility and that gastrin-induced contraction of the lower oesophageal sphincter may help reduce gastro-oesophageal reflux. Intravenous bolus injections of gastrin raised the basal closure tension in the lower oesophageal sphincter (Giles *et al.*, 1969b), but dose–response relationships were not established. Castell and Harris (1970) found that pentagastrin 1 μg kg^{-1} s.c. raised sphincteric pressures, and this effect was later confirmed by other workers (Cohen and Lipshutz, 1971a; Nebel and Castell, 1972, 1973). Furthermore, intragastric instillation of alkali, peptone broth or the ingestion of ground beef can increase sphincter closure tension. These procedures release endogenous gastrin but they also induce various other neural, biochemical or hormonal effects. Antral acidification inhibits gastrin secretion, and this could help explain why intragastric instillation of HCl reduced the sphincteric closure tension (Castell and Harris, 1970). The effect of gastrin *in vivo* on the lower oesophageal sphincter does not appear to be mediated through cholinergic nerves, since in a double-blind study by Jensen *et al.* (1978), intravenous atropine did not significantly inhibit the sphincter stimulation by intravenous gastrin. Anticholinergic effects such as dry mouth and tachycardia were common after atropine, indicating that pharmacologically effective concentrations of the drug were achieved.

It is accepted that exogenous gastrin can contract the lower oesophageal sphincter, but it seems unlikely that normal endogenous blood gastrin levels have this effect (Grossman, 1974). Several studies have revealed no relationship between fasting serum gastrin and basal sphincter pressure (Dodds *et al.*, 1974; Morris *et al.*, 1974; Boesby *et al.*, 1976), and pentagastrin (0.9 mg kg^{-1} h^{-1} i.v.) did not increase the lower oesophageal sphincter pressure significantly despite producing maximum gastric acid secretion (Frank *et al.*, 1973). Henderson *et al.* (1978) found that instillation of protein into the stomach did not significantly change the sphincter pressure despite a stimulation of gastrin release. Dent and Hansky (1976) found that the rise of serum gastrin after a test meal preceded the increase in lower oesophageal sphincter pressure by 30 min, and that sphincter pressure also increased with a control which did not raise serum gastrin levels. Since exogenous gastrin has an immediate effect on sphincter pressure, this temporal dissociation is further evidence against gastrin having a physiological role in regulating lower oesophageal sphincter pressure. However, before a firm conclusion can be made, studies are required on the many gastrins which may be released, their relative potencies on the sphincter and their possible interactions with other stimuli.

Secretin

Secretin does not seem to have been studied on human isolated lower oesophageal sphincter. *In vivo* neither exogenous secretin (as a bolus injection or as a constant intravenous infusion) nor acidification of the duodenum, which releases endogenous secretin, significantly changed sphincteric closure tension (Cohen and Lipshutz, 1971a; Nebel and Castell, 1972). However, secretin antagonises sphincter stimulation by gastrin. Intravenous infusions or bolus injection of secretin reduced the response to bolus injections of gastrin I, and bolus injection of secretin transiently reduced the sphincteric closure tension during gastric alkalinisation, which releases gastrin. A continuous intravenous infusion of secretin caused a parallel shift to the right of the dose–response curve for gastrin without depressing the maximal attainable response. Cohen and Lipshutz (1971a) therefore concluded that secretin competitively antagonises gastrin, but although these characteristics of the inhibition are consistent with a competitive effect, they are not firm proof. Other important information desirable to evaluate such a claim is the actions of secretin on other excitatory substances and receptor binding studies.

Cholecystokinin

Cholecystokinin does not seem to have been studied on the isolated lower oesophageal sphincter. *In vivo,* bolus intravenous injections of moderately pure cholecystokinin reduced the resting sphincteric closure tension (Fisher *et al.,* 1973a), and the pure synthetic C-terminal octapeptide of cholecystokinin produced a similar dose-related effect (Resin *et al.,* 1973). Although Sturdevant and Kun (1974) confirmed that bolus injection of cholecystokinin octapeptide (5 and 20 ng kg^{-1}) reduced lower oesophageal sphincter pressure, cholecystokinin (40 ng kg^{-1} h^{-1} i.v.) did not significantly reduce the basal sphincter pressure, although it reduced the increase caused by pentagastrin. Since it is not known whether this infusion rate established physiological blood levels, the role of cholecystokinin in the regulation of lower oesophageal sphincter pressure is not known. Grossman (1970) postulated that because the C-terminal pentapeptides of gastrin and cholecystokinin are similar, both hormones might have an affinity for the same receptor sites.

Ingested fats release endogenous cholecystokinin, and this may explain why in normal subjects a fatty meal or intraduodenally instilled corn oil reduced the sphincteric closure tension (Nebel and Castell, 1972). However, certain fats are precursors for prostaglandins. The synthesis of prostaglandin E_2, for example, could account partially for their effects. A fatty meal shifted the dose–response curve to bolus intravenous injections of pentagastrin to the right in parallel (Nebel and Castell, 1973). This is consistent with competitive antagonism, a view also favoured by others.

Fisher *et al.* (1973a) considered that gastrin, cholecystokinin and secretin can act at the same receptors, but the roles of these substances in the physiological control of the sphincter have not been established. As with secretin, it is important to know whether or not cholecystokinin inhibits sphincteric contractions to other agonists.

Glucagon

There is a chemical similarity between glucagon and secretin—14 of the 27 amino acids occupy the same position as in glucagon, which has 29 amino acids. Since secretin antagonises the stimulant effect of gastrin on the lower oesophageal sphincter, similar studies were made with glucagon. Glucagon reduced the resting lower oesophageal pressure by about a half with pharmacological doses of 60 μg kg^{-1} i.v. (Jennewein *et al.*, 1973), 20 μg kg^{-1} i.v. (Christiansen and Borgeskov, 1974) or 10 μg kg^{-1} i.m. (Jaffer *et al.*, 1974). These groups also showed that glucagon reduced the stimulation of lower oesophageal pressure by pentagastrin.

Whereas secretin caused a parallel shift to the right of the gastrin dose–response curve (Cohen and Lipshutz, 1971a), glucagon flattened the dose–response curve to pentagastrin without any lateral shift (Jennewein *et al.*, 1973), which is indicative of non-competitive inhibition. Cholecystokinin can release endogenous glucagon (Unger *et al.*, 1967), and this might contribute to the relaxation of the lower oesophageal sphincter by cholecystokinin (Jennewein *et al.*, 1973).

Oesophageal sphincters of patients with achalasia are thought to be supersensitive to gastrin (Cohen *et al.*, 1971), and this might explain why glucagon decreased the elevated resting pressure of such patients. L-1-arginine 0.6 g kg^{-1} infused intravenously in healthy volunteers raised the plasma concentration of pancreatic glucagon to levels obtained after a protein meal, and inhibited stimulation of the lower oesophageal pressure by pentagastrin (Christiansen *et al.*, 1977).

Glucagon (1.6 kg^{-1} h^{-1}) i.v. resulted in plasma glucagon concentrations three times higher, but a smaller inhibition of the sphincter pressure, than after arginine infusion. Perhaps arginine exerts an effect on the sphincter or affects the release of other substances. Although these results are consistent with a physiological role for pancreatic glucagon in the regulation of lower oesophageal pressure, it must be remembered that the effect has been demonstrated with pentagastrin as a pharmacological stimulus.

Vasoactive Intestinal Peptide (VIP)

Intravenously infused VIP (0.8, 1.6 and 3.2 μg kg^{-1} h^{-1}) dose-dependently inhibited the increase in lower oesophageal sphincter pressure caused by pentagastrin, but did not significantly decrease the basal pressure (Domschke *et al.*, 1978). The plasma levels of VIP achieved were substantially higher than the levels normally encountered, and the effect of physiological amounts is not known.

Motilin

Debas (1975) suggested that motilin might have a physiological role in the control of the lower oesophageal sphincter pressure in certain situations. Intravenous bolus injection of the synthetic analogue 13-norleucine-motilin, which is biologically as active as the natural polypeptide in causing contractions of gastroduodenal muscle (Strunz *et al.*, 1976), increased oesophageal sphincter pressure in normal subjects (Lux *et al.*, 1976) at doses equivalent to those of physiological concentrations of the natural hormone. Domschke *et al.* (1976) instilled acid intraduodenally to release motilin, and found that sphincter pressure and plasma motilin levels rose. Basal values were exceeded by about 80 per cent and 90 per cent, respectively, at 3–4 min, and sphincter pressure returned to basal levels within approximately 5 min, during which time plasma motilin decreased to a plateau about 50 per cent above baseline. Domschke *et al.* (1976) considered that some other neural or hormonal factor activated by duodenal acidification may antagonise the effects of motilin on the sphincter so that the pressure returns to basal more rapidly than plasma motilin levels. They suggest that such a substance could be secretin, which is also released by duodenal acidification.

However, if motilin plays an important role in controlling lower oesophageal sphincter pressure, the motilin levels and the pressure changes should be correlated in different situations. Hellemans *et al.* (1976) used various conditions which would be expected to alter motilin levels—e.g. alkalinisation and subsequent acidification of the antrum and duodenum. The lower oesophageal sphincter pressure did not correlate significantly with the fasting or with the evoked motilin levels in 31 subjects. Thus, no physiological role has been established in the contribution of motilin to the control of lower oesophageal sphincter pressure.

The numerous hormones and other substances discussed may have various actions and interactions, some of which may not be apparent in the fasting state. For example, different substances which on their own are insufficient to have an effect might co-operate to produce a response under physiological conditions.

Pregnancy

While most authorities have suggested that the increased frequency of reflux oesophagitis during pregnancy is due to upward displacement and compression of the stomach by the enlarging uterus, combined with decreased gastrointestinal motility, others have questioned this conclusion and have suggested that some as yet undetermined hormone change occurring during pregnancy is responsible for the reflux in pregnant women (Pope, 1973).

Van Thiel *et al.* (1976) found that the resting lower oesophageal sphincter pressure was similar during menstruation when no medication was taken, and during the rest of the cycle while oral ethinyloestradiol was taken. However, the pressure was less when the oral progestational agent dimethisterone was given with ethinyloestradiol. There were not significant differences in gastric pH and basal plasma gastrin during the various phases of the menstrual cycle which would account for the pressure changes.

In four pregnant women Van Thiel *et al.* (1977) found that lower oesophageal sphincter pressure was less during pregnancy, reaching its lowest at 36 weeks, but was normal post-partum. Acid reflux was detected in all four patients during, but not after, pregnancy. Plasma concentrations of progesterone, oestrone and oestradiol increased during pregnancy, and fell post-partum. Basal gastric pH, plasma gastrin levels, and basal and peak acid secretory responses to pentagastrin during pregnancy were comparable with post-partum measurements. Such data support the hypothesis that hormonal changes in pregnancy reduce lower oesophageal sphincter pressure, allowing reflux to occur which results in heartburn.

In eight women during the first 20 weeks of pregnancy, when serum oestrogen and progesterone levels were high, basal sphincter pressures were within normal limits and there were no symptoms of reflux, but the increases of sphincter contraction with pentagastrin, edrophonium, methacholine or a protein meal were less than at 6 weeks after pregnancy had been terminated (Fisher *et al.*, 1978). These results also support an association of elevated plasma levels of female sex hormones with reduced lower oesophageal sphincter activity.

Prostaglandins

Prostaglandin $F_{2\alpha}$ given intravenously increased lower oesophageal sphincter pressure (Dilawari *et al.*, 1975). Prostaglandin E_2 alone had no effect, but it inhibited pentagastrin-induced sphincter contraction. These results are consistent with the findings that prostaglandin F compounds usually contract the circular muscle of the gastrointestinal tract, whereas prostaglandin E compounds usually cause a relaxation (Bennett and Fleshler, 1970). Dilawari *et al.* (1975) also obtained an increase of sphincter pressure when the prostaglandin synthesis inhibitor indomethacin was given rectally. This is consistent with an inhibitory role of prostanoids (prostaglandins and related substances) in the lower oesophageal sphincter, and suggests that inhibitors of prostaglandin synthesis may be of value in reducing gastro-oesophageal reflux. In contrast, perhaps some antisecretory or 'cytoprotective' (Robert, 1979) prostanoids, which may be used to treat peptic ulceration, might have the disadvantage of increasing oesophageal reflux by relaxing the lower oesophageal sphincter.

Metoclopramide

Justin-Besancon and colleagues (Justin-Besancon *et al.*, 1964; Justin-Besancon and Laville, 1964) described the antiemetic properties of metoclopramide (2-methoxy-5-chloro-procainamide) and its ability to stimulate upper gastrointestinal motility. Metoclopramide 20 mg infused i.v. in healthy subjects increased the resting lower oesophageal sphincter pressure, without interfering with either sphincter relaxation on swallowing or elevation of resting pressure in response to increased abdominal pressure (Heitmann and Moller, 1970). The drug also increased the strength and duration of peristaltic waves in the lower oesophagus. There were no changes in oesophageal spontaneous activity, the percentage of non-peristaltic waves, or the gastric fundus or corpus pressures. This combination of properties seems advantageous for the treatment of gastro-oesophageal incompetence, and, unlike derivatives of acetylcholine, anticholinesterases or gastrin, metoclopramide does not increase gastric secretion (Connell and George, 1969; Cohen et al., 1976). Metoclopramide 10 mg orally increased the lower oesophageal sphincter pressure in patients suffering from symptoms of gastro-oesophageal reflux. The drug increased the amplitude of oesophageal peristaltic waves, but gastric motility was only sometimes stimulated (Dilawari and Misiewicz, 1973). Stanciu and Bennett (1972) reported that intravenous infusions of metoclopramide diminished the frequency of reflux and increased the rate at which the oesophagus expelled an acid load. The increase in sphincter pressure caused by metoclopramide was blocked by atropine, but was unaffected in vagotomised patients.

It should be remembered, however, that truncal vagotomy probably does not denervate the lower oesophageal sphincter. The authors concluded that metoclopramide may act via the intramural cholinergic nerves, but another possibility is that atropine merely inhibited basal cholinergic nerve activity.

McCallum et al. (1975) found that orally administered metoclopramide increased the lower oesophageal sphincter pressure in patients with symptoms of gastro-oesophageal reflux, without altering serum gastrin I concentrations. Cohen et al. (1976) established dose–response relationships for the decrease of gastro-oesophageal reflux with oral and intravenous metoclopramide. Metoclopramide contracted the circular muscle from human small intestine and colon, but did not affect gastric and colonic longitudinal muscle, except that contractions to acetylcholine were enhanced (Eisner, 1968). However, in vivo metoclopramide does not seem to affect the human intestine.

In vitro metoclopramide weakly contracted two out of eight strips of circular muscle from the lower oesophageal sphincter of five patients; the remaining strips were unaffected (Burleigh, 1979). One factor in this weak effect in vitro may have been the high resting tone of the muscle strips.

Histamine and Histamine Antagonists

Ash and Schild (1966) first suggested the concept of different types of histamine receptor on the basis that drugs such as mepyramine antagonise contraction of gastrointestinal muscle (H_1 receptors) but not gastric acid secretion induced by histamine. Black *et al.* (1972) defined H_2 receptors which mediate gastric secretion in response to histamine, gastrin, pentagastrin or food (Black *et al.*, 1973; Wood and Simpkins, 1973).

Oesophageal inhibitory histamine H_1 and H_2 receptors occur in the Australian opossum (De Carle and Glover, 1974), whereas in the North American opossum there are histamine H_1 excitatory and H_2 inhibitory receptors (Cohen and Snape, 1975; De Carle *et al.*, 1976). Histamine $2-40$ μg kg^{-1} h^{-1} infused intravenously into human subjects caused graded increases in acid secretion and lower oesophageal pressure which were unaffected by intravenous diphenhydramine, a histamine H_1 receptor antagonist (Kravitz *et al.*, 1978). Cimetidine, a histamine H_2 receptor antagonist (Wood and Simpkins, 1973), did not alter basal sphincter pressure, or the increase in lower oesophageal pressure with intravenous pentagastrin or oral beef hydrolysate, but prevented the increase caused by histamine. Cimetidine $50-400$ mg orally did not affect the lower oesophageal pressure in normal subjects (Freeland *et al.*, 1977), and a 90 minute intravenous infusion of cimetidine (100 mg h^{-1}) did not modify the sphincter contraction to an intravenous bolus of pentagastrin (Osborne *et al.*, 1977).

Endogenous histamine therefore seems to play no significant role in the control of basal sphincter pressure.

Ethanol

Hogan *et al.* (1972) reported a decrease in lower oesophageal sphincter pressure in normal subjects drinking 103.5 g ethanol (as whisky in divided doses) or infused intravenously with ethanol 1.13 g per kg body weight over a 90 minute period. Plasma ethanol concentrations were, respectively, 66–344 mg per 100 ml and 134–205 mg per 100 ml. Kaufman and Kaye (1978) found that 180 ml vodka, sipped slowly during a meal, increased the incidence of reflux in healthy volunteers; peak blood ethanol concentrations were 63–129 mg per 100 ml. The mechanisms by which ethanol causes gastro-oesophageal reflux could include an effect on the lower oesophageal sphincter by stimulating the synthesis of prostaglandin E_2 (Collier *et al.*, 1976), stimulation of gastric acid secretion and impairment of gastric emptying. Kaufman and Kaye (1978) considered that ethanol may contribute to the development of reflux oesophagitis in some individuals, and that patients with gastro-oesophageal reflux or oesophagitis should avoid alcohol.

Tobacco Smoking

During the period of tobacco smoking, the lower oesophageal sphincter pressure fell in healthy volunteers who were chronic cigarette smokers

(Dennish and Castell, 1971). In smokers who complained of heartburn, and who in many cases had radiologically proved gastro-oesophageal reflux, smoking reduced the sphincter pressure and tended to increase acid reflux (Stanciu and Bennett, 1972; Chattopadhyay et al., 1977). The effect may be caused by nicotine, which relaxes circular muscle of the lower oesophageal sphincter in vitro (Ellis et al., 1960), and nicotine can facilitate the formation of prostaglandin E_2 (Wennmalm, 1978).

Nitrites

Since nitrites relax smooth muscle, they have been studied in oesophageal spasm. Swamy (1977), using manometric measurements, pH recordings and subjective assessment, found that sublingually administered nitroglycerin did not change oesophageal motility in control subjects. Sublingually administered nitroglycerin or orally administered long-acting nitrites relieved spasm in patients who had little gastro-oesophageal reflux, but nitrites were not generally beneficial in patients with acid reflux.

Diazepam, Morphine and Pethidine

These drugs are given prior to endoscopic procedures and for sedation before and after surgery. Their effect on regurgitation and pulmonary aspiration is therefore important. Hall et al. (1975) reported that diazepam, morphine or pethidine given intravenously reduced the lower oesophageal sphincter pressures and increased the rate of gastro-oesophageal reflux. Unfortunately, these authors relied on the lack of effect of intravenous saline injections reported in other studies for their controls. By contrast, in a controlled double-blind cross-over study on healthy volunteers, diazepam 70–280 μg kg^{-1} i.v. (corresponding to a total dose of 5–20 mg) did not lower sphincter pressure significantly over a period of 2 h, and the largest dose increased sphincter pressure 40–80 min after administration (Weihrauch et al., 1979). This finding casts some doubt on the above results with morphine and pethidine.

Achalasia

Achalasia is a condition in which oesophageal peristalsis is absent, the resting lower oesophageal sphincter is elevated and there is incomplete sphincteric relaxation with swallowing (Cohen and Lipshutz, 1971b). This combination of factors produces dysphagia. The lack of peristalsis is probably due to a deficiency of ganglion cells in the myenteric plexus throughout the oesophagus (Trounce et al., 1957). Nicotine and DMPP relax circular strips of sphincter tissue from non-achalasic patients but not from patients with achalasia (Adams *et al.*, 1961; Misiewicz *et al.*, 1969a). In accordance with Cannon's law of denervation supersensitivity (Cannon, 1939), the achalasic oesophagus and sphincter are particularly sensitive to cholinergic stimulation with methacholine (Cohen and Guelrod, 1971). According to Cohen *et al.* (1971), the sphincter in achalasia is also supersensitive to gastrin, and this may explain its hypertonicity. However, Corazziari *et al.* (1978) found that pentagastrin did not significantly alter achalasic sphincter pressure, but the basal pressure in their achalasic patients was similar to the maximally stimulated sphincter in normal subjects, and therefore the sphincter may have been incapable of responding to further stimulation.

THE PYLORIC RING

The thick ring of muscle at the gastroduodenal junction is often referred to as the pyloric sphincter. Its function is not clear, and since there is some doubt that it is a true sphincter, we refer to it as the pyloric ring. Gaskell (1920) suggested on the basis of experiments by Cannon (1911) that the pyloric ring has a special nerve supply, different from that of the stomach and duodenum, and the idea was created that pyloric function was distinct from that of the rest of the gastric muscle. Thomas and Wheelon (1922) refuted the suggestion, since in dogs the sphincter and the adjacent muscle (antrum and duodenal bulb) responded similarly to stimulation of the extrinsic nerves.

Thomas (1957) reviewed the mechanics and regulation of gastric emptying and concluded that the pylorus, while helping to prevent duodenogastric reflux, was not the primary controlling mechanism for emptying. Whereas the lower oesophageal sphincter is normally closed, this may not be so with the pyloric ring. Atkinson *et al.* (1957) found that the pylorus closed only intermittently with peristaltic waves from the stomach. In contrast, Fisher and Cohen (1973), using a perfused catheter system which they regarded as better than balloons for sensing pressure, found that the human pylorus *in vivo* is characterised by a high-pressure zone which relaxes with peristalsis, contracts in response to acid, fats, amino acids or glucose, and prevents duodenal reflux. Secretin and cholecystokinin augmented pyloric sphincter pressure, but gastrin had no effect (Lipshutz and Cohen, 1972; Fisher *et al.*, 1973b). Cohen and his collaborators suggested that the pylorus functions as an anti-reflux mechanism, and possibly as a regulator of gastric emptying.

Studies of the Autonomic Nervous System

Bennett and Whitney (1966b) found that circular or longitudinal muscle strips of pyloric ring contracted weakly to acetylcholine. Various sympathomimetic drugs (noradrenaline, adrenaline, phenylephrine and isoprenaline) inhibited spontaneous contractions and caused relaxations or reduced contractions to acetylcholine or potassium. The ganglion stimulants dimethylphenylpiperazinium and nicotine usually caused relaxation, although occasionally there was no response. Antral and duodenal tissue behaved similarly: acetylcholine always caused contraction, whereas sympathomimetic amines always caused relaxation, a finding confirmed by Bass *et al.* (1970). As with the pyloric ring, DMPP or nicotine relaxed the circular or longitudinal muscles from the first part of the duodenum (Bennett and Whitney, 1966a), but in contrast these drugs sometimes contracted the antral muscle. Valenzuela *et al.* (1976) found that basal pyloric pressure *in vivo* decreased when one cigarette was smoked, possibly because of the nicotine.

Annuras *et al.* (1974) examined electrically induced responses of strips from one human specimen, but they did not analyse the mechanisms involved. Stimulation relaxed two strips of pyloric ring; two strips more distally located relaxed only slightly. They obtained similar responses with tissue from cats, opossums and some dogs, and produced evidence for the presence of non-adrenergic inhibitory nerves. Although the anatomy and much of the pharmacology of the opossum oesophagus and lower oesophageal sphincter are similar to that of man (Christensen and Lund, 1969; Lund and Christensen, 1969; Christensen, 1970; Tuch and Cohen, 1973), it is important to remember that they are not identical.

Valenzuela *et al.* (1976) found that duodenal perfusion with acid doubled the pyloric sphincter pressure. Atropine inhibited this effect, presumably by blocking muscarinic receptors on the muscle and/or by inhibiting the release of duodenal hormones.

Hormones and Autacoids

The mechanisms by which the human pylorus contracts in response to intraduodenal stimuli such as HCl, olive oil and amino acids are not understood, but these substances can release secretin and cholecystokinin. Fisher *et al.* (1973a) found that secretin or cholecystokinin infused i.v. alone or together increased the pyloric pressure with similar maximum responses. Gastrin I did not increase pyloric pressure significantly at any dose, but it antagonised the increase caused by duodenal perfusion with 0.1 M HCl (G. Bennett, 1973). Gastrin I, gastrin II or pentagastrin contracted some circular or longitudinal muscle strips from the antrum (apparently by a direct action on the muscle), but not from the duodenum; but the pyloric ring was not studied.

5-Hydroxytryptamine (5-HT) or histamine either inhibited or had no effect on circular or longitudinal muscle strips of pyloric ring. The antrum was affected similarly by 5-HT, but histamine caused relaxation, contraction or no effect (Bennett and Whitney, 1966b). In the first part of the duodenum both amines produced variable responses (Bennett and Whitney, 1966a).

Metoclopramide

Metoclopramide 10 mg i.v. increased the pyloric 'sphincter' pressure in control subjects, in patients with duodenal ulcer and in patients with gastric ulcer who had low resting pyloric pressure (Valenzuela *et al.*, 1976). The mode of action was not explored.

CHOLEDOCHODUODENAL AND PANCREATIC DUCT SPHINCTERS

The human common bile duct and pancreatic duct share a common entrance into the duodenum. The annular muscle fibres at the end of the bile duct form a sphincter which can obstruct bile flow without closing the pancreatic duct, although annular muscle fibres sometimes also surround the lower end of the main pancreatic duct. The passage of bile or pancreatic juice may also be influenced by the tone of the duodenal muscle around the openings of the ducts. Resistance to flow is due principally to the sphincters, since the biliary and pancreatic ducts contain little muscle.

Effect of Drugs on Pancreatic Intraductal Pressure

Little information is available on pancreatic intraductal pressure. Duval (1958) reported that its average resting value after overnight fasting was 10.3 cm water in patients provided with pancreatic fistulas. An average pressure of 17.6 cm water was necessary to overcome sphincteric resistance to the flow of saline through the fistula and pancreatic duct. Morphine increased the pancreatic ductal pressure in a patient from 9 to 36 cm water (White *et al.*, 1964). As discussed later regarding the biliary sphincter, morphine may cause this increase by eliminating duodenal peristalsis and enhancing non-propulsive muscle tone.

We have not found other human drug data, but in dogs the cholinergic agonist pilocarpine increased, and atropine decreased, the pancreatic intraductal pressure and sphincteric resistance; continuous intravenous administration of adrenaline had only a small effect (usually a slight reduction) on either aspect, and papaverine or nitrites sometimes reduced the intraductal pressure slightly and briefly (Duval, 1958).

Effects of Drugs on the Biliary Sphincter

Oddi (1887) measured the resistance to opening of the muscle surrounding the end of the common bile duct in several animal species. This sphincteric region was named after him, although he was not the first to examine its structure (Tansy and Kendall, 1975). Some workers, however, consider that the sphincter of Oddi is part of the duodenal musculature and not a separate sphincter. It is generally accepted that the passage of bile through the choledochoduodenal junction may involve both the sphincter of Oddi and the state of contraction of contiguous duodenal muscle.

Ashkin *et al.* (1978) collected bile proximally and distally to the sphincter of Oddi in subjects with and without gall bladders to determine the relative contribution of the sphincter and gall bladders to the delivery of bile to the duodenum. A functional sphincter of Oddi significantly reduced the delivery and appeared to be the most important factor regulating transport of bile to the duodenum. The relatively poor accessibility of the sphincter of Oddi for experimental purposes in man partly explains why only limited data are available. Measurements of drug effects have been possible in patients requiring intubation of the common bile duct. The pressure in the bile duct has been measured in patients immediately following gall bladder excision, by determining the pressures required to overcome sphincter resistance and initiate the flow of saline solution into the common bile duct. Bergh (1942) found that the human sphincter of Oddi yielded at pressures of 9–23 cm water.

Studies of the Autonomic Nervous System

In patients who had undergone cholecystectomy and cannulation of the common bile duct, the resistance of the biliary sphincter did not change after subcutaneous injection of pilocarpine, methacholine or neostigmine (Bergh, 1942). Curreri and Gale (1950) thought that the cholinergic agonist bethanechol might relax the sphincter, and gave the drug subcutaneously after inducing spasm with the opiate preparation dilaudid. Instead, intraductal pressure increased. This misleading expectation presumably arose from the belief that sympathetic activity produces sphincteric contraction and parasympathetic activity produces relaxation—effects opposite to those on intestinal muscle. Some data support this view, such as the increased tone of the canine sphincter of Oddi on stimulation of the splanchnic sympathetic nerves (Doyon, 1894), and the relaxation with vagal stimulation (Westphal, 1923). However, other data, reviewed by Bergh (1942), are contradictory; for example, atropine was reported to decrease sphincteric resistance in anaesthetised dogs, and this probably led clinicians to believe that atropine would relax the sphincter of Oddi by blocking the response to parasympathetic activity. Various drugs such as atropine and hyoscine in doses sufficient to produce unwanted effects (e.g. dryness of the mouth) do not significantly alter sphincter pressure, and do not relieve sphincter spasm induced by opiates (Butsch et al., 1936; Doubilet and Colp, 1937; Bergh, 1942; Curreri and Gale, 1950). Following elevation of the pressure in the common bile duct in normal subjects by subcutaneously injected morphine, administration of adrenaline or ephedrine either had no effect (Butsch et al., 1936) or variably altered the sphincter resistance in normal subjects (Bergh, 1942).

In another study isoprenaline, given to patients in doses which raised the pulse rate and caused tremor, did not relieve spontaneous or opiate-induced sphincter spasm (Gaensler and McGowan, 1950).

Hormones

Nebel (1975) determined the effect of pentagastrin, cholecystokinin, secretin and glucagon on sphincter pressure using a non-operative manometric technique. Separate studies were performed for each substance on five normal volunteers, who received only intravenous diazepam and pharyngeal anaesthesia. In all subjects the sphincter pressure decreased after intravenous cholecystokinin (0.5 u kg^{-1}) or glucagon (1 mg), and increased after intravenous pentagastrin (0.1 μg kg^{-1}) or secretin (0.5 u kg^{-1}).

Smooth Muscle Relaxants

Theophylline ethylenediamine (aminophylline) given intravenously reduced the elevation of biliary pressure by codeine (Butsch et al., 1936; Curreri and Gale, 1950) but did not affect the unstimulated sphincter (Bergh, 1942). Aminophylline and other xanthines inhibit cyclic AMP phosphodiesterase, and the elevated amounts of cyclic AMP presumably relax the spastic sphincter. Inhalation of amylnitrite or sublingual administration of glyceryltrinitrate promptly but temporarily alleviated opiate-induced spasm of the biliary tract (Butsch et al., 1936; Curreri and Gale, 1950; Kewenter and Kock, 1971).

The smooth muscle relaxant papaverine (30–60 mg) did not reduce normal or morphine-elevated intrabiliary pressure (Butsch et al., 1936; Doubilet and Colp, 1937; Bergh, 1942), although Curreri and Gale (1950) found that a much larger dose (120 mg) was as effective as 1.2 mg glyceryltrinitrate.

Morphine and Related Drugs

Butsch et al. (1936) concluded their paper with the statement: 'It is significant that all the alkaloids of opium commonly used as analgesics cause a rise in intrabiliary pressure and may actually prolong the pain for which they are given.' These authors observed that morphine given subcutaneously to human volunteers increased the intrabiliary pressure from the normal of 0–2 cm water to 20–30 cm water, and increased the perfusion pressure needed to overcome sphincteric resistance from the normal of 15–20 cm water to 40–50 cm water. The elevation in pressure began 2.5–5 min after the injection of morphine, reached its maximum in 15 min, lasted up to 2 h, and produced an attack of biliary colic in some subjects. Other opiates, including codeine, also raised intrabiliary and perfusion pressures, though less rapidly and extensively. Radiographic studies have conclusively shown spasm of the common bile duct sphincter after giving morphine (Caroli et al., 1960; Myers et al., 1962). Smooth muscle relaxants such as nitrites, which have no direct effect on human gall bladder muscle in vitro (Mack and Todd, 1968), temporarily reduced the pressure and relieved the pain, whereas anticholinergic drugs were ineffective. These observations have been generally confirmed by other authors (Doubilet and Colp, 1937; Bergh, 1942; Curreri and Gale, 1950; Gaensler and McGowan, 1950), but Boulter (1961) found that atropine 1.2 mg or another anticholinergic, propantheline 15 mg, relieved morphine-induced spasm, and Kewenter and Kock (1971) showed a similar effect with intravenous hyoscine butylbromide 10 mg, but not with atropine 0.5 mg.

Jacobsson et al. (1961) compared the action of codeine and pholcodine on duodenal motility and choledochal pressure. Pholcodine had no effect in antitussive doses, but codeine 20 mg given orally or intraduodenally to fasting patients increased the pressure in the common bile duct by 4–18 cm water. A further increase occurred when the bile duct was perfused, mimicking a situation where bile flow would be stimulated by feeding, and pain similar to biliary colic was reported. Codeine, but not pholcodine, also caused periodic intestinal activity with frequent non-propulsive contractions. Pethidine 50 mg i.v. reduced flow in the common bile duct in most subjects (Boulter, 1961). The peak effect was sometimes as great as with morphine 10 mg i.v., but the duration of spasm, about 8 min, was considerably less than with morphine. Hopton and Torrance (1967) confirmed that pethidine was less effective than morphine in raising the pressure in the human common bile duct; dextropropoxyphene or phenacozine did not cause a rise in biliary pressure.

The exact site of action of the opiates in their effect on biliary drainage is not known. In contrast to its effects on the sphincter, morphine has no direct action on human isolated gall bladder muscle (Mack and Todd, 1968). The common bile duct has a mainly fibrous wall, with little smooth muscle, which presumably makes only a small contribution to the intrabiliary pressure (Myers *et al.*, 1962).

Sphincterotomy only partly lessens opiate-induced spasm (Boulter, 1961), probably because duodenal muscles at the site of entry of the ducts contribute to the resistance to bile flow. Duodenal peristalsis appears to enhance intermittent passage of bile into the lumen by a 'milking' action which is inhibited by narcotic analgesics (Hallenbeck, 1968).

Ethanol

Ethanol may affect the sphincter of Oddi. Bergh (1942) reported a very slight relaxation of the sphincter in two out of three experiments when 50 ml of 28.5–47.5 per cent ethanol was given intraduodenally. Subsequent reports, however, mention an opposite effect. Nossel and Efron (1955) found increased choledochal pressure in four patients who had drunk 30 ml whisky.

Intragastric infusion of 48 g ethanol increased the resistance by the sphincter of Oddi to flow in the common bile duct (Capitaine and Sarles, 1971); and ethanol, 300–600 mg per kg body weight infused i.v. over 20 min, increased common bile duct pressure to the same extent as did 10–15 mg parenteral morphine (Pirola and Davis, 1968). An increased rate of bile flow was considered unlikely to cause the pressure change, and the reduction of pressure with inhalation of amylnitrite supports the idea that ethanol or morphine increased resistance to flow. Pirola and Davis (1970) noted that intravenous ethanol reduced the volume of pancreatic secretion and increased duodenal motility, whereas dextrose was ineffective; they postulated that systemic ethanol contracts the sphincteric musculature at the junction of the pancreatic and common bile ducts with the duodenum. The mode of action of ethanol is not known, but it can stimulate prostaglandin synthesis (Collier *et al.*, 1976).

THE ILEOCAECAL SPHINCTER

The junction of the human ileum and caecum is marked by a well-defined anatomical structure which, because of its relative inaccessibility, has had limited experimental investigation. Elliott (1904) mentioned that in man (as opposed to laboratory animals) the arrangement '... is quite exceptional, being so highly differentiated that it does employ the mechanical advantages resulting from an oblique entry of the ileum through the wall of the colon. But the fundamental control is by a muscular sphincter. Hence it is erroneous to emphasise the mechanical adjunct in man and postulate its generalisation in the mammalian viscera by the term "ileo caecal valve". In its stead should be employed the name ileo-colic sphincter.'

In vitro **Studies**

Gazet and Jarrett (1964) studied circular and longitudinal muscle strips from specimens of human ileocaecal junction obtained at operation from patients undergoing right hemicolectomy for carcinoma of the colon. Acetylcholine caused a contraction which was potentiated by the anticholinesterase eserine and blocked by atropine. Adrenaline or noradrenaline contracted circular muscle from the most terminal intracaecal portion of the ileum, considered to be the sphincter; the α-adrenoceptor antagonist phentolamine blocked the contractions. Strips from the more proximal (non-sphincteric) regions relaxed with adrenaline or noradrenaline. Isoprenaline caused only relaxations of sphincter strips, as in other muscles, and nicotine had little or no effect. Bennett and Whitney (1966b) cite unpublished experiments that confirm the ability of noradrenaline and adrenaline to contract the ileocaecal sphincter, and Bass *et al.* (1970) also found that acetylcholine or adrenaline contracted isolated circular muscle strips from the human caecal junction.

In vivo **Studies**

White *et al.* (1934) performed balloon studies on a female patient provided with a caecostomy. Adrenaline, given subcutaneously or locally, decreased the sphincter tone, whereas subcutaneous pilocarpine increased the rhythmic activity of the sphincter. Buirge (1944) confirmed these results on another female patient with a caecostomy and, among several other incidental observations, noted that atropine abolished the increased activity caused by neostigmine. However, Liotta *et al.* (1957) found that adrenaline sometimes increased and sometimes decreased sphincteric tone. Distension of the ileum with a balloon through a colostomy relaxed the caecal junction, whereas distension of the caecum caused sphincter contraction (Cohen *et al.*, 1968). Subcutaneously administered pentagastrin decreased ileocaecal pressure within 15 min of the injection (Castell *et al.*, 1970). Consistent with this are the findings that gastric acidification, a procedure expected to inhibit gastrin release, increased the ileocaecal sphincter pressure; gastric alkalinisation, which would release gastrin, decreased sphincter pressure. It is tempting to attribute these effects to gastrin, but it must be remembered that entry of acid into the duodenum may affect the response (Misiewicz *et al.*, 1967). The relaxation of the ileocaecal sphincter with gastrin and pentagastrin is opposite to the contraction of the lower oesophageal sphincter described previously. Gastrin or pentagastrin increases gastric motility (Smith and Hogg, 1966; Bennett *et al.*, 1967; Misiewicz *et al.*, 1967, 1969b), but the effect on the small intestine is disputed. Smith and Hogg (1966) reported an increase, whereas others report no effect of gastrin or pentagastrin on the small intestine (Logan and Connell, 1966; Bennett *et al.*, 1967; Misiewicz *et al.*, 1967), although there may be a stimulation of colonic motility. Castell *et al.* (1970) speculated that gastrin released by food in the antrum might, by producing the combined motility effects described, speed the passage of small intestinal contents into the colon.

THE RECTOSIGMOID JUNCTION

The existence of a sphincter at the rectosigmoid junction has been proposed by some investigators (Martin and Burden, 1927; Didio and Anderson, 1968; Mann, 1975), whereas others have not detected sphincteric activity in the sigmoid colon or rectum of healthy subjects (Hill *et al.*, 1960; Bacon, 1941). Chowdhury *et al.* (1976) recorded colonic and rectal intraluminal pressures in subjects with colonic motor disorders and in healthy controls. Constipated patients, but rarely controls, had hyperactivity at the rectosigmoid junction with spontaneous complex waves of activity. This segment was not a true sphincter, since there was neither a significant elevation of the basal pressure nor a pressure gradient proximally or distally. Secretin or cholecystokinin 1 u kg^{-1} h^{-1} infused i.v. for 30 min inhibited the hyperactive segment, but secretin depressed and cholecystokinin stimulated motor activity of the adjacent sigmoid colon (Chowdhury *et al.*, 1976). Neither substance significantly influenced rectal activity. Glucagon 10 μg kg^{-1} h^{-1} or atropine 12 μg kg^{-1} h^{-1} infused i.v. markedly inhibited all wave activity of the hyperactive segment and of the adjacent colon and rectum. The effect of atropine suggests that the hyperactivity involves cholinergic nerve activity.

THE INTERNAL AND EXTERNAL ANAL SPHINCTERS

The combined action of several muscles helps to maintain anal continence. The angulation between the axis of the rectum and that of the anal canal results from the tonic activity of the puborectalis portion of the levator ani muscles. The anal canal itself is surrounded by the internal (smooth muscle) and external (striated muscle) sphincters.

Normally both internal and external anal sphincters are in a constant state of tone (Schuster *et al.*, 1963, 1965; Alva *et al.*, 1967; Bennett and Duthie, 1964). The tone of the internal anal sphincter is considerably greater than that of the external sphincter, and contributes most to the pressure recorded from the anal canal (Alva *et al.*, 1967; Bennett and Duthie, 1964). The exact origin of the stimulus for internal anal sphincter tone is uncertain, but it persists after interruption of spinal nervous connections (Frenckner, 1975).

The internal anal sphincter receives sacral parasympathetic and thoracolumbar sympathetic innervation. There is histochemical evidence for both parasympathetic and sympathetic innervation of the internal sphincter (Baumgarten *et al.*, 1971), but there are few, if any, ganglion cells in the rectum (Baumgarten *et al.*, 1971, 1973; Howard, 1975).

According to the ideas discussed by Gaskell (1920), the sympathetic nerves would be expected to be excitatory, and the parasympathetic inhibitory, to the sphincter. Evidence for excitatory sympathetic nerves to the internal anal sphincter is the loss of sphincter tone caused by high spinal anaesthesia (Frenckner and Ihre, 1976), or α-adrenoceptor blockade (Guiterrez and Shah, 1975). However, Shepherd and Wright (1968) reported that stimulation of the hypogastric (sympathetic) presacral nerves in patients caused sphincter relaxation which was unaffected by 1 mg atropine. These authors were not convinced that adrenergic nerves subserve an inhibitory function in the internal anal sphincter, because the presacral outflow might contain functionally mixed nerves rather than just adrenergic fibres, and the concentration of atropine in tissues might have been less than that needed to block a cholinergic effect.

In vitro preparations develop higher tone than strips of adjacent rectal circular muscle. This tone is unaffected by phentolamine or tetrodotoxin (Burleigh *et al.*, 1979). The existence of sympathetic excitatory nerves is supported by evidence that noradrenaline contracts isolated strips of internal anal sphincter muscle (Parks and Fishlock, 1967; Friedmann, 1968; Parks *et al.*, 1969; Burleigh *et al.*, 1973). The contraction was antagonised by α-adrenoceptor blocking agents, and prevention of contraction unmasked a relaxation which, with isoprenaline, was antagonised by β-adrenoceptor blocking agents.

The proximal and distal parts of the sphincter respond to acetylcholine with either contraction, relaxation or no response (Friedmann, 1968; Parks *et al.*, 1969). Burleigh *et al.* (1979) found that out of 250 strips from about 30 patients the majority (84 per cent) relaxed in response to acetylcholine. Bethanechol, which selectively stimulates muscarinic receptors (Rand and Stafford, 1967; Burleigh, 1978a), also relaxed most sphincter strips. Burleigh *et al.* (1979) considered that previous authors may have obtained inconsistent responses to acetylcholine (and to electrical field stimulation: Friedmann, 1968) because of damage to intrinsic nerves during preparation of muscle strips. Burleigh *et al.* (1979) found that relaxations to acetylcholine were blocked by hyoscine, partly inhibited by the nerve-blocking drug tetrodotoxin, but not significantly affected by hexamethonium. Thus, the response probably involved muscarinic receptors on nerves and muscle, but not nicotinic receptors on ganglia. Muscarinic receptors have been demonstrated in autonomic ganglia, although they did not seem essential for normal neurotransmission (Volle and Koelle, 1975). There are few, if any, ganglion cells in the sphincter muscle (Baumgarten *et al.*, 1971, 1973; Howard, 1975), but many occur in the enteric plexuses which would be at least partly retained in the isolated muscle strips.

Tetrodotoxin reduced the effect of acetylcholine more on proximal than on distal strips of internal anal sphincter (Burleigh *et al.*, 1979). This may be because acetylcholine stimulated the non-cholinergic, non-adrenergic inhibitory nerves which Baumgarten *et al.* (1973) detected much more frequently in the proximal than in the distal region of the internal anal sphincter. Nicotine or DMPP, which stimulate ganglia at nicotinic sites, relaxed strips of proximal and distal sphincter muscle (Burleigh *et al.*, 1979). The relaxations were blocked by tetrodotoxin, hexamethonium, guanethidine or propranolol (Burleigh, 1978b; Burleigh *et al.*, 1979), which suggests that nicotinic receptors in adrenergic nerves were stimulated and a sympathomimetic amine was released, causing relaxation by activating β-adrenoceptors. Burleigh (1978) preincubated sphincter strips with ^{3}H-noradrenaline, and found that relaxations to DMPP were accompanied by an increase in the release of ^{3}H material. This agrees with the suggestion by Parks *et al.* (1969) that nicotine relaxes sphincter strips by releasing an adrenergic neurotransmitter close to β-adrenoceptors. However, sympathetic ganglia are thought to lie outside the gut and would not be expected to occur in the muscle strips. An explanation of the catecholamine release may be that nicotine and DMPP can also stimulate adrenergic nerve terminals (Thompson, 1958; Daniel, 1968; Muscholl, 1970).

Burleigh *et al.* (1979) found that electrical field stimulation always relaxed strips from the proximal or distal part of the internal anal sphincter. These relaxations were unaffected by hyoscine, propranolol or hexamethonium, but were prevented by concentrations of tetrodotoxin selective for blockade of nerves. The responses were therefore thought to arise from stimulation of inhibitory intrinsic nerves which were neither adrenergic nor cholinergic. The existence of such nerves in human gastrointestinal muscle is accepted, although the transmitter is not characterised (Bucknell, 1966; Daniel, 1973; Bennett and Stockley, 1975). Burleigh *et al.* (1979) thought that the transmitter was unlikely to be histamine or prostaglandin E_2, since mepyramine or indomethacin did not affect the relaxations. Prostaglandin $F_{2\alpha}$, 5-hydroxytryptamine and dopamine seem unlikely candidates, since they contracted the tissue. However, vasoactive intestinal peptide (VIP) (0.6 nM–0.75 μM) relaxed sphincter strips, and in a brief report it has been claimed that human internal anal sphincter contains a rich supply of VIP-containing nerves (Alumets *et al.*, 1978). Burleigh *et al.* (1979) examined the possible involvement of purinergic nerves (Burnstock, 1975) in the response to electrical stimulation. Adenosine triphosphate (ATP) relaxed sphincter strips. Higher concentrations of ATP (causing desensitisation) or the ATP antagonist 2,2'-pyridylisatogen (Hooper *et al.*, 1974) reduced the response to ATP and electrical stimulation, but both procedures non-selectively reduced control responses to isoprenaline.

Hirschsprung's disease usually presents as an acute intestinal obstruction in infants, and chronic obstruction in children. The rectum is constricted and the colon appears dilated. Myenteric ganglion cells are few or absent in the constricted portion of the bowel, and there are large abnormal nerve trunks between the longitudinal and the circular muscle (Whitehouse and Kernohan, 1948). Since these large fibres give a strongly positive reaction for acetylcholinesterase, they are regarded as cholinergic parasympathetic nerves (Kamijo et al., 1953; Adams et al., 1960; Garrett et al., 1969).

When the rectum is distended, the internal anal sphincter normally relaxes by a rectoanal reflex independent of spinal nervous connections (Duthie and Bennett, 1963), and is believed to involve intraneural nervous pathways. In Hirschsprung's disease rectal distension causes contraction of the internal anal sphincter (Lawson and Nixon, 1967; Tobon et al., 1968).

In normal bowel most of the fluorescent adrenergic nerves are found in close association with ganglia, with only a few in the muscle layers (Baumgarten, 1967; Bennett et al., 1968). The aganglionic constricted segment in Hirschsprung's disease contains an increased number of adrenergic nerves which are distributed throughout the muscle layers. This region normally relaxes to adrenergic stimuli, but the spasm of the affected segment may be related to the abnormal distribution of the adrenergic nerves.

In the cat relaxation of the internal sphincter is thought to be mediated by parasympathetic nerves which include the intramural ganglia (Davenport, 1961; Smith, 1967). The lack of ganglia in Hirschsprung's disease may interrupt the afferent parasympathetic pathway, thus preventing normal sphincteric relaxation. Perhaps the absence of normal parasympathetic innervation in Hirschsprung's disease results in unopposed sympathetic stimulation, which causes contraction of the internal anal sphincter following rectal distension.

GENERAL CONCLUSIONS

Evidence from *in vitro* experiments has revealed that excitation of cholinergic muscarinic receptors causes contraction in the lower oesophageal sphincter, the pyloric ring and the ileocaecal sphincter. In contrast, acetylcholine relaxes the internal anal sphincter. Excitation of β-adrenoceptors always relaxes sphincter tissue, whereas excitation of α-adrenoceptors can contract lower oesophageal, ileocaecal and internal anal sphincter muscle *in vitro*. However, a role *in vivo* for these receptors has not been established in every case.

Non-cholinergic non-adrenergic inhibitory nerves are probably important, but poorly understood, contributors to the control of gastrointestinal motility, and these nerves probably occur in the lower oesophageal and internal anal sphincters.

Exogenous hormones affect the tone of some of the sphincters, but there is no convincing evidence that they have a physiological role in regulating pressure.

Drugs can improve the function of incompetent sphincters (e.g. metoclopramide alleviating the symptoms of gastro-oesophageal reflux) or adversely affect sphincter pressure (e.g. ethanol, which should be avoided by patients with gastro-oesophageal reflux). Drugs can also cause spasm of sphincters (e.g. opiate-induced spasm of the biliary sphincter).

REFERENCES

Adams, C. W. M., Brain, R. H. F., Ellis, F. G., Kauntze, R. and Trounce, J. R. (1961). Achalasia of the cardia. *Guy's Hospital Report*, **110**, 191-236

Adams, C. W. M., Marples, E. A. and Trounce, J. R. (1960). Achalasia of the cardia and Hirschsprung's disease. The amount and distribution of cholinesterase. *Clin. Sci.*, **19**, 473-481

Alumets, J., Hakanson, R., Sundler, F. and Uddman, R. (1978). VIP innervation of sphincters. *Scand. J. Gastroenterol.*, **13**, Suppl. 49, 6

Alva, J., Mendeloff, A. I. and Schuster, M. M. (1967). Reflex and electromyographic abnormalities associated with fecal incontinence. *Gastroenterology*, **53**, 101-106

Ambache, N. and Freeman, M. A. (1968). Atropine-resistant longitudinal muscle spasm due to excitation of non-cholinergic neurones in Auerbach's plexus. *J. Physiol., Lond.*, **199**, 705-727

Annuras, S., Cooke, A. R. and Christensen, J. (1974). An inhibitory innervation at the gastroduodenal junction. *J. Clin. Invest.*, **54**, 529-535

Ash, A. S. F. and Schild, H. O. (1966). Receptors mediating some actions of histamine. *Br. J. Pharmacol.*, **27**, 427-439

Ashkin, J. R., Lyon, D. T., Shull, S. D., Wagner, C. I. and Soloway, R. D. (1978). Factors affecting delivery of bile to the duodenum in man. *Gastroenterology*, **74**, 560-565

Atkinson, M., Edwards, D. A. W., Honor, A. J. and Rowlands, E. M. (1957). Comparison of cardiac and pyloric sphincters: a manometric study. *Lancet*, **273**, 918-922

Bacon, H. E. (1941). *Anus-Rectum-Sigmoid Colon, Diagnosis and Treatment*, 3rd edn, Vol. 1, Lippincott, Philadelphia, pp. 1-50

Bass, D. D., Ustach, T. J. and Schuster, M. M. (1970). In vitro pharmacologic differentiation of sphincteric and non-sphincteric muscle. *Johns Hopkins Med. J.*, **127**, 185-191

Baumgarten, H. G. (1967). Uber die verteilung von catecholaminen im darm des menschen. *Z. Zellforsch. Mikroskop. Anat.*, **83**, 133-146

Baumgarten, H. F., Holstein, A. F. and Stelzner, F. (1971). Differences in the innervation of the large intestine and internal anal sphincter in mammals and humans. *Verhandl. Anat. Ges.*, **56**, 43-47

Baumgarten, H. F., Holstein, A. F. and Stelzner, F. (1973). Nervous elements in the human colon of Hirschsprung's disease (with comparative remarks on neuronal profiles in the normal human and monkey colon and sphincter ani internus). *Virchows Arch. Abt. A, Path. Anat.*, **358**, 113-136

Bennett, A. (1964). An improved isolated organ bath. *J. Sci. Technol.*, **10**, 176-177

Bennett, A. (1968). Relationship between in-vitro studies of gastrointestinal muscle and motility of the alimentary tract in vivo. *Am.J. Dig. Dis.*, **13**, 410-414

Bennett, A. (1973). The pharmacology of isolated gastrointestinal muscle. In *Pharmacology of Gastrointestinal Motility and Secretion*, Vol III (ed. Pamela Holton), Pergamon Press, Oxford, pp. 399-432

Bennett, A. and Fleshler, B. (1970). Prostaglandins and the gastrointestinal tract. *Gastroenterology*, **59**, 790-800

Bennett, A., Garrett, J. R. and Howard, E. R. (1968). Adrenergic myenteric nerves in Hirschsprung's disease. *Br. Med. J.*, **1**, 487-489

Bennett, A., Misiewicz, J. J. and Waller, S. L. (1967). Analysis of the motor effects of gastrin and pentagastrin on the human alimentary tract in vitro. *Gut*, **8**, 470-474

Bennett, A. and Posner, J. (1971). Studies on prostaglandin antagonists. *Br. J. Pharmacol.*, **42**, 584-594

Bennett, A. and Stockley, H. L. (1974). Effect of electrode positions on contractions of guinea-pig isolated ileum to electrical stimulation. *Br. J. Pharmacol.*, **50**, 453p-454p

Bennett, A. and Stockley, H. L. (1975). The intrinsic innervation of the human alimentary tract and its relation to function. *Gut*, **16**, 443-453

Bennett, A. and Whitney, B. (1966a). A pharmacological study of the motility of the human gastrointestinal tract. *Gut*. **7**, 307-316

Bennett, A. and Whitney, B. (1966b). A pharmacological investigation of human isolated stomach. *Br. J. Pharmacol.*, **27**, 286-298

Bennett, R. C. and Duthie, H. L. (1964). Functional importance of internal anal sphincter. *Br. J. Surg.*, **51**, 355-357

Bergh, G. S. (1942). The sphincter mechanism of common bile duct in human subjects: Its reactions to certain types of stimulation. *Surgery*, **11**, 299-330

Bettarello, A., Tuttle, S. G. and Grossman, M. I. (1960). Effect of autonomic drugs on gastro-esophageal reflux. *Gastroenterology*, **39**, 340-346

Black, J. W., Duncan, A. M., Durant, C. W., Durant, C. J., Ganellin, C. R. and Parsons, E. M. (1972). Definition and antagonism of histamine H_2 receptors. *Nature*, **236**, 385-390

Black, J. W., Duncan, W. A. M., Emmett, J. C., Ganellin, C. R., Hesselbo, T., Parsons, E. M. and Wyllie, J. H. (1973). Metiamide—an orally active histamine H_2-receptor antagonist. *Agents Actions*, **3**, 133-137

Boesby, S., Brandsborg, M., Brandsborg, O., Larsen, N. K. and Pedersen, S. A. (1976). The effect of carbachol on resting gastro-oesophageal sphincter pressure and serum gastrin in normal human subjects. *Scand. J. Gastroenterol.*, **11**, 171-175

Boulter, P. S. (1961). The effects of analgesics and antispasmodics on flow through the human common bile duct. *Guy's Hospital Reports*, **110**, 246-262

Bucknell, A, (1965). Effects of direct and indirect stimulation on isolated colon. *J. Physiol., Lond.*, **177**, 58-59

Bucknell, A. (1966). Studies of the physiology and pharmacology of the colon of man and other mammals. Ph.D. Thesis, University of London

Buirge, R. E. (1944). Experimental observations on the human ileocecal valve. *Surgery*, **16**, 356-369

Burleigh, D. E. (1978a). Selectivity of bethanechol on muscarinic receptors. *J. Pharm. Pharmacol.*, **30**, 398-399

Burleigh, D. E. (1978b). Dimethylphenylpiperazinium (DMPP) causes an increase in ^3H overflow from superfused strips of human internal anal sphincter. In *Abstracts of the 7th International Congress of Pharmacology*, Pergamon Press, Oxford, p.773

Burleigh, D. E. (1979). The effects of drugs and electrical field stimulation on the human lower oesophageal sphincter. *Arch. Int. Pharmacodyn. Therap.*, **240**, 169-176

Burleigh, D. E., D'Mello, A. and Parks, A. G. (1973). An in vitro pharmacological investigation of the human internal anal sphincter. *Naunyn-Schmiedebergs Arch. Pharmacol.*, **279**, 59 (in supplement)

Burleigh, D. E., D'Mello, A. and Parks, A. G. (1979). Responses of isolated human internal anal sphincter to drugs and electrical field stimulation. *Gastroenterology*, **77**, 484-490

Burnstock, G. (1975). Purinergic transmission. In *Handbook of Psychopharmacology*, Vol. 5 (ed. L. L. Iversen, S. D. Iversen and S. H. Snyder), Plenum Press, New York, pp. 131-134

Butsch, W. L., McGowan, J. M. and Walters, W. (1936). Clinical studies on the influence of certain drugs in relation to biliary pain and to the variations in intrabiliary pressure. *Surg., Gyn. Obst.*, **63**, 451-456

Cannon, W. B. (1911). *The Mechanical Factors of Digestion*, Longmans, New York

Cannon, W. B. (1939). A law of denervation (abstract). *Am. J. Med. Sci.*, **198**, 739

Capitaine, Y. and Sarles, H. (1971). Action of ethanol on the tonicity of Oddi's sphincter in humans. *Biol. Gastroenterol. (Paris)*, **3**, Suppl. 3, 231-235

Caroli, J., Porcher, P., Pequignot, G. and Delattre, M. (1960). Contribution of cineradiography to study of the function of the human biliary tract. *Am. J. Dig. Dis.*, **5**, 677-696

Castell, D. O., Cohen, S. and Harris, L. D. (1970). Response of human ileocecal sphincter to gastrin. *Am. J. Physiol.*, **219**, 712-715

Castell, D. O. and Harris, L. D. (1970). Hormonal control of gastro-esophageal sphincter strength. *New Engl. J. Med.*, **282**, 886-889

Chattopadhyay, D. K., Greaney, M. G. and Irvin, T. T. (1977). Effect of cigarette smoking on the lower oesophageal sphincter. *Gut*, **18**, 833-835

Chowdhury, A. R., Dinoso, V. P. and Lorber, S. H. (1976). Characterization of a hyperactive segment at the rectosigmoid junction. *Gastroenterology*, **71**, 584-588

Christiansen, J. and Borgeskov, S. (1974). The effect of glucagon and the combined effect of glucagon and secretin on lower oesophageal sphincter pressure in man. *Scand. J. Gastroenterol.*, **9**, 615-618

Christiansen, J., Lauritzen, K., Moesgaard, J. and Holst, J. J. (1977). Effect of endogenous and exogenous glucagon on pentagastrin-stimulated lower esophageal sphincter pressure in man. *Scand. J. Gastroenterol.*, **12**, 33-36

Christensen, J. (1970). Patterns and origins of some esophageal responses to stretch and electrical stimulation. *Gastroenterology*, **59**, 909-916

Christensen, J. (1975). Pharmacology of the esophageal motor function. *Ann. Rev. Pharmacol.*, **15**, 243-258

Christensen, J. and Lund, G. F. (1969). Esophageal responses to distension and electrical stimulation. *J. Clin. Invest.*, **48**, 408-419

Cohen, S., Fisher, R., Lipshutz, W., Turner, R., Myers, A. and Schumacher, R. (1972). The pathogeneseis of esophageal dysfunction in scleroderma and Raynaud's disease. *J. Clin. Invest.*, **51**, 2663-2668

Cohen, B. R. and Guelrod, M. (1971). 'Cardiospasm' in achalasia: demonstration of supersensitivity of the lower oesophageal sphincter. *Gastroenterology*, **60**, 769

Cohen, S., Harris, L. D. and Levitan, R. (1968). Manometric characteristics of the human ileocaecal junctional zone. *Gastroenterology*, **54**, 72-75

Cohen, S. and Lipshutz, W. (1971a). Hormonal regulation of human lower esophageal sphincter competence: interaction of gastrin and secretin. *J. Clin. Invest.*, **50**, 449-454

Cohen, S. and Lipshutz, W. (1971b). Lower oesophageal sphincter dysfunction in achalasia. *Gastroenterology*, **61**, 814-819

Cohen, S., Lipshutz, W. and Hughes, W. (1971). Role of gastrin supersensitivity in the pathogenesis of lower esophageal sphincter hypertension in achalasia. *J. Clin. Invest.*, **50**, 1241-1247

Cohen, S., Morris, D. W., Schoen, H. J. and Di Marino, A. J. (1976). The effect of oral and intravenous metoclopramide on human lower oesophageal sphincter pressure. *Gastroenterology*, **70**, 484-487

Cohen, S. and Snape, W. J. (1975). Action of metiamide on the lower oesophageal sphincter. *Gastroenterology*, **69**, 911-919

Collier, H. O. J., McDonald-Gibson, W. J. and Saeed, S. A. (1976). Stimulation of prostaglandin biosynthesis by drugs: effects in vitro of some drugs affecting gut function. *Br. J. Pharmacol.*, **58**, 193-199

Connell, A. M. and George, J. D. (1969). Effect of metoclopramide on gastric function in man. *Gut*, **10**, 678-680

Corazziari, E., Pozzessere, C., Dani, S., Anzini, F. and Torsoli, A. (1978). Lower oesophageal sphincter response to intravenous infusions of pentagastrin in normal subjects, antrectomised and achalasic patients. *Gut*, **19**, 1121-1124

Crema, A., Del Tacca, M., Frigo, G. M. and Lecchini, S. (1968). Presence of non-adrenergic inhibitory system in the human colon. *Gut*, **9**, 633-637

Curreri, A. R. and Gale, J. W. (1950). Effect of analgesics and antispasmodics on common duct pressures. *Ann. Surg.*, **132**, 348-361

Daniel, E. E. (1968). Pharmacology of the gastrointestinal tract. In *Handbook of Physiology, Section 6: Alimentary Canal*, Vol. 4 (ed. C. F. Code), American Physiological Society, Washington, D.C., pp. 2276-2287

Daniel, E. E. (1973). A conceptual analysis of the pharmacology of gastrointestinal motility. In *Pharmacology of Gastrointestinal Motility and Secretion*, Vol. II (ed. Pamela Holton),

Pergamon Press, Oxford, pp. 457-545

Davenport, H. W. (1961). *Physiology of the Digestive Tract: An Introductory Text,* Year Book Medical, Chicago, p. 67

Debas, H. T. (1975). The LES merry-go-round. *Gastroenterology,* **68,** 615-616

De Carle, D. J., Brody, M. J. and Christensen, J. (1976). Histamine receptors in esophageal smooth muscle of the opossum. *Gastroenterology,* **70,** 1071-1075

De Carle, D. J. and Glover, W. E. (1974). Independence of gastrin and histamine receptors in the lower oesophageal sphincter of the monkey and possum. *J. Physiol., Lond.,* **245,** 78-79

Dennish, G. W. and Castell, D. O. (1971). Inhibitory effect of smoking on the lower esophageal sphincter. *New Engl. J. Med.,* **284,** 1136-1137

Dent, J. and Hansky, J. (1976). Relationship of serum gastrin response to lower oesophageal sphincter pressure. *Gut,* **17,** 144-146

Didio, L. J. A. and Anderson, M. C. (1968). *The 'Sphincters' of the Digestive System,* 1st edn, Williams and Wilkins, Baltimore, pp. 204-209

Dilawari, J. B. and Misiewicz, J. J. (1973). Action of oral metoclopramide on the gastro-oesophageal junction in man. *Gut,* **14,** 380-382

Dilawari, J. B., Newman, A., Poleo, J. and Misiewicz, J. J. (1975). Response of the human cardiac sphincter to circulating prostaglandins $F_{2\alpha}$ and E_2 and its anti-inflammatory drugs. *Gut,* **16,** 137-143

Dodds, W. J., Hogan, W. J., Miller, W. N., Arndorfer, R. C. and Barreras, R. R. (1974). Relationship between serum gastrin levels and lower oesophageal sphincter pressure in fasting subjects. *Gastroenterology,* **66,** 686

Domschke, W., Lux, G., Domschke, S., Strunz, U., Bloom, S. R. and Wünsch, E. (1978). Effects of vasoactive intestinal peptide on resting and pentagastrin-stimulated lower oesophageal sphincter pressure. *Gastroenterology,* **75,** 9-12

Domschke, W., Lux, G., Mitznegg, P., Rösch, W., Domschke, S., Bloom, S. R., Wünsch, E. and Demling, L. (1976). Relationship of plasma motilin response to lower esophageal sphincter pressure in man. *Scand. J. Gastroenterol.,* **11,** Suppl. 39, 81-84

Doubilet, H. and Colp, R. (1937). Resistance of the sphincter of Oddi in the human. *Surg., Gynec. Obst.,* **64,** 622-633

Douglas, W. W. and Ritchie, J. M. (1957). On the frequency of firing of mammalian non-medullated nerve fibres. *J. Physiol., Lond.,* **139,** 400-407

Doyon, M. (1894). Del action exercee par le systeme nerveux sur l'appareil excreteur de la bile. *Arch. Physiol. Norm. Path.,* **6,** 19

Dunne, J. F. (1967). Designing a clinical trial. *Hospital Med.,* **1,** 336-341

Duthie, H. L. and Bennett, R. C. (1963). The relation of sensation in the anal canal to the functional anal sphincter: a possible factor in anal incontinence. *Gut,* **4,** 179-182

Duval, M. K. Jr. (1958). The effect of chronic pancreatitis on pressure tolerance in the human pancreatic duct. *Surgery,* **43,** 798-801

Eakins, K. E., Karim, S. M. M. and Miller, J. D. (1970). Antagonism of some smooth muscle actions of prostaglandins by polyphloretin phosphate. *Br. J. Pharmacol.,* **39,** 556-563

Eisner, M. (1968). Gastrointestinal effects of metoclopramide in man. In vitro experiments with human smooth muscle preparations. *Br. Med. J.,* **IV,** 679-680

Elliott, T. R. (1904). On the innervation of the ileo-colic sphincter. *J. Physiol.,* **31,** 157-168

Ellis, F. G., Kauntze, R. and Trounce, J. R. (1960). The innervation of the cardia and lower oesophagus in man. *Br. J. Surg.,* **47,** 466-472

Farrell, R. L., Roling, G. T. and Castell, D. O. (1973). Stimulation of the incompetent lower oesophageal sphincter. A possible advance in therapy of heartburn. *Am. J. Dig. Dis.,* **18,** 646-650

Farrell, R. L., Roling, G. T. and Castell, D. O. (1974). Cholinergic therapy of chronic heartburn. A controlled trial. *Ann. Int. Med.,* **80,** 573-576

Fisher, R. and Cohen, S. (1973). Physiological characteristics of the human pyloric sphincter. *Gastroenterology,* **64,** 67-75

Fisher, R., Di Marino, A. J. and Cohen, S. (1973a). Mechanism of cholecystokinin-induced inhibition of lower oesophageal sphincter pressure. *Clin. Res.,* **21,** 825

Fisher, R. S., Lipshutz, W. and Cohen, S. (1973b). The hormonal regulation of pyloric sphincter function. *J. Clin. Invest.,* **52,** 1289-1296

Fisher, R. S., Malmud, L. S., Roberts, G. S. and Lobis, I. F. (1977). The lower oesophageal sphincter as a barrier to gastroesophageal reflux. *Gastroenterology,* **72,** 19-22

Fisher, R. S., Roberts, G. S., Grabowski, C. J. and Cohen, S. (1978). Altered lower oesophageal sphincter function during early pregnancy. *Gastroenterology*, **74**, 1233-1237

Fishlock, D. J. and Parks, A. G. (1963). Nicotine and colonic muscle. *Br. Med. J.*, **2**, 1528

Folkow, B. (1952). Impulse frequency in sympathetic vasomotor fibres correlated to the release and elimination of the transmitter. *Acta Physiol. Scand.*, **25**, 49-76

Frank, S. A., Walker, C. O. and Fordtran, J. S. (1973). The effect of continuous pentagastrin infusion on lower oesophageal sphincter pressure. *Gastroenterology*, **64**, 728

Freeland, G. R., Higgs, R. H. and Castell, D. O. (1977). Lower oesophageal sphincter response to oral administration of cimetidine in normal subjects. *Gastroenterology*, **72**, 28-30

Frenckner, B. (1975). Function of the anal sphincter in spinal man. *Gut*, **16**, 638-644

Frenckner, B. and Ihre, T. (1976). Influence of autonomic nerves on the internal anal sphincter in man. *Gut*, **17**, 306-312

Friedmann, C. A. (1968). The action of nicotine and catecholamine on the human internal anal sphincter. *Am. J. Dig. Dis.*, **13**, 428-431

Furness, J. B. (1970). An examination of nerve-mediated hyoscine-resistant excitation of the guinea-pig colon. *J. Physiol., Lond.*, **207**, 803-821

Gaensler, E. A. and McGowan, J. M. (1950). Activity of some newer spasmolytic agents on the biliary tract of man. *J. Pharmacol. Expl Therap.*, **99**, 304-311

Garrett, J. R., Howard, E. R. and Nixon, H. H. (1969). Autonomic nerves in rectum and colon in Hirschsprung's disease. *Arch. Dis. Childhood*, **44**, 406-417

Gaskell, W. H. (1920). *The Involuntary Nervous System*, Longmans, London

Gazet, J. C. and Jarrett, R. J. (1964). The ileocaeco-colic sphincter. Studies in vitro in man, monkey, cat and dog. *Br. J. Surg.*, **51**, 368-370

Giles, G. R., Humphries, C., Mason, M. C. and Clark, C. G. (1969a). Effect of pH changes on the cardiac sphincter. *Gut*, **10**, 852-856

Giles, G. R., Mason, M. C., Humphries, C. and Clark, C. G. (1969b). Action of gastrin on the lower oesophageal sphincter in man. *Gut*, **10**, 730-734

Grossman, M. I. (1970). Gastrin and its activities. *Nature*, **228**, 1147-1150

Grossman, M. I. (1974). A continuation of 'what is physiological?' *Gastroenterology*, **67**, 1303

Guiterrez, J. G. and Shah, A. N. (1975). Autonomic control of the internal anal sphincter in man. In *5th International Symposium of Gastrointestinal Motility* (ed. G. Vantrappen), Typoff Press, pp. 363-373

Hall, A. W., Moossa, A. R., Clark, J., Cooley, G. R. and Skinner, D. B. (1975). The effects of premedication drugs on the lower oesophageal high pressure zone and reflux status of Rhesus monkeys and man. *Gut*, **16**, 347-352

Hallenbeck, G. A. (1968). Biliary and pancreatic intraductal pressures. In *Handbook of Physiology, Section 6: Alimentary Canal*, Vol. 2 (ed. C. F. Code), American Physiological Society, Washington, D.C., pp. 1007-1025

Heitmann, P. and Moller, N. (1970). The effect of metoclopramide on the gastroesophageal functional zone and the distal oesophagus in man. *Scand. J. Gastroenterol.*, **5**, 621-625

Hellemans, J., Vantrappen, G. and Bloom, S. R. (1976). Endogenous motilin and the LES pressure. *Scand. J. Gastroenterol.*, **11**, Suppl. 39, 67-73

Henderson, J. M., Lidgard, G., Osborne, D. H., Carter, D. C. and Heading, R. C. (1978). Lower oesophageal sphincter response to gastrin—pharmacological or physiological? *Gut*, **19**, 99-102

Hill, J. R., Kelley, M. Jr., Schlegel, J. F. and Code, C. F. (1960). Pressure profile of the rectum and anus of healthy persons. *Dis. Colon Rectum*, **4**, 203-209

Hogan, W. J., Viegas de Andrade, S. R. and Winship, D. H. (1972). Ethanol-induced acute oesophageal motor dysfunction. *J. Appl. Physiol.*, **32**, 755-760

Hooper, M., Spedding, M., Sweetman, A. J. and Weetman, D. F. (1974). 2,2'-pyridylisatogen tosylate: an antagonist of the inhibitory effects of ATP on smooth muscle. *Br. J. Pharmacol.*, **50**, 458p-459p

Hopton, D. S. and Torrance, H. B. (1967). Action of various new analgesic drugs on the human common bile duct. *Gut*, **8**, 296-300

Howard, E. R. (1975). Personal communication

Humphries, T. J., Farrell, R. L., Castell, D. O. and McGuigan, J. E. (1974). Serum gastrin response to oral bethanechol. *Gastroenterology*, **66**, 714

Jacobsson, B., Kewenter, J. and Kock, N. G. (1961). Action of codeine and some other antitussive drugs on choledochal pressure and duodenal activity. A study in cholecystectomised patients. *Acta Chir. Scand.*, **122**, 407-413

Jaffer, S. S., Makhlouf, G. M., Schorr, B. A. and Zfass, A. M. (1974). Nature and kinetics of inhibition of lower oesophageal sphincter pressure by glucagon. *Gastroenterology*, **67**, 42-46

Jennewein, H. M., Waldeck, F., Siewert, R., Weiser, F. and Thimm, R. (1973). The interaction of glucagon and pentagastrin on the lower oesophageal sphincter in man and dog. *Gut*, **14**, 861-864

Jensen, D. M., McCallum, R. and Walsh, J. H. (1978). Failure of atropine to inhibit gastrin-17 stimulation of the lower oesophageal sphincter in man. *Gastroenterology*, **75**, 825-827

Justin-Besancon, L., Grivaux, M. and Waltez, E. (1964). L'Epreuve au métoclopramide en radiologie digestive. *Bull. Soc. Med. Hop. Paris*, **114**, 721-726

Justin-Besancon, L. and Laville, C. (1964). Action anti-emetique du métoclopramide vis-à-vis de l'apomorphine et de l'hydergine. *C.R. Soc. Biol. (Paris)*, **158**, 723-727

Kamijo, K., Hiatt, R. B. and Koelle, G. B. (1953). Congenital megacolon: a comparison of the spastic and hypertrophied segments with respect to cholinesterase activities and sensitivities to acetylcholine, DFP, and the barium ion. *Gastroenterology*, **24**, 173-185

Kantrowitz, P. A., Siegel, C. I. and Hendrix, T. R. (1966). Differences in motility of the upper and lower esophagus in man and its alteration by atropine. *Bull. Johns Hopkins Hospital*, **18**, 476-491

Kao, C. Y. (1966). Tetrodotoxin, saxitoxin and their significance in the study of excitation phenomena. *Pharmac. Rev.*, **18**, 997-1049

Kaufman, S. E. and Kaye, M. D. (1978). Induction of gastro-oesophageal reflux by alcohol. *Gut*, **19**, 336-338

Kewenter, J. and Kock, N. G. (1971). The effect of some spasmolytic drugs on the choledocho-duodenal function in man. *Scand. J. Gastroenterol.*, **6**, 401-405

Kravitz, J. J., Snape, W. J. and Cohen, S. (1978). Effect of histamine and histamine antagonists on human lower oesophageal sphincter function. *Gastroenterology*, **74**, 435-449

Krebs, H. A. and Henseleit, K. (1932). Untersuchungen über die Harnstoffbildung im Tierkörper. *Hoppe-Seyler's Z. Physiol. Chem.*, **210**, 33-66

Lawson, J. O. N. and Nixon, H. H. (1967). Anal canal pressures in the diagnosis of Hirschsprung's disease. *J. Paediat. Surg.*, **2**, 544-552

Liebermann-Meffert, D., Allgower, M., Schmid, P., Math, D. and Blum, A. (1979). Muscular equivalent of the lower oesophageal sphincter. *Gastroenterology*, **76**, 31-38

Lind, J. F., Crispin, J. S. and McIver, D. W. (1968). The effect of atropine on the gastroesophageal sphincter. *Can. J. Physiol. Pharmac.*, **46**, 233-238

Lionel, N. D. W. and Herxheimer, A. (1970). Assessing reports of therapeutic trials. *Br. Med. J.*, **3**, 637-640

Liotta, D., Zuppone, V. and Giffoniello, A. H. (1957). Estudios sobre la motilidad y la farmacología del esfinter ileocaecal y del ileon terminal en el hombre. *Pren. Med. Argent.*, **44**, 3093-3096

Lipshutz, W. and Cohen, S. (1972). Interaction of gastrin I and secretin on gastrointestinal circular muscle. *Am. J. Physiol.*, **222**, 775-781

Logan, C. J. H. and Connell, A. M. (1966). The effect of a synthetic gastrin-like peptide (I.C.I. 50, 123) on intestinal motility in man. *Lancet*, **i**, 996-999

Lund, G. F. and Christensen, J. (1969). Electrical stimulation of esophageal smooth muscle and effects of antagonists. *Am. J. Physiol.*, **217**, 1369-1374

Lux, G., Rösch, W., Domschke, S., Domschke, W. and Wünsch, E. (1976). Intravenous 13-Nle-motilin increases the human lower esophageal sphincter pressure. *Scand. J. Gastroenterol.*, **11**, Suppl. 39, 75-79

McCallum, R. W., Kline, M. M., Curry, N. and Sturdevant, A. L. (1975). Comparative effects of metoclopramide and bethanechol on lower esophageal pressure in reflux patients. *Gastroenterology*, **68**, 1114-1118

Mack, A. J. and Todd, J. K. (1968). A study of the human gall bladder muscle in vitro. *Gut*, **9**, 546-549

Mann, C. V. (1975). Recent evidence for a sphincteric mechanism at the rectosigmoid junction zone. *Mayo Clinic Proc.*, **50**, 529

Martin, E. and Burden, V. G. (1927). The surgical significance of the recto-sigmoid sphincter. *Ann. Surg.*, **86**, 86-93

Misiewicz, J. J., Holdstock, D. J. and Waller, S. L. (1967). Motor responses of the human alimentary tract to near-maximal infusions of pentagastrin. *Gut*, **8**, 463-469

Misiewicz, J. J., Waller, S. L., Anthony, P. P. and Gummer, J. W. P. (1969a). Achalasia of the cardia: pharmacology and histopathology of isolated cardiac sphincteric muscle from patients with and without achalasia. *Quart. J. Med.*, **38**, 17-30

Misiewicz, J. J., Waller, S. L. and Holdstock, D. J. (1969b). Gastrointestinal motility and gastric secretion during intravenous infusions of gastrin II. *Gut*, **10**, 723-729

Morris, D. W., Schoen, H., Brook, F. P. and Cohen, S. (1974). Relationship of serum gastrin and lower oesophageal sphincter pressure in normals and patients with antrectomy. *Gastroenterology*, **66**, 750

Muscholl, E. (1970). Cholinomimetic drugs and release of the adrenergic transmitter. In *New Aspects of Storage and Release Mechanisms of Catecholamines* (ed. H. J. Schuman and G. Kroneberg), Springer, New York, pp. 168-186

Myers, R. N., Haupt, G. J., Birkhead, N. C. and Deaver, J. M. (1962). Cinefluorographic observations of common bile duct physiology. *Ann. Surg.*, **156**, 442-450

Nebel, O. T. (1975). Effect of enteric hormones on the human sphincter of Oddi. *Gastroenterology*, **68**, 962

Nebel, O. T. and Castell, D. O. (1972). Lower esophageal sphincter pressure changes after food ingestion. *Gastroenterology*, **63**, 778-783

Nebel, O. T. and Castell, D. O. (1973). Kinetics of fat inhibition of the lower oesophageal sphincter. *J. Appl. Physiol.*, **35**, 6-8

Nossel, H. L. and Efron, G. (1955). The effect of morphine on the serum and urinary amylase and the sphincter of Oddi: with some preliminary observations on the effect of alcohol on the serum amylase and the sphincter of Oddi. *Gastroenterology*, **29**, 409-416

Oddi, R. (1887). D'une disposition à sphincter speciale de l'ouverture du canal choledoque. *Arch. Ital. Biol.*, **8**, 317-322

Osborne, D. H., Lennon, J., Henderson, M., Lidgard, J., Creel, R. and Carter, D. C. (1977). Effect of cimetidine on the human lower oesophageal sphincter. *Gut*, **18**, 99-105

Parks, A. G. and Fishlock, D. J. (1967). Catecholamines. *Proc. R. Soc. Med.*, **60**, 217

Parks, A. G., Fishlock, D. J., Cameron, J. D. H. and May, H. (1969). Preliminary investigation of the pharmacology of the human internal anal sphincter. *Gut*, **10**, 674-677

Paton, W. D. M. (1955). The response of the guinea-pig ileum to electrical stimulation by coaxial electrodes. *J. Physiol., Lond.*, **27**, 40p-41p

Pirola, R. C. and Davis, A. E. (1968). Effects of ethylalcohol on sphincteric resistance at the choledocho-duodenal junction in man. *Gut*, **9**, 557-560

Pirola, R. C. and Davis, A. E. (1970). Effect of intravenous alcohol on motility of the duodenum and of the sphincter of Oddi. *Australas. Ann. Med.*, **19**, 24-29

Pope, C. E. II (1973). Reflux oesophagitis. In *Gastrointestinal Diseases* (ed. M. H. Sleisenger and J. S. Fordtran), Saunders, Philadelphia, p. 432

Rand, M. H. and Stafford, A. (1967). Cardiovascular effects of choline esters. In *Physiological Pharmacology* (ed. W. S. Root and F. G. Hofmann), Academic Press, New York, pp. 1-95

Resin, H., Stern, D. H., Sturdevant, R. A. L. and Isenburg, J. I. (1973). Effect of the C-terminal octapeptide of cholecystokinin on lower esophageal sphincter pressure in man. *Gastroenterology*, **64**, 946-949

Robert, A. (1979). Cytoprotection by prostaglandins. *Gastroenterology*, **77**, 761-767

Roling, G. T., Farrell, R. L. and Castell, D. O. (1972). Cholinergic response of the lower esophageal sphincter. *Am. J. Physiol.*, **222**, 967-972

Sanger, G. J. and Bennett, A. (1981). In vitro techniques for studying gastrointestinal motility. In *Handbook of Experimental Pharmacology. Gastrointestinal Motility: Mediators and Drugs* (ed. G. Bertaccini), Springer-Verlag, Berlin, in press

Sanner, J. H. (1969). Antagonism of prostaglandin E_2 by 1-acetyl-2-(8-chloro-10, 11-dihydrodibenz (b, f) (1,4)-oxazepine-10-carbonyl) hydrazine (SC-19220). *Arch. Int. Pharmacodyn. Therap.*, **180**, 46-50

Schuster, M. M., Hendrix, T. R. and Mendeloff, A. I. (1963). Internal anal sphincter response: Manometric studies on its normal physiology, neural pathways, and alteration in bowel disorders. *J. Clin. Invest.*, **42**, 196-207

Schuster, M. M., Hookman, P., Hendrix, T. R. and Mendeloff, A. I. (1965). Simultaneous manometric recording of internal and external anal sphincter reflexes. *Bull. Johns Hopkins Hospital*, **116**, 79-88

Shepherd, J. J. and Wright, P. G. (1968). The response of the internal anal sphincter in man to stimulation of the presacral nerve. *Am. J. Dig. Dis.*, **13**, 421-427

Skinner, D. B. and Camp, T. F. (1968). Relation of esophageal reflux to lower esophageal sphincter pressure decreased by atropine. *Gastroenterology*, **54**, 543-551

Smith, A. N. and Hogg, D. (1966). Effect of Gastrin II on the motility of the gastrointestinal tract. *Lancet*, **i**, 403-404

Smith, B. (1967). Myenteric plexus in Hirschsprung's disease. *Gut*, **8**, 308-312

Stanciu, C. and Bennett, J. R. (1972). Smoking and gastro-oesophageal reflux. *Br. Med. J.*, **3**, 793-795

Stanciu, C. and Bennett, J. R. (1973). Metoclopramide in gastrointestinal reflux. *Gut*, **14**, 275–279

Stockley, H. L. (1974). Pharmacological studies on the innervation of human and guinea-pig isolated alimentary smooth muscle. Ph.D. Thesis, University of London

Strunz, U., Domschke, W., Domschke, S., Mitznegg, P., Wünsch, E., Jaeger, E. and Demling, L. (1976). Gastroduodenal motor response to natural motilin and synthetic 13-substituted motilin analogues: a comparative in vitro study. *Scand. J. Gastroenterol*, **11**, 199-203

Sturdevant, R. A. and Kun, T. (1974). Interaction of pentagastrin and the octapeptide of cholecystokinin on the human lower oesophageal sphincter. *Gut*, **15**, 700-702

Swamy, N. (1977). Esophageal spasm: Clinical and manometric response to nitroglycerine and long acting nitrites. *Gastroenterology*, **72**, 23-27

Tansy, M. F. and Kendall, F. M. (1975). Choledochoduodenal junction. In *Functions of the Stomach and Intestine* (ed. M. F. H. Friedman), H.M. & M. Medical and Scientific Publishers, pp. 93-120

Thomas, J. E. (1957). Mechanisms and regulation of gastric emptying. *Physiol. Rev.*, **37**, 453-474

Thomas, J. E. and Wheelon, H. (1922). The nervous control of the pyloric sphincter. *J. Lab. Clin. Med.*, **7**, 375-391

Thompson, J. W. (1958). Studies in the response of the isolated nictitating membrane of the cat. *J. Physiol.*, **141**, 46-72

Tobon, F., Reid, N. C. R. W., Talbert, J. L. and Schuster, M. M. (1968). Nonsurgical test for the diagnosis of Hirschsprung's disease. *New Engl. J. Med.*, **278**, 188-194

Torgerson, S. A., Precup, J. W., Juniper, K. Jr. and Farrell, R. (1979). Oral anticholinergic effect on the human lower oesophageal sphincter. *Gut*, **20**, 904

Trounce, J.R., Deuchar, D. C., Kauntze, R. and Thomas, G. A. (1957). Studies in achalasia of the cardia. *Quart. J. Med.*, **26**, 433-456

Tuch, A. and Cohen, S. (1973). Lower esophageal sphincter relaxation: Studies on the neurogenic inhibitory mechanism. *J. Clin. Invest.*, **52**, 14-20

Unger, R. H., Ketterer, H., Dupre, J. and Eisentraut, A. M. (1967). The effects of secretin, pancreozymin and gastrin on insulin and glucagon secretion in anaesthetised dogs. *J. Clin. Invest.*, **46**, 630-645

Valenzuela, J. E., Defilippi, C. and Csendes, A. (1976). Manometric studies on the human pyloric sphincter: effect of cigarette smoking, metoclopramide and atropine. *Gastroenterology*, **70**, 481-483

Van Derstappen, G. and Texter, E. C. (1964). Response of physiologic gastroesophageal sphincter to increased intra-abdominal pressure. *J. Clin. Invest.*, **43**, 1856-1868

Van Thiel, D. H., Gavaler, J. S., Joshi, S. N., Sara, R. K. and Stremple, J. (1977). Heartburn of pregnancy. *Gastroenterology*, **72**, 666-668

Van Thiel, D. H., Gavaler, J. S. and Stremple, J. (1976). Lower oesophageal sphincter pressure in women using sequential oral contraceptives. *Gastroenterology*, **71**, 232-234

Vatn, M. H., Schrumpf, E. and Myren, J. (1975). The effect of carbachol and pentagastrin on the gastric secretion of acid, pepsin and intrinsic factor (IF) in man. *Scand. J. Gastroenterol.*, **10**, 55-58

Volle, R. L. and Koelle, G. B. (1975). Ganglion stimulating and blocking agents. In *The Pharmacological Basis of Therapeutics* (ed. L. S. Goodman and A. Gilman), Macmillan, New York, pp. 565-575

Weihrauch, T. R., Förster, C. F., Köhler, H., Ewe, K. and Krieglstein, J. (1979). Effect of intravenous diazepam on human lower oesophageal sphincter pressure under controlled double blind crossover conditions. *Gut,* **20,** 64-67

Wennmalm, A. (1978). Effects of nicotine on cardiac prostaglandin and platelet thromboxane synthesis. *Br. J. Pharmacol.,* **64,** 559-563

Westphal, K. (1923). Muskelfunktion, nervensystem u. pathologie der gallenwege. I. Untersuchungen uber den schmerzanfall der gallenwege und seine austrahlended reflexe. *Z. Klin. Med.,* **96,** 22

White, H.L., Rainey, W. R., Monaghan, B. and Harris, A. S. (1934). Observations on the nervous control of the ileocaecal sphincter and on intestinal movements in an unanaesthetised human subject. *Am. J. Physiol.,* **108,** 449-457

White, T. T., Elmslie, R. G. and Magee, D. F. (1964). Observations of the human intraductal pancreatic pressure. *Surg., Gyn. Obst.,* **118,** 1043-1045

Whitehouse, F. R. and Kernohan, J. W. (1948). Myenteric plexus in congenital megacolon. *Arch. Int. Med.,* **82,** 75-111

Wood, C. J. and Simpkins, M. A. (Eds) (1973). *International Symposium on Histamine H$_2$ Receptor Antagonists,* Smith, Kline and French Laboratories, Welwyn Garden City

Zfass, A. M., Prince, R., Allen, F. N. and Farrar, J. T. (1970). Inhibitory beta adrenergic receptors in the human distal esophagus. *Am. J. Dig. Dis.,* **15,** 303-310

3
The Cricopharyngeal Sphincter

C. E. Gabriel and P. McKelvie

ANATOMY

In a study of the anatomy of this region it is usual to consider thyropharyngeus and cricopharyngeus muscles as the two parts of the inferior constrictor of the pharynx, although there is doubt whether the upper part of this muscle plays any part in the mechanism of the cricopharyngeal sphincter. The thyropharyngeus muscle arises from the oblique line of the thyroid cartilage, from a strip of the surface behind this line and from a fine tendinous band which is thrown across the cricothyroid muscle from the inferior thyroid tubercle to the cricoid cartilage. In addition, there is a small slip of muscle arising from the inferior cornu of the thyroid. Its fibres spread backwards and medially to be inserted with the muscle of the opposite side into a fibrous raphe in the midline of the posterior wall of the pharynx. The lower fibres are thinned out and lack the support of the underlying middle and superior constrictor muscles below the level of the vocal cords.

Valsalva described cricopharyngeus in 1717. The muscle is rounder and thicker than the flatter structure of the other constrictor muscles. It extends uninterruptedly from one side of the cricoid arch to the other around the pharynx and is continuous with the circular muscle fibres of the oesophagus. There is, however, dispute as to whether or not the circle of the fibres of the cricopharyngeus muscle exist as a continuous circular sheet or whether, as has been suggested, they meet posteriorly in a raphe which is visible only microscopically. The weak area above cricopharyngeus produced by thinning of the lower margin of thyropharyngeus is known as the dehiscence of Killian.

The cricopharyngeal sphincter therefore consists of a combination of circular fibres of the cricopharyngeus muscle and the circular fibres of the cervical or upper oesophagus—with the latter being the more prominent

(Zaino *et al.*, 1970). At both sites the muscle is striated. The sphincter so formed is about 1–2 cm in length. It is difficult to separate anatomically its two components, but any circular fibres at the upper end of the oesophagus which are thickened are considered to be oesophageal in origin if they do not arise from the cricoid cartilage. The longitudinal muscle of the oesophagus is attached anteriorly to the larynx by the suspensory ligament and by a few strands to the lateral edge of the cricoid lamina, while posteriorly there is a very close mingling of its fibres.

At the beginning of a swallow both the hyoid and cricoid cartilages move upwards with the cricopharyngeal sphincter. The sphincter may only be seen by an indentation posteriorly with a thickness of 1–2 cm. This appearance can be accentuated by a Valsalva manoeuvre. This mound is called the oesophageal lip; it is positioned at any level from C6 to C7 but is always at the same level in each patient. The older the patient the more prominent and more frequently this lip is seen. It is not related to osteophytes in the cervical vertebrae and it does not appear to be of pathological importance, although it is not necessarily visible in normal healthy young people.

There is also a plexus of veins in the region of the sphincter and this has been suggested as a cause of oesophageal lip, but it is extremely unlikely that the mound represents veins alone, particularly as some people have suggested that the veins are present only anteriorly. It is clear, therefore, that there is still doubt about the exact anatomical composition of the oesophageal lip.

The average figures for the distance from the upper incisors to the cricopharyngeal sphincter are: at birth 7 cm, at 3 years 10 cm, at 14 years 14 cm and in adult life 16 cm.

Cricopharyngeus receives its nerve supply from the recurrent laryngeal nerve and the external laryngeal nerve branch of the vagus. The central connection is in the nucleus ambiguus in the medulla close to the respiratory centre in the reticular formation and to the fourth ventricle. Thus, lesions in the medulla may interfere with the swallowing reflex, and the fact that respiration usually stops during swallowing suggests that there is connection between the two centres.

PHYSIOLOGY

The function of the oesophagus is to transmit food from the mouth to the stomach. Entry of food into the oesophagus depends on the opening of the cricopharyngeal sphincter. The following theoretical modes of action of the cricopharyngeal sphincter have been proposed. At rest the sphincter is normally closed. Opening begins with relaxation of the cricopharyngeus muscle in response to an afferent stimulus from the base of the tongue. The ingested bolus then pushes it open and the lumen is enlarged by elevation and forward movement of the larynx—an action which is helped by the sphincter being fixed to the prevertebral fascia.

There is general agreement that the sphincter at rest is normally closed, and that it remains closed even when subjected to raised pressure both from above and below (Lund, 1965). No satisfactory manometric or cineradiographic evidence has been produced to support the remainder of the above theoretical modes of action. For example, it has been demonstrated in some individuals that swallowing together with relaxation of the sphincter can occur without elevation of the hyo-laryngo-pharyngeal complex. In addition, it has been observed that during vomiting and retching the sphincter can open without laryngeal elevation.

Cricopharyngeal occlusion at rest and relaxation in response to a swallow were originally thought to be a passive phenomenon. Resting closure was attributed to compression of the pharyngo-oesophageal region by extrinsic tissues or by the prominent extramural venous plexuses of the oesophagus. There is, however, experimental evidence to show that opening and closing of the upper sphincter reflects muscular activity, although the elasticity of surrounding tissues is responsible in part for the cricopharyngeal sphincter pressure (Asoh and Goyal, 1978).

There is a segment of slightly pale striated muscle about 3 cm long in the upper oesophagus where the resting wall tension is high. The length of this segment may vary between 2 and 6 cm but the band of maximal pressure is usually only 1 cm wide. The resting pressure varies between 15 and 60 cm of water, both between individuals and in any one individual at different times. It has been suggested that both radial and axial asymmetry exist and that the greatest pressures are recorded anteriorly (Winans, 1972; Asoh and Goyal, 1978). Evidence that this band of high pressure is due to muscle tone is provided by the finding of tonic discharges of electrical potentials recorded from electrodes implanted in the muscle wall of the upper oesophageal sphincter when the sphincter is closed (Andrew, 1956; Vantrappen and Hellemans, 1970). In addition, abolition of electrical activity by motor nerve section or administration of D-tubocurarine causes a marked reduction in cricopharyngeal sphincter pressure (Asoh and Goyal, 1978). When the sphincter opens on swallowing, these action potentials disappear transiently for a period which corresponds to the period of relaxation of the upper oesophageal sphincter.

Normal swallowing begins with a voluntary movement, but after this it is completed by means of a series of involuntary reflex arcs. The impact of the food bolus against the posterior wall of the pharynx acts as the stimulus which initiates the reflex movements of swallowing. Anaesthesia of the posterior pharyngeal wall prevents normal swallowing, and there is experimental evidence to suggest that the most sensitive area in this trigger action is the posterior pillar of fauces. Afferent stimuli are conveyed by fibres of the second division of the trigeminal nerve, the glossopharyngeal nerve and the pharyngeal branches of the superior laryngeal nerves to the swallowing centre in the medulla. Efferent impulses to the tongue muscles are conveyed via the hypoglossal nerves, to the mylohyoid by means of the trigeminal nerve, and to the fauces and pharynx by the ninth, tenth and eleventh cranial nerves.

The cricopharyngeal sphincter usually opens 0.2–0.3 s after the beginning of a swallow and can remain open for 0.5–1 s before it closes. At the same time the gastro-oesophageal sphincter relaxes, so that the on-coming bolus can pass unimpeded into the stomach. Electrical recording of cricopharyngeal activity has shown inhibition of reflex activity for several hundred milliseconds at the onset of swallowing (Car and Roman, 1970). In the opossum, however, the degree of fall in pressure is more than one would expect from that observed after experimental abolition of sphincteric myogenic activity, and it is suggested that the geniohyoid muscle may have a role in the pressure changes associated with deglutition (Asoh and Goyal, 1978).

Ingested material enters the oesophagus when the sphincter relaxes and is then swept down the oesophagus by peristaltic waves which travel at the speed of approximately 4 cm s^{-1}. The force and velocity of this wave may differ appreciably, according to the volume and temperature of the bolus swallowed (Dodds et al., 1973). This probably implies the presence of both mechano- and thermoreceptors in the oesophagus—indeed, the former have been identified in the cat (Mei, 1965).

The nerve supply of the cricopharyngeal sphincter is the recurrent laryngeal nerve and the pharyngeal branch of the vagus working through nicotinic receptors common to those of other skeletal muscle. However, the role of these nerves is unclear, because in man recurrent laryngeal nerve paralysis does not affect relaxation of the cricopharyngeal sphincter.

Finally, while in the majority of people the opening of the cricopharyngeal sphincter occurs subconsciously, some people appear to have voluntary control. This is demonstrated when sword swallowers or beer drinkers who are 'pourers' practice their art.

MEDICAL AND SURGICAL THERAPEUTIC IMPLICATIONS IN DISEASE

Upper oesophageal sphincter dysfunction produces a symptom complex of oropharyngeal dysphagia characterised by hesitation in initiation of swallows, food or liquid sticking in the throat, nasal or oral regurgitation and post-deglutitive cough. Causes of such a symptom complex are multiple but basically fall into two groups—those associated with a neuromuscular disorder involving either the central or peripheral nervous system, or the presence of local structural lesions (Hurwitz *et al.*, 1975). In this chapter only four of these conditions will be discussed—namely globus hystericus, pharyngeal pouch, cricopharyngeal achalasia and post-cricoid web.

Globus Hystericus

In contrast to true organic dysphagia, if identical symptoms occur in the absence of fluid or food ingestion, the condition is usually termed globus hystericus. If one takes the analogy of patients with muscle spasm in other parts of the digestive tract who complain of a lump, it is possible that a raised pressure in the cricopharyngeal sphincter is responsible for at least some of the cases of globus hystericus. Cricopharyngeal sphincter pressure measurements in 9 patients with globus hystericus when compared with 22 controls have been shown to differ significantly (Watson and Sullivan, 1974), although there is no universal agreement about this.

In addition, a proportion of patients with globus sensations can be shown to be suffering from gastro-oesophageal reflux with or without a hiatus hernia. Manometrically there may be high cricopharyngeal sphincter pressure which returns to normal when the hiatus hernia is repaired. In the majority of globus patients, however, there is no demonstrable evidence of radiological or manometric abnormalities. However, no patient should be labelled hysterical until oesophageal manometry, barium swallow, a trial of antacids or oesophagoscopy has been carried out.

Pharyngeal Pouch (Zenker's Diverticulum)

This is a rare disease affecting men more than women over the age of 50. A detailed discussion of the theories of the anatomical defects associated with this condition is available in Chapter 1. The symptoms consist basically of upper end dysphagia, occasionally noisy swallowing or gurgling and more rarely hoarseness. The size of the diverticulum (which is more frequently seen on the left) varies, and in a large diverticulum a plain X-ray of the neck may show the presence of a fluid level. There is a small but definite increased incidence of carcinoma arising in such pouches.

It has long been suggested that this condition occurs as a result of a disorder of cricopharyngeal sphincter function. However, the aetiology of this disease is still unclear. Hypotheses include cricopharyngeal spasm, delayed onset of relaxation on swallowing, premature contraction which shortens the period of swallow-induced relaxation of the cricopharyngeal sphincter and, lastly, the occurrence of a second swallow against a closed sphincter.

There is no manometric evidence to support a failure of the sphincter to relax in this condition, although it may be a factor in other causes of upper oesophageal sphincter dysfunction (Hurwitz and Duranceau, 1978). Cineradiology has shown occasional definite premature closures of the sphincter, and if this occurs, filling of the pouch is seen to occur when the sphincter is contracting.

Perhaps more important is the small but definite association between other oesophageal diseases and a pharyngeal pouch. Higher upper oesophageal sphincter pressures are recorded in patients with hiatus hernia and this could increase resistance to entry of food and liquid into the upper oesophagus. In 8 per cent of a series of pharyngeal diverticula other oesophageal diseases, including hiatus hernia, oesophageal traction diverticula, oesophageal varices, achalasia and dysphagia lusoria, were seen. In addition, two cases of carcinoma of the lower oesophagus were found to be present coincidentally with a pharyngeal diverticulum. It seems wise, therefore, in all cases of such diverticula to ensure that the oesophagus is shown to be normal.

On the premise, as yet not conclusively proven, that dysfunction of the upper oesophageal sphincter is partly responsible for the formation of a pharyngeal pouch, some workers have advocated that a cricopharyngeal sphincteric myotomy should form part of the treatment of such pouches. Myotomy has been performed either alone or coupled with excision of the pouch. The evidence for doing so is unclear and is largely circumstantial. In some cases division of the sphincter alone without excision of the pouch has led to regression in size of the pouch (Blakely et al., 1968). In addition, there is a suggestion that in patients with pharyngeal pouches who also have gastro-oesophageal reflux or higher than normal resting upper sphincteric pressures, there is a higher incidence of re-occurrence of pharyngeal pouch after excision if the sphincter is not divided.

In summary, the evidence supporting myotomy as forming part of the routine surgical treatment of pharyngeal pouches is probably not sufficiently strong to justify recommending its use as a routine procedure.

This having been said, it is evident that every clinician operating on pharyngeal pouches in any number has experienced the obvious tightness of cricopharyngeus at rest, indeed under relaxation. The 'sphincter' may well have become fibrous. When a pouch is opened at operation, or when the beaked speculum is introduced at Dohlmann's endoscopic diathermisation of the party wall between pouch and oesophagus, this is only too obvious. Hence, there is a natural inclination to do a myotomy, or similar procedure, to relieve an obstruction which seemingly must have evoked the development of this pulsion diverticulum.

Post-cricoid Web

The Paterson–Brown–Kelly syndrome has been defined as the presence of dysphagia and hypochromic microcytic anaemia with a post-cricoid web in middle-aged females. Radiology demonstrates the presence of a post-cricoid web at the level of the cricopharyngeal sphincter. Its interest is magnified by the definite association between post-cricoid webs and carcinoma of the hypopharynx. Pathologically this lesion appears to be acquired as the result of mucosal changes (Chisholm *et al.*, 1971), although the muscle itself is not inflamed (Entwhistle and Jacobs, 1965). In common with other lesions in this region, the syndrome has also been noted in patients with hiatus herniae and who have had a partial gastrectomy. There is no evidence to show that malfunction of the cricopharyngeal sphincter plays any part in the aetiology of this disease.

Cricopharyngeal Achalasia

Doubt exists as to whether this is a real entity. By definition it results from failure of the cricopharyngeal sphincter to relax during swallowing, and it is often accompanied by a pharyngeal diverticulum. Often, however, there is an element of early closure of the sphincter before the pharynx has completed its contraction. Outflow resistance between the pharynx and the upper oesophagus causes dilatation of the hypopharynx, stagnation in the valleculae and pyriform fossae and overflow of the food into the respiratory tree. Cricopharyngeal achalasia may be associated with anterior poliomyelitis, thyrotoxicosis affecting the pharyngeal muscles, bilateral recurrent laryngeal nerve paralysis and bulbar paralysis in the aged (Ascherson, 1950). Cricopharyngeal myotomy is the logical treatment, although operative experience and results of such treatment are not extensive.

REFERENCES

Andrew, B. L. (1956). The nervous control of the cervical oesophagus of the rat during swallowing. *J. Physiol., Lond.,* **134**, 729-740
Ascherson, N. (1950). Achalasia of the cricopharyngeal sphincter. *J. Laryng.,* **64**, 747-758
Asoh, R. and Goyal, R. K. (1978). Manometry and electromyography of the upper oesophageal sphincters in the opossum. *Gastroenterology,* **74**, 514-520
Blakely, W. R., Garety, E. J. and Smith, D. E. (1968). Section of the crico-pharyngeus muscle for dysphagia. *Arch. Surg.,* **96**, 745-762
Car, A. and Roman, C. (1970). L'Activité spontane du sphincter oesophagieu superieur chez le mouton. Ses variations au cours de la deglutition et de la rumination. *J. Physiol. (Paris),* **62**, 505-511
Chisholm, M., Ardran, G. M., Callender, S. T. and Wright, R. (1971). Iron deficiency and autoimmunity in post-cricoid webs. *Quart. J. Med.,* **40**, 421-433
Dodds, W. J., Hogan, W. J., Reid, D. P., Stewart, E. T. and Arndorfer, R. C. (1973). A comparison between primary peristalsis following wet and dry swallows. *J. Appl. Physiol.,* **35**, 851-857
Entwhistle, C. C. and Jacobs, A. (1965). Histological findings in the Paterson–Kelly syndrome. *J. Clin. Path.,* **18**, 408-413
Hurwitz, A. L. and Duranceau, A. (1978). Upper oesophageal sphincter dysfunction. Pathogenesis and treatment. *Am. J. Dig. Dis.,* **23**, 275-281

Hurwitz, A. L., Nelson, J. A. and Haddad, J. K. (1975). Oropharyngeal dysphagia. Manometric and cine oesophagraphic findings. *Am. J. Dig. Dis.*, **20**, 313-324

Lund, W. S. (1965). A study of the crico-pharyngeal sphincter in man and in the dog. *Ann. R. Coll. Surg. Engl.*, **37**, 225-246

Mei, N. (1965). *C. R. Acad. Sci. (Paris)*, **260**, 307-315

Vantrappen, G. and Hellemans, J. (1970). Oesophageal motility. *Rend. R. Gastroenterol.*, **2**, 7-19

Watson, W. C. and Sullivan, S. N. (1974). Hypotonicity of the crico-pharyngeal sphincter: a cause of globus sensation. *Lancet*, **ii**, 1417-1419

Winans, C. S. (1972). The pharyngo-oesophageal closure mechanism: a manometric study. *Gastroenterology*, **63**, 768-777

Zaino, C., Jacobson, H. G., Lepow, H. and Ozturk, C. H. (1970). *Pharyngo-oesophageal Sphincter*, Thomas, Springfield, Ill.

4
The Gastro-oesophageal Sphincter

Paul A. Thomas

INTRODUCTION

An anti-reflux mechanism is essential at the gastro-oesophageal junction because of the pressure difference between the fundus of the stomach and the body of the oesophagus, which would otherwise force gastric contents, including acid, up into the oesophagus. This mechanism has several components—most of which are anatomical. These include the length of intra-abdominal oesophagus, the right crus of the diaphragm, the gastric sling fibres and the redundant mucosa lining the oesophagogastric junction. In addition, there is now general acceptance that a 'physiological sphincter' mechanism separates these two cavities. All of the above are important components of the anti-reflux mechanism but as yet their relative contributions to the competence of the junction are unclear. It is plain, however, that an abnormal anatomical configuration, as shown by the presence of a hiatus hernia radiologically, is not always associated with oesophageal reflux (Price and Castell, 1978).

This chapter therefore is concerned primarily with a review of the physiological sphincter. In particular, it is an attempt to relate basic physiological and pharmacological data on this sphincter to the pathophysiology and treatment of certain sphincter disorders. It is not intended as an exhaustive review of oesophageal motility disorders. This information is already available (Atkinson, 1976).

ANATOMY

The oesophagus is a hollow muscular tube. In man the proximal one-third of both layers of the muscularis propria is striated muscle. The remainder is smooth muscle. There are species differences in muscle distribution. Some

75

marsupials and primates share the human proportions. Dogs have a striated muscle oesophagus, while in amphibia, birds and reptiles the whole of the oesophagus is smooth muscle. In all species the muscularis mucosa is smooth muscle. In man an anatomical smooth muscle sphincter cannot be demonstrated at the gastro-oesophageal junction (Ingelfinger, 1958), although it is visible in the dog (Mann and Shorter, 1964).

The lumen of the oesophagus is lined by stratified squamous epithelium, but either within, or just below, the lower oesophageal sphincter (LOS) the epithelial lining changes, in most people, to the columnar glandular type.

The oesophagus receives its nerve supply from the vagus nerves and the sympathetic outflow tracks (figure 4.1). In general, the wall of the gastrointestinal tract contains two nerve plexuses. Auerbach's or the myenteric plexus lies between the outer longitudinal and inner circular muscle layers. Its main function is to control motor activity. The submucosal or Meissner's plexus has mainly a sensory function. In the wall of the oesophagus, which has a purely motor function, the latter plexus is absent.

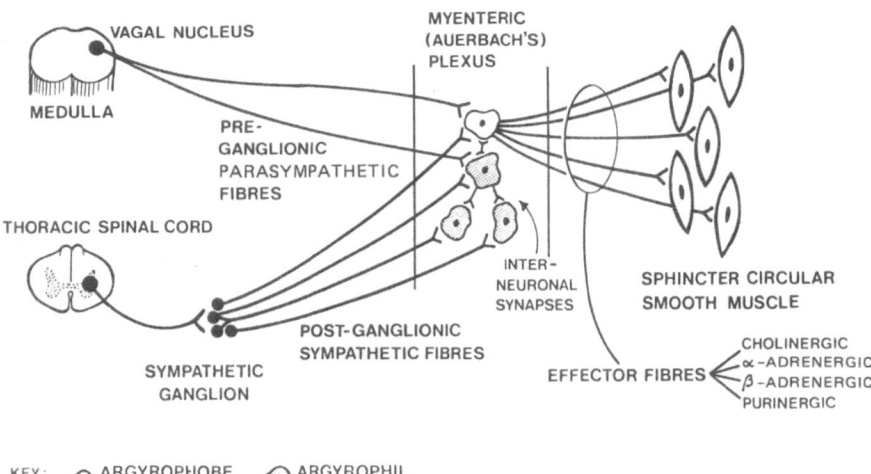

Figure 4.1 The efferent oesophageal autonomic fibres synapse within the myenteric plexus linking both argyrophobic and argyrophilic neurons, before the four types of effector fibres are given off to the lower oesophageal sphincter smooth muscle cells.

In the oesophagus and LOS the myenteric plexus is distributed throughout both striated and smooth muscle portions. It contains a large number of neurons connected by nerve trunks. The neurons connect with both post-ganglionic sympathetic and pre-ganglionic vagal fibre synapses. The final common pathway fibres of the autonomic nervous system are anatomically indistinguishable. (See figure 4.1.)

Silver stain techniques demonstrate two populations of neurons. Argyrophobe neurons are seen to supply the muscle fibres. Argyrophil neurons communicate with other neurons in the myenteric plexus (both argyrophobe and argyrophil). They are thought to function as transmitting neurons and may be involved as a control pathway for intrinsic mural reflexes.

PHYSIOLOGY

The two generally well-accepted criteria used as evidence of a physiological sphincter mechanism at the gastro-oesophageal junction are, first, a zone of elevated pressure separating the stomach from the body of the oesophagus, and second, that it relaxes in response to a swallow (Fyke et al., 1956). A third, less well-accepted, criterion is the response of this zone to an increase in intragastric pressure. It has been demonstrated by some workers that the sphincter responds to an increase in gastric pressure with an even greater increase in sphincter pressure (Lind et al., 1966).

Sphincter Tone

At rest the LOS is tonically contracted. It has a resting pressure of 10–15 cm of water when measured by an open-tip catheter (see later for a discussion of methods of pressure measurement). This pressure is variable and has been used as a means of differentiating groups of people with and without gastro-oesophageal reflux (Atkinson et al., 1957).

Tonic contraction of the LOS is a function of its smooth muscle rather than its control mechanism. Studies on isolated strips of smooth muscle taken from the LOS show an increased length–tension relationship when compared with adjacent smooth muscle taken from the fundus of the stomach or the body of the oesophagus (Christensen et al., 1973b; Christensen and Conklin, 1974). Tetrodotoxin, an agent which abolishes nerve action potentials, does not change these length–tension characteristics, which proves them to originate in a mechanism intrinsic to the smooth muscle. As expected, muscle depolarisation agents do interfere with these length–tension characteristics. This raises the possibility that different myogenic characteristics of the LOS smooth muscle may be due to differing resting membrane potentials.

It is possible that the LOS control mechanisms—both nervous and hormonal—act by altering the myogenic responsiveness of the sphincter. Such control could be mediated by varying the level of the resting membrane potential.

Neural Control of Tone

Innervatory mechanisms are thought to effect LOS tone in a number of ways (Diament and El-Sharkawy, 1977). Circulating hormones can stimulate nerve pathways. For example, gastrin may act via post-ganglionic cholinergic nerves (Lipshutz *et al.*, 1971), although this has recently been disputed in man (Jensen *et al.*, 1977a). Second, tonic efferent discharges have been recorded in the canine vagus nerves supplying the cardia (Miolan and Roman, 1973). Finally, some evidence shows that α-adrenergic receptor excitation alters resting tone (DiMarino and Cohen, 1973). The pathway for this is unknown (Rattan and Goyal, 1974). Stimulation of the cervical sympathetic trunk has no effect on the LOS; the excitatory effect may lie in the lower thoracic sympathetic outflow.

In addition to efferent control, recordings from vagal afferent fibres demonstrate the presence of mechanoreceptors which are sensitive to tonic and phasic changes in the sphincter (Mei *et al.*, 1972). Such activity could provide feedback to a central control mechanism.

Hormonal Control of Tone

Since Giles and colleagues first demonstrated in 1969 that gastrin altered the LOS pressure in man, many workers have studied the relationship between a variety of polypeptide gastrointestinal hormones and the LOS pressure. Despite an abundance of information, it still remains a field where the significance of the results is debated. In particular, the argument relates to whether their effects are physiological or pharmacological (Grossman, 1973; Cohen, 1974).

Most work has tested the effect of gastrin. Data obtained from *in vitro* and animal experiments suggest a physiological role for this hormone. *In vitro* studies on the opossum (an animal with an oesophageal muscle distribution similar to that of man) demonstrates a specific effect of gastrin on sphincteric circular smooth muscle strips (Lipshutz and Cohen, 1971). The dose threshold for a gastrin contractile effect on LOS muscle is lower than that required to contract muscle strips taken from the body of the oesophagus, gastric fundus or antrum. In addition, the maximal tension produced by sphincteric muscle strips in response to gastrin was twice that found in muscle from other neighbouring regions. Its site of action is at post-ganglionic parasympathetic fibres. Cholecystokinin has also been shown to act here.

Animal studies using rabbit anti-human gastrin antiserum (Lipshutz *et al.*, 1972) also seemed to suggest a physiological role for gastrin. Following passive transfer of antiserum into the opossum, there was a marked diminution in LOS pressure. Also, the increases in LOS pressure induced by gastric alkalinisation (which was assumed to be gastrin mediated) and exogenous intravenous administration of gastrin 1 were abolished, although later work has disputed this (Goyal and McGuigan, 1975).

Earlier human studies also supported a physiological role for the polypeptide hormones. Castell and Harris (1970) demonstrated changes in LOS pressure in response to gastric alkalinisation, acidification and feeding. Dose–response curves for gastrin have been plotted (Cohen and Lipshutz, 1971a) and secretin has been shown to inhibit competitively the gastrin contractile effect. Similarly, the C-terminal octapeptide of cholecystokinin and glucagon both reduced the tone of the LOS (Jennewein *et al.*, 1973; Resin *et al.*, 1973). Reductions in LOS pressure following fatty meals were thought to result from release of cholecystokinin (Nebel and Castell, 1972).

At that point in time the case for an LOS hormonal control mechanism seemed strong. However, since circulating levels of hormones have been measured, the picture has changed. Dodds *et al.* (1975a) showed no correlation between resting sphincter tone and serum gastrin levels as measured by radio-immunoassay. Serum gastrin levels were similar in control subjects and people with gastro-oesophageal reflux, despite differences in the LOS pressure (Farrell *et al.*, 1974). Furthermore, it has always been assumed that increases in LOS pressure following gastric alkalinisation are related to gastrin release. Total radio-immunoassayable serum gastrin, however, does not appear to alter under these circumstances (Higgs *et al.*, 1974; Kline *et al.*, 1975), even though increases in LOS

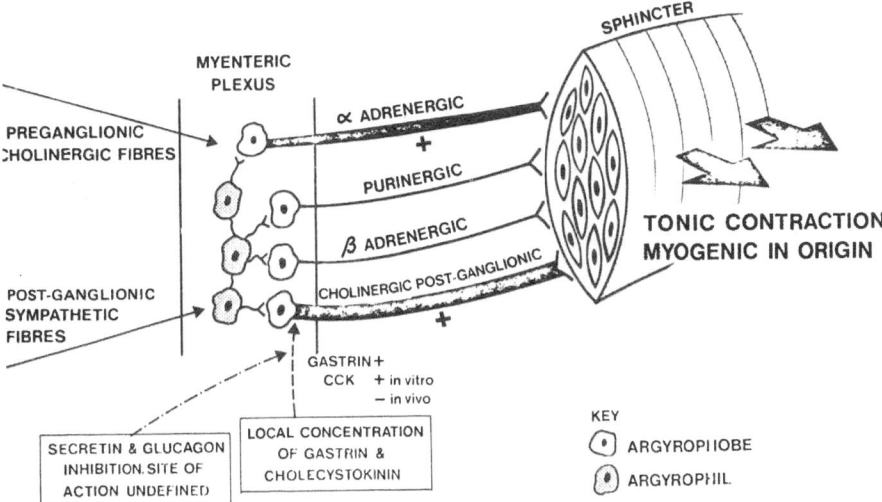

Figure 4.2 Basic sphincter tone is myogenic in origin but is also controlled by both the autonomic nervous system and probably the effect of local hormone concentrations.

pressure are recorded (Higgs *et al.*, 1974). In addition, specific release of gastrin from the antrum does not appear to alter the LOS pressure (Koelz *et al.*, 1978). As it stands at present, then, the case made out for gastrin being the dominant hormonal controller of LOS tone is less convincing than it seemed at first. One reaction to this type of data was for it to be suggested that the different molecular species of gastrin may have a different biological effect. Work comparing the effects of human big gastrin (G34) and gastrin 1 (G17) does not support this concept (Jensen *et al.*, 1977b).

It is possible that too much stress is being laid upon the lack of correlation between serum levels of gastrin and LOS pressure. Pharmacological studies do show that the LOS smooth muscle is more sensitive to the hormone than surrounding smooth muscle, and there presumably must be a reason for this. Serum hormone levels are likely to turn out to be a very inaccurate measurement of a substance whose main function may be as a local control mechanism. Measurement of local tissue concentrations are more relevant. The concept of the paracrine effect of gastrointestinal hormones has been discussed more fully (Wingate, 1976).

A visual concept of the control of sphincter tone is seen in figure 4.2.

Sphincteric Relaxation

Deglutition is characterised by a peristaltic wave passing the length of the oesophagus associated with relaxation of the gastro-oesophageal high-pressure zone. Classically there are two types of normal oesophageal peristaltic waves, depending on their mode of initiation (Meltzer, 1899). Primary waves are induced by swallowing, while a secondary wave arises in response to a local oesophageal stimulus such as fluid within its lumen. Relaxation of the LOS is associated with both types. The arrival of the peristaltic waves at the relaxed sphincter is followed by a wave of contraction passing through the proximal but not distal half of the LOS.

It has been argued that the basis for sphincteric relaxation is mechanical but it seems more likely that it is dependent on nerves. The original mechanical concept was that in response to a swallow the oesophagus would shorten, pulling the gastro-oesophageal junction away from the buttressing effect of the diaphragmatic hiatus, with the result of a fall of pressure. This seems unlikely, because relaxation is observed even when the oesophagogastric junction lies at rest well within the thorax.

Electrical field stimulation of LOS smooth muscle strips produces relaxation, while adjacent muscle strips from the stomach and oesophagus contract. In contrast to its lack of effect on sphincteric tone, tetrodotoxin abolishes this response, thereby demonstrating that nerves control relaxation (Christensen *et al.*, 1973a). Pharmacological studies, using specific blocking agents, show that relaxation is produced by an inhibitory peripheral post-ganglionic, non-cholinergic, non-adrenergic pathway (Tuch and Cohen, 1973; Goyal and Rattan, 1975). Neither dopamine (Rattan and Goyal, 1976; de Carle and Christensen, 1976) nor histamine receptors appear to be involved in sphincteric relaxation. The transmitter substance was thought to be a purine nucleotide and the nerve fibres responsible for it were termed 'purinergic' (Burnstock, 1972). More recently, though, it has been suggested that the transmitter may be a polypeptide hormone secreted by 'peptidergic nerves'.

This inhibitory nerve pathway can be excited by local intramural pathways from as far away as the striated muscle portion of the oesophagus (Mann *et al.*, 1964). In response to afferent impulses, efferent discharges destined for the inhibitory neurons would follow. In addition, tonic excitatory discharges to the LOS are temporarily inhibited (Miolan and Roman, 1973).

Response of LOS to Increased Intragastric Pressure

The pressure in the unstimulated LOS is not large and it might be expected to be insufficiently high to withstand the increase in intra-abdominal pressure associated with straining. Canadian workers showed, however, that the normal sphincter responds to an increase of intragastric pressure of up to 80 cm of water by raising its pressure to maintain a barrier between the stomach and the oesophagus (Wankling *et al.*, 1965). There is no general agreement as to whether this reflex exists—a later paper found no relationship between sphincteric and intragastric pressure (Dodds *et al.*, 1975b).

This response was originally thought to be a cholinergic reflex arc involving the vagus nerves (Crispin *et al.*, 1967; Lind *et al.*, 1969; Behar and Kastendieck, 1974). More recent work suggests that it is independent of the vagus (Behar *et al.*, 1976), as it does exist in an isolated, extrinsically denervated sphincter preparation (Thomas, 1977).

The afferent stimulus for the reflex is presumably the increase in intragastric pressure producing local stretch forces on the smooth muscle of the sphincter. In response, the LOS muscle contracts to counteract the stretch forces and thereby increases its pressure. There is some evidence to support this concept. Higher sphincter pressures are recorded as the diameter of the intraluminal pressure recording unit is increased or when the rate of infusion of water through the unit is increased (Kaye and Showalter, 1974; Biancini *et al.*, 1975; Holly, 1977). Studies on normal sphincter diameter—pressure curves demonstrate that the normal response to stretch is an increase in LOS intraluminal pressure (Biancini *et al.*, 1975). The basis of this response is either the smooth muscle itself or its local controlling mechanism.

Relatively little information on the control of the reflex is available.

Cohen and Harris (1969) suggested that LOS in those patients with low basal pressures could be made to respond normally to increases in intragastric pressure, provided that the LOS pressure was raised first to normal levels by pharmacological means. Similarly, LOS pressure–diameter curves can be altered (Biancini *et al.*, 1975). Urecholine returns the pressure–diameter curve to normal in patients with reflux. On the other hand, probanthine converted a normal pressure–diameter curve to that typical of reflux. Gastrin has also been shown to enhance the sphincteric response to an increased intragastric pressure (Thomas, 1977).

METHODS OF INVESTIGATION IN MAN

Radiology and endoscopy are the two most frequently used investigations. The former enables the anti-reflux function of the gastro-oesophageal junction to be assessed in addition to defining motility patterns. Endoscopy is now used widely because of fibre optic advances, and provides a visual assessment of the lining of the lower oesophagus.

Additional tests are available but are not used extensively in clinical practice. They do, however, provide useful information about this junction. Gastro-oesophageal pressure recordings have enabled the LOS to be defined in terms of its pressure and motility characteristics. Attempts have been made to characterise these findings in both health and disease. Other tests include potential difference and pH gastro-oesophageal profiles, acid perfusion tests and oesophageal acid-clearing assessments. These are used generally as marker tests of gastro-oesophageal reflux.

Radiology

Details of technique and interpretation are not relevant in this review. Barium studies enable function of the gastro-oesophageal junction to be studied and such studies should include cine filming in addition to spot films (Dodds *et al.*, 1976). Liquid barium appears to be the liquid of choice (Zboralske and Dodds, 1969).

Such methods enable the relationship between oesophageal peristalsis and gastro-oesophageal relaxation to be visualised. In addition, the efficacy of the cardia as an anti-reflux mechanism can be assessed. One of its main drawbacks is that it is not a direct measure of sphincter function. The presence of radiological reflux is indicative of a weak barrier, but this is not necessarily sphincteric in origin.

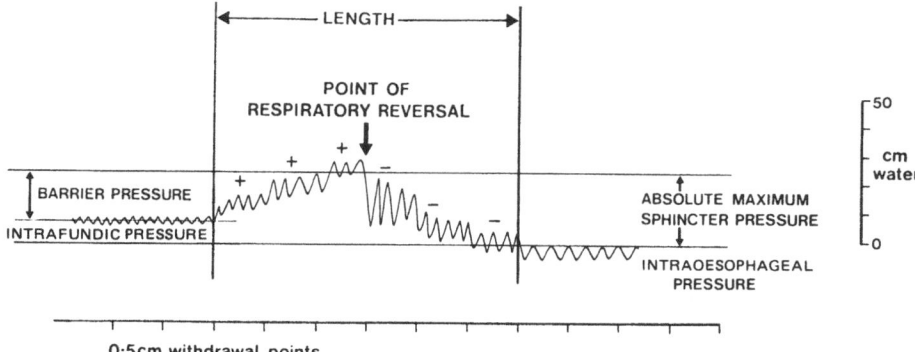

Figure 4.3 A diagrammatic representation of a pressure profile of a normal gastro-oesophageal junction demonstrating the various parameters which can be measured.

Manometry (figure 4.3)

Pressure measurements at the gastro-oesophageal junction provide information on:

(1) The level of the pressure barrier (ZEP = zone of elevated pressure) between the stomach and oesophagus. This can be expressed in relation to atmospheric pressure or as the difference between the gastro-oesophageal sphincter and the mean fundic pressures. The latter is called the barrier pressure.

(2) The relationship of the ZEP to the diaphragm. Respiratory deflections are seen in pressure recordings. Below the diaphragm these show a positive deflection with inspiration. Above the diaphragm the pattern of the deflections is exactly reversed, becoming negative on inspiration. The point of change of 'respiratory reversal' marks the diaphragmatic hiatus.

(3) The length of the pressure zone.

(4) Its response to swallowing.

(5) Its response to increasing intragastric pressure.

(6) Its response to drugs.

The usual way of recording LOS pressures is to pass the catheter assembly into the stomach and then to withdraw it into the body of the oesophagus using a station pull-through technique. The unit is withdrawn at 0.5 cm intervals through the ZEP while pausing for pressure equilibration with 4–5 cycles of respiration. This technique enables various criteria such as pressure and length of LOS and point of respiratory reversal to be measured. More recently there has been support for a more rapid pull-through profile (Dodds *et al.*, 1975c). This is claimed to give more reproducible results than the above. There may be less interference by spontaneously occurring swallows and minute-by-minute monitoring of the LOS pressure can be obtained, although a recent study does not substantiate this (Goodal *et al.*, 1980).

The manometric features of a normal gastro-oesophageal junction were first described by Fyke *et al.* (1956). Using small pressure transducers, they recorded a ZEP of 10–15 cm water above atmospheric, 2–4 cm long, straddling the diaphragm, and which relaxed in response to a swallow. They noted that while the whole ZEP relaxed in response to a swallow, only the proximal half showed an after-contraction. This coincided with the arrival of the oesophageal peristaltic wave. From such recordings it was concluded that the ZEP had the characteristics of a physiological sphincter mechanism. There is general agreement about these basic characteristics. There has, however, been considerable discussion about the methods of pressure measurement and their relevance in both health and disease.

It is interesting to study the evolution of manometric studies of the LOS. The lessons which have been learnt are applicable to pressure recording throughout the gastrointestinal tract.

Before the methods of measurement are discussed, it should be realised at the outset that it is not possible to measure true resting sphincter pressure. The LOS is tonically contracted at rest. Any method of measurement which involves opening the lumen will alter the pressure within it. Biancini *et al.* (1975) have shown that sphincteric muscle gives a reproducible response to local stretch forces. It increases its pressure as the diameter of the probe enlarges. This precludes the use of an intraluminal pressure probe for measuring 'true' resting pressure.

The most commonly used manometer probe has been the water-filled polyvinyl tube which is attached externally to a transducer. Earlier studies used non-infused units. Dissatisfaction with these resulted in the introduction of water-filled tubes infused continuously with small quantities of water. Non-infusion manometry did not separate adequately groups of people with and without gastro-oesophageal reflux. It was felt that the non-infused catheter tip became blocked by the mucosa lining the lumen of the stomach. As a result, the subsequent pressure recording reflected the last pressure to which the catheter tip was exposed prior to entering the sphincter region.

The use of an infused system was tested initially on anal sphincter pressure measurements (Harris *et al.*, 1966). It was noted that the intrasphincteric pressures measured in this way were greater than when a non-infused system was used. These workers realised that the parameter being measured was not 'resting' pressure but the 'yield' or 'sphincteric force of closure' pressures. It was, in fact, the sphincteric response to local stretch which was being recorded. By extending this technique to the LOS a better separation of the LOS in normals and reflux patients was obtained (Pope, 1967; Winans and Harris, 1967). It is not altogether surprising that subsequent work has shown that 'force of closure' measurements vary with the diameter of the manometer probe (Lyndon *et al.*, 1975) and with the rate of infusion (Stef *et al.*, 1974). It is, therefore, imperative that if comparisons of absolute results between studies are being made, such variables are taken into account. With this in mind, a low-compliance manometer system (Arndorfer *et al.*, 1977), requiring very low perfusion rates (0.6 ml min^{-1} or less), has been introduced. More widespread use of this system or the sleeve system introduced by Dent and Chir (1976) may allow series from different centres to be compared.

An alternative technique is to use an intraluminal transducer. These are superior, the main drawbacks being cost and fragility of the instruments. Their frequency responses are better than those of open-tip assemblies. Other advantages include a small assembly diameter, and the facts that they are not sensitive to position change and that the calibration is more stable (Millhon *et al.*, 1968; Stef *et al.*, 1974). They seem to be particularly useful in studies on oesophageal peristalsis (Hollis and Castell, 1972; Humphries and Castell, 1977).

In addition to the above variables, there is still discussion as to what the ZEP represents. Pressure profiles would seem to be measuring more than the radial squeeze of the sphincter muscle. Several studies reveal radial asymmetry of the ZEP (Kaye and Showalter, 1971; Winans, 1977), the highest pressure occurring in the left posterior quadrant of the sphincter. Posture seems to affect the ZEP—being highest when the subject lies on his left side (Babka and Castell, 1973). It is highly likely that some of the ZEP derives from a diaphragmatic contribution. A small pressure zone is found at the hiatus even when the LOS lies within the thorax (Habibulla, 1972), while at the same time the displaced extrathoracic LOS has a reduced pressure profile.

What, then, can one conclude about the validity of using gastro-oesophageal pressure measurements either clinically or in research projects? Bearing in mind the above variables, the results obtained in any one individual cannot safely be relied upon. When applied to groups, better separation seems to be possible. It seems at present that clinical manometric recordings give more reliable information in dealing with motility patterns in the body of the oesophagus. Assessment of the gastro-oesophageal junction by pressure recordings alone are less reliable.

Potential Difference (PD)

Donne (1834) first demonstrated a potential difference between the skin and gastric mucosa. The potential appears to be dependent upon the integrity of the mucosa (Rehm, 1946), and its electrochemical basis seems to be the mucosal handling of sodium (Dobson, 1959; Davenport *et al.*, 1964) and chloride ions (Hogben, 1955).

The electrode system which is generally used to record PD is a metal–metal salt–salt combination. A salt–tissue junction is preferable to a metal–tissue one because the latter creates a junction potential. The most commonly used electrode is a mercury–mercuric chloride–potassium chloride combination. The exploring electrode is passed through the mouth into the stomach and then withdrawn through the gastro-oesophageal junction. This profile is usually obtained in combination with pressure recording through a separate perfused open-tip recording assembly. The reference electrode is sited subcutaneously. Skin reference sites are less reliable (Geall *et al.*, 1970; Grantham *et al.*, 1970).

Intragastric potential difference is negative with reference to the skin and varies between −10 and −80 mV. The body of the oesophagus has a slightly positive potential. The change of polarity occurs within the ZEP at the gastro-oesophageal junction, and is maximal at the point of respiratory reversal (Helm *et al.*, 1965). In two-thirds of people the reversal seemed related to the columnosquamous epithelial junction. Closer study of the type of mucosa demonstrated the reversal point to be correlated with the absence of parietal cells (Meckeler and Ingelfinger, 1967). There is evidence that the negative intragastric potential difference is largely the result of the transfer of negatively charged chloride ions (Hogben, 1955). The electromotive forces (the pump mechanism) responsible are likely to be a function of the parietal cell.

Clinically, this test is used to relate the mucosal change to the ZEP. This usually occurs within the ZEP near the hiatus. It has been used in the diagnosis of hiatus hernia (Helm *et al.*, 1965).

pH Measurements

Regurgitation into the oesophagus of acid–pepsin mixtures is accepted as the important factor in the pathogenesis of oesophagitis. In an attempt to quantify regurgitation, an array of tests designed to measure H^+ ion concentrations in the lower oesophagus has evolved.

The intragastric pH lies between 1.0 and 2.8 (Helm *et al.*, 1965). In the absence of gastro-oesophageal reflux, the pH of the oesophageal mucosa 5 cm above the LOS should be higher than 4.0. Any pH less than this indicates reflux. Some degree of reflux, however, is physiological. On swallowing, the pH in the LOS prior to the arrival of the primary oesophageal peristaltic wave becomes more acidic—reflux occurring while the sphincter is relaxed and awaiting the peristaltic wave. This oncoming wave then wipes the oesophagus clean. In addition, if reflux should occur for any other reason, acid in the lower oesophagus would be expected to be cleared by a secondary peristaltic wave.

Simultaneous pH and pressure profiles have been used to define a weak anti-reflux barrier (Tuttle and Grossman, 1958; Tuttle *et al.*, 1960, 1961). Reflux has been determined by relating pH to distance above the hiatus—the latter being marked by the point of respiratory reversal. Most people would regard a pH of lower than 4 within 5 cm of the hiatus as evidence of reflux. The Tuttle test, however, is unphysiological, because the stomach is pre-loaded with 0.1 N hydrochloric acid—a manoeuvre which itself can lower LOS pressure. False negative tests are sometimes obtained with this test, and it is regarded only as a rough and ready discriminator for the presence or absence of oesophagitis (Johnson *et al.*, 1974).

An alternative technique is to record intra-oesophageal pH over longer periods of up to 24 h (Johnson and Demester, 1974). From such studies, it appears that the period when acid–pepsin mixtures are in contact with the lower oesophagus for longest are at night (Atkinson and Van Gelder, 1977). Nocturnal records would seem likely to give more information.

Comparatively little work has been carried out on the oesophageal response to the presence of refluxed material within its lumen. The type of reflux material and the time it is in contact with the lower oesophagus would seem to be two critical factors in the pathogenesis of the disease.

There is some evidence to suggest disordered primary peristaltic wave activity in patients with reflux and associated inefficient oesophageal clearing of acid (Booth *et al.*, 1968; Boesby, 1977). Normally, 15 ml of 0.1 N HCl should be cleared from the oesophagus in less than ten swallows. This is not the case when reflux is present. It is possible that the clearing ability is normal but that the HCl is returned to the oesophagus by instantaneous reflux. However, abnormal motility patterns have been recorded in patients with oesophagitis (Siegel and Hendrix, 1963; Olsen and Schlegel, 1965; Donner *et al.*, 1966)—viz. motor inco-ordination, feeble contractions with loss of peristalsis, and even total paralysis. If stimulated by the instillation of acid or acid–barium (Siegel and Hendrix, 1963; Donner *et al.*, 1966), spontaneous non-peristaltic segmental contractions and regurgitations are seen.

Little is known about secondary peristaltic wave activity in patients with reflux. These waves arise spontaneously in response to intra-oesophageal fluid and are more important than the primary waves in reducing the oesophageal contact time of refluxed acid–pepsin mixtures.

Instead of measuring H^+ ion concentration, it is possible to instil acid into into the oesophagus and reproduce the pain of oesophagitis (Bernstein and Baker, 1958). This was originally a fairly non-specific test when HCl was placed into the body of the oesophagus. It was not always possible to be sure that the sensory receptors being stimulated were in the oesophagus or stomach (de Moraer-Filho and Bettarello, 1974). The accuracy of the test has been improved by placing the infusion tube at a predetermined distance above the LOS and at the same time infusing alkali into the stomach (Earlam, 1972). This test is used to help differentiate oesophageal and cardiac pain.

Endoscopy

With the exception of radiology, the previously described tests were developed to help manage patients with reflux. They were necessary because direct visualisation of the oesophagus with the rigid oesophagoscope was hazardous. Since the introduction of the flexible fibrescope, endoscopy and biopsy have now probably superseded other tests in clinical practice. Its chief advantage is that it enables the lower oesophageal mucosa to be seen and biopsied and reflux can be observed to occur.

Details of the technique and interpretation of biopsies are not relevant here. Recent reviews are available (Gibbs, 1976; Thompson, 1976).

The investigatory criteria for normal anti-reflux function of the gastro-oesophageal junction have been tabulated (table 4.1). Obviously, the multiplicity of tests indicate that the situation is not as clear-cut as it would seem from the dogmatic type of list. The difficulties arising will be recognised and discussed in the following section.

Table 4.1   Investigatory criteria of a normal gastro-oesophageal junction

---

(1) No reflux of barium seen on radiological studies.

(2) No oesophagitis seen on endoscopy.

(3) A ZEP with an absolute pressure in excess of 15 cm water, as measured by infused open-tip catheter assembly. ZEP straddles the hiatus.

(4) Mucosal change-over occurring within the ZEP at the hiatus.

(5) Intra-oesophageal pH > 4 at 5 cm above hiatus.

(6) Oesophagus clears 15 ml 0.1 N HCl in ten swallows.

(7) No positive pain reproduction test on acid perfusion of oesophagus.

DISORDERS OF SPHINCTER FUNCTION

This section will deal with the pathophysiology and possible therapeutic implications of three groups of sphincter disorders—the common problem of oesophageal reflux, the rarer group of achalasia-type disorders and, finally, the hypertensive lower oesophageal sphincter.

Oesophageal Reflux

Pathophysiology

Oesophagitis has been defined as 'an oesophageal response to injury caused by gastro-duodenal contents making adequate contact with the oesophageal mucosa' (Pope, 1976). The fault lies in the anti-reflux mechanism—whether it be a low-pressure barrier or an inability of the lower oesophagus to keep its lumen clear of refluxed gastric contents. There has been a tendency to regard the LOS as the most important component of the reflux barrier, based on plentiful comparative studies of LOS pressure levels in groups of people with and without reflux. However, the overall evidence suggests that the LOS by itself should not override other components of the anti-reflux mechanisms (Dodds *et al.*, 1976).

Measurements of LOS pressure in groups of patients with reflux show an overall lower level, although there can be considerable overlap with normal values (Pope, 1967). In addition, the response of the LOS to increased intragastric pressure is abnormal. A barrier pressure between stomach and oesophagus is not maintained (Lind *et al.*, 1966). There does not, however, appear to be any disorder of sphincteric relaxation.

Some doubt exists over the validity of correlating LOS pressure measurements with reflux. First, there is the overlap of pressure levels, as mentioned above. Second, pharmacologically produced increases in LOS pressure do not always prevent reflux occurring (Miller *et al.*, 1974). Third, surgical repair of hiatus herniae can stop reflux without altering pressures in the LOS (Brennan *et al.*, 1974). Such findings, however, need not necessarily be compatible. It is realised from radiological studies (Tumen *et al.*, 1960) that hiatus hernia and oesophageal reflux, although they commonly exist together, can occur separately. It is probable that the zone of elevated pressure has a diaphragmatic pressure component in addition to that of the LOS (Habibulla, 1972). It follows, then, that people with a hiatus hernia and no reflux are likely to have a competent LOS. Vice versa, those without a hiatus hernia but who reflux have an incompetent LOS. The third, and largest, group have both reflux and a hiatus hernia. It is not possible in this group to identify the weak component of the anti-reflux mechanism. The LOS is probably at fault, but the anatomical mechanisms may be as well. It would seem that a more accurate correlation between LOS pressure and reflux (if it should exist) is likely to be obtained from a study of those cases with reflux but no hiatus hernia.

An alternative explanation of the overlap in pressure has been provided by animal studies (Eastwood *et al.*, 1975). When oesophagitis was induced experimentally, it was found that LOS pressure varied inversely with the degree of inflammation. Provided that stricture formation did not occur, the process was reversible and LOS pressures returned to normal as the inflammation settled. In man the degree of damage induced by reflux is variable, and on this basis an overlap of LOS pressure in the two groups would not be surprising. Human studies support this idea (Siewart *et al.*, 1974). People with clinical reflux but no endoscopic signs of oesophagitis had normal LOS pressure and responded normally to pentagastrin. In those people with endoscopic oesophagitis the LOS pressures were lower and there was a diminished response to pentagastrin. It is not yet clear whether the LOS pressure changes are the cause or the effect of the oesophagitis.

While it is accepted that the evidence is not clear-cut, there does seem to be sufficient to conclude that a disorder of the LOS can be responsible for oesophageal reflux. The cause for this lies in either the smooth muscle of the LOS or its control mechanisms.

Pressure–tension–force of closure characteristics of 'incompetent' sphincters differ from normal (Biancini *et al.*, 1975). As the internal lumen of the LOS decreases and approaches closure conditions, the pressure increases in the competent and decreases in the incompetent LOS. In addition, in response to local stretch exerted by manometer tubing of increasing diameter, pressure rises are greater in competent sphincters. The defect seemed to be in smooth muscle control. Urecholine reversed the response to stretch of an incompetent LOS. Probanthine had the opposite effect by rendering a sphincter incompetent.

Other work suggests that there may be a defect in the smooth muscle itself. The LOS in patients with reflux responded less well to gastrin (Siewart *et al.*, 1974) and to drugs such as Tensilon and bethanechol (Farrell *et al.*, 1973). The response seemed to depend on the level of unstimulated resting pressure—the lower the pressure the less the response. There is no evidence at present that the level of LOS resting pressure is dependent on circulating gastrin levels (Farrell *et al.*, 1974; Wright *et al.*, 1975). This is not to say that manoeuvres which alter the circulating level of gastrin will not alter the LOS pressure. This, in fact, does happen and is used in the therapy of oesophageal reflux.

Scientific Basis for Treatment Regimen

Customary medical therapy for oesophageal reflux includes antacids, decreasing the intake of fat and abolition of smoking. Subsequent studies on the effect these manoeuvres have on the LOS pressure have demonstrated advantageous effects in terms of reflux protection.

Antacids were thought originally to act solely by neutralising acid gastric contents. However, LOS pressure is elevated by intragastric alkali working through a non-gastrin-mediated mechanism (Higgs *et al.*, 1974). Similarly, the frequent association between heartburn and the intake of fatty foods can be explained by the effects fats have on the LOS. The pressure is reduced (Babka and Castell, 1973) either by release of cholecystokinin or on other enterogastrones apart from secretin (Nebel and Castell, 1972). Cigarette smoking, presumably by its nicotine action, reduces LOS pressure and for this reason should be avoided (Dernish and Castell, 1971; Stanciu and Bennett, 1972). Anticholinergic drugs have often been included in preparations used for relieving dyspepsia. In patients with heartburn these should be avoided because atropine reduces LOS pressure (Kantrowitz *et al.*, 1966).

More recently, attempts have been directed to finding therapeutic agents which can directly stimulate the LOS. Metoclopramide has been shown to increase LOS pressure when given both intravenously and orally (Dilwari and Misiewicz, 1973; Stanciu and Bennett, 1973). It was originally thought to also improve the acid-clearing capacity of the oesophagus but this is now being questioned (Behar and Biancini, 1976). Unfortunately, it appears that the response to any drug is directly related to the level of baseline pressure and the LOS pressure responses obtained with metoclopramide or bethanechol are poor.

There are other possibilities. Prostaglandin $F_{2\alpha}$ infusion produces a sustained increase in LOS pressure. Prostaglandin E_2 does not affect the LOS pressure but does diminish pentagastrin-induced sphincter contractions. Inhibition of prostaglandin synthetase by intrarectal indomethacin increases sphincteric pressure (Dilwari *et al.*, 1973). As yet, no commercially useful preparation is available but it is possible that prostaglandin analogues may prove useful.

It has been demonstrated that the LOS has H_2 histamine receptors. The histamine H_2 receptor antagonist metiamide increases the LOS pressure in the opossum (Cohen and Snape, 1975). In man the LOS receptors appear more sensitive to histamine than are gastric acid secretory receptors. They seem to control the response of the sphincter to histamine, but play no part in the control of basal LOS pressure (Krawitz *et al.*, 1977). Following withdrawal of metiamide from clinical usage, cimetidine has recently been tested and shown to have no effect on LOS pressure in normal people (Freeland *et al.*, 1977).

At present there is no entirely satisfactory stimulant of LOS function which is useful in the treatment of oesophageal reflux. There does, however, appear to be good scientific backing for most medical therapy which is now in use. Until a better stimulant is found, this will continue to be the basis of present-day medical therapy. Surgery will continue to be used to deal with complications and when medical therapy fails. Its success is based on returning the anatomy to normal and perhaps by doing that to compensate for a weak sphincter. The multitude of operations and inevitable small proportion of recurrence only serve to stress the importance of finding a satisfactory sphincter stimulant.

Achalasia and Chagas' Disease

Pathophysiology

The aetiology of achalasia is unknown. Chagas' disease is due to parasitic infection with *Trypanosoma cruzi*. In both diseases the myenteric nerve plexus are damaged. In achalasia there is also evidence of damage to the vagus nerve (Cassella *et al.*, 1965; Smith, 1970). The loss of myenteric neurons may be variable but the cells which escape are argyrophobe (Smith, 1970). Loss of argyrophil cells results in loss of co-ordinative reflexes, while the presence of some remaining argyrophobe cells allows some motor activity to remain. The motor features of achalasia and Chagas' disease are multiple simultaneous contractions of the body of the oesophagus with a varying degree of intensity combined with absence of sphincteric relaxation. Peristaltic waves disappear from the oesophagus in achalasia but are seen in Chagas' disease.

Intrinsic denervation of the LOS produces a higher than normal LOS pressure when measured by an infused open-tip catheter assembly (Cohen and Lipshutz, 1971). Although sphincter tone is largely myogenic in origin, this finding is unlikely to be caused by changes in the muscle itself. Histological studies show patchy sclerosis of smooth muscle (Harrison, 1969). This would be unlikely to increase the LOS pressure. The pressure change probably results from changes in the control mechanisms. Evidence from studies with gastrin suggest that the muscle is supersensitive to this hormone. This probably represents denervation supersensitivity (Cohen *et al.*, 1971).

As sphincter relaxation is neurally mediated, it would be expected to be affected in achalasia. The pathway responsible for relaxation forms part of the purigenic–peptidergic nervous system and this seems to be affected by destruction of myenteric neurons. Partial or complete loss of relaxation is one of the early manometric signs of achalasia and Chagas' disease (Cohen and Lipshutz, 1971b; Csendes *et al.*, 1975).

As yet, there are no available data about the reaction of the LOS affected by these diseases to increase in intragastric pressure. If one were to speculate, the response is likely to be exaggerated. The higher resting pressures obtained with infusion manometry suggest that the smooth muscle response to local stretch is exaggerated. Also, clinical oesophageal reflux is not a feature of achalasia.

Scientific Basis of Treatment

Widespread neuronal damage with loss of co-ordination reflexes makes it unlikely that achalasia or Chagas' disease will respond to any form of medical treatment. This is the case with both diseases. Management is largely surgical, involving a sphincteric myotomy. This permits the oesophagus to empty but subsequent gastro-oesophageal reflux is more likely.

The Hyperactive Lower Oesophageal Sphincter

Retrospective studies of several series of oesophageal motility recordings have revealed a very small group of people with a hyperactive LOS. There are three different types, all of which tend to accompany other oesophageal disorders—in particular, diffuse spasm and hiatus hernia. Little is known about their aetiology. The types are as follows:

Hypertensive lower oesophageal sphincter. The criteria used for establishing this diagnosis depend on the method of pressure measurement. Pressures in excess of 40 cm water as measured by open-tip units, or 140 cm water with balloon-covered transducers, have been designated to indicate a hypertensive sphincter (Code *et al.*, 1960). There is a frequent association with diffuse spasm of the oesophageal body but it is rare in achalasia. In addition, half of these sphincters showed poor relaxation and a quarter contracted with excessive vigour after swallowing.

Hyperreactive lower oesophageal sphincter. This is characterised by an exaggerated sphincteric contraction with a high amplitude. It may or may not be associated with a hypertensive LOS, but is commonly associated with a hiatus hernia or diffuse spasm.

Hypercontracting lower oesophageal sphincter. This is represented by an unusually prolonged sphincteric contraction which may or may not be of excessive pressure. Similar to the above, it is most commonly found in association with the motility patterns of hiatus hernia and diffuse spasm (Garrett and Goodwin, 1969).

Little is known about these disorders. They seem to be interrelated and probably form part of an associated group of disorders. Smooth muscle hypertrophy is seen with diffuse spasm and occasionally this can be localised to the LOS. Its cause is unknown. No pharmacological studies on sphincter smooth muscle are available.

FUTURE ADVANCES

Physiology

The smooth muscle sphincter has been shown to differ in its basic myogenic properties from neighbouring muscle. It is possible that this is the result of a low negative hypopolarised membrane potential. Intracellular potential recordings are required. It is also possible that the gastrointestinal hormones and other controlling mechanisms act by altering this potential.

Lower Oesophageal Sphincter Pressure and Measurement

(1) Infusion open-tip manometry would seem to be the most satisfactory generally available manometric system. The inherent defects and variables are recognised. For the sake of comparison, the systems in use need to be standardised.

(2) Most reliable information on LOS pressure in reflux patients is likely to be obtained from studying those people with reflux but without a hiatus hernia.

(3) A better test of relating intragastric to sphincteric pressure in man is required. As reflux is most likely to occur at times when intragastric pressure is raised, the sphincteric response to it is important. The results produced by Canadian workers (Lind *et al.*, 1966) have been difficult to reproduce. There are, however, enough experimental data (Biancini *et al.*, 1975; Thomas, 1977) to support the concept that such a reflex exists.

(4) Lower oesophageal sphincter and sleep. Twenty-four hour pH recordings demonstrate that reflux occurs most commonly at night. Nocturnal pressure measurements within the LOS are required to see whether such reflux can be correlated with a reduced LOS pressure at night. Cyclical interdigestive activity has been recorded in the LOS (Itoh *et al.*, 1978), and disorganisation of relative pressure levels in the LOS and fundus at times of high activity may be a cause of reflux.

Hormone Studies

Relating circulating levels of hormones to LOS pressures seems to be of little practical use. Pharmacological data suggest that sphincter muscle is more sensitive to hormones than surrounding muscle, with the existence in the LOS of specific hormone receptors (Goyal and Rattan, 1978). The critical factor would seem to be the tissue hormone concentrations. At present there is no available technique enabling these to be measured.

Investigations

Recent introduction of scintiscanning and measurement of the reflux of technetium introduced into the stomach seems a promising non-invasive way of qualitating reflux (Fisher *et al.*, 1976, 1977). More experience using this technique is required.

Therapy

The search for a sphincteric smooth muscle stimulant continues. At the moment it seems that the responses of such drugs are related inversely to the level of unstimulated LOS pressure. The use of electrical stimuli may be a possible way of improving sphincteric tone and reactivity.

REFERENCES

Arndorfer, R. C., Stef, J. J., Dodds, W. J., Linehan, J. H. and Hogan, W. J. (1977). Improved infusion system for intraluminal oesophageal manometry. *Gastroenterology*, 73, 23-27

Atkinson, M. (1976). Disorders of oesophageal motility. *Clinics in Gastroenterology*, January 1976

Atkinson, M., Edwards, D. A. W., Horow, A. J. and Rowlands, E. N. (1957). The oesophago-gastric sphincter in hiatus hernia. *Lancet*, ii, 1138-1142

Atkinson, M. and Van Gelder, A. (1977). Oesophageal intraluminal pH recording in the assessment of gastro-oesophageal reflux and its consequences. *Am. J. Dig. Dis.*, 22, 365

Babka, J. C. and Castell, D. O. (1973). On the genesis of heartburn. The effect of specific foods on the lower oesophageal sphincter. *Am. J. Dig. Dis.*, 18, 391-397

Babka, J. C., Hage, G. W. and Castell, D. O. (1973). The effect of body position on lower oesophageal sphincter pressure. *Am. J. Dig. Dis.*, 18, 441-442

Behar, J. and Biancini, P. (1976). Effect of oral metoclorpramide on gastro-oesophageal reflux in the post cibal state. *Gastroenterology*, 70, 331

Behar, J., Biancini, P. and Kerstein, M. (1976). Mechanism of lower oesophageal sphincter pressure increases in response to gastric pressure increments. *Gastroenterology*, 70, A-5 863

Behar, J. and Kastendieck, J. (1974). Studies on sphincter competence. *Gastroenterology*, 66, 834A

Bernstein, L. M. and Baker, L. A. (1958). A clinical test for oesophagitis. *Gastroenterology*, 34, 760

Biancini, P., Zabinski, M. P. and Behar, J. (1975). Pressure, tension and force of closure of the human lower oesophageal sphincter and oesophagus. *J. Clin. Invest.*, 56, 476-483

Boesby, S. (1977). Gastro-oesophageal sphincter pressure, motility and acid clearing. *Scand. J. Gastroenterol.*, 12, 407-416

Booth, D. J., Kemmerer, W. T. and Skinner, D. B. (1968). Acid clearing from the distal oesophagus. *Arch. Surg.*, 96, 731

Brennan, T. G., Trindade, L. M., Rozycki, Z. J. and Giles, G. R. (1974). The influence of lower oesophageal sphincter pressure on the outcome of hiatus hernia repair. *Br. J. Surg.*, 61, 201-205

Burnstock, G. (1972). Purinergic nerves. *Pharm. Rev.*, 24, 509-581

Cassella, R. R., Ellis, F. H. Jr. and Brown, A. L. (1965). Fine structure changes in achalasia of the oesophagus. 1. Vagus nerves. *Am. J. Pathol.*, 46, 279-288

Castell, D. O. and Harris, L. D. (1970). Hormonal control of gastro-oesophageal sphincter strength. *New Engl. J. Med.*, 282, 886-890

Christensen, J. and Conklin, J. (1974). Studies on the origin of the distinctive mechanics of smooth muscle at the oesophago-gastric junction. In *Proceedings of the IVth International Symposium on Gastro-Intestinal Motility*, Mitchell Press, Vancouver, pp. 63-71

Christensen, J., Conklin, J. L. and Freeman, B. W. (1973a). Physiological specialisation at the oesophago-gastric junction in the opossum. *Am. J. Physiol.*, 225, 1265-1270

Christensen, J., Freeman, B. W. and Miller, J. K. (1973b). Some physiological characteristics of the oesophago-gastric junction in the opossum. *Gastroenterology*, 64, 1119-1125

Code, C. F., Schlegel, J. F., Kelley, M. L. Jr., Olsen, A. M. and Ellis, F. H. (1960). Hypertensive gastro-oesophageal sphincter. *Proc. Staff Meetings Mayo Clinic*, 35, 391-399

Cohen, S. (1974). What is physiological? An answer! *Gastroenterology*, 66, 497

Cohen, S. and Harris, L. (1969). The adaptive response of the lower oesophageal sphincter. *Clin. Res.*, 17, 3000

Cohen, S. and Lipshutz, W. (1971a). Hormonal regulation of human lower oesophageal sphincter competence: interaction of gastrin and secretin. *J. Clin. Invest.*, 50, 449-454

Cohen, S. and Lipshutz, W. (1971b). Lower oesophageal sphincter dysfunction in achalasia. *Gastroenterology*, 61, 814

Cohen, S., Lipshutz, W. and Hughes, W. (1971). Role of gastrin supersensitivity in the pathogenesis of lower oesophageal sphincter hypertension in achalasia. *J. Clin. Invest.*, 50, 1241

Cohen, S. and Snape, W. J. Jr. (1975). Action of metiamide on the lower oesophageal sphincter. *Gastroenterology*, 69, 911-919

Crispin, J. S., McIver, D. K. and Lind, D. F. (1967). Manometric study of the effect of vagotomy on the gastro-oesophageal sphincter. *Can. J. Surg.*, **10**, 299-303

Csendes, A., Stramszer, T. and Uribe, P. (1975). Alterations in normal oesophageal motility in patients with Chagas' disease. *Am. J. Dig. Dis.*, **20**, 437

Davenport, H. W., Warner, H. A. and Code, C. F. (1964). Functional significance of gastric mucosal barrier to sodium. *Gastroenterology*, **47**, 142

de Carle, D. J. and Christensen, J. (1976). A dopamine receptor in oesophageal smooth muscle of the opossum. *Gastroenterology*, **70**, 216-219

de Moraer-Filho, J. P. P. and Bettarello, A. (1974). Lack of specificity of the acid perfusion test in duodenal ulcer patients. *Am. J. Dig. Dis.*, **19**, 785

Dent, J. and Chir, B. (1976). A new technique for continuous sphincter pressure measurement. *Gastroenterology*, **71**, 263–267

Dernish, G. W. and Castell, D. O. (1971). Inhibitory effect of smoking on the lower oesophageal sphincter. *New Engl. J. Med.*, **284**, 1136

Diament, N. E. and El-Sharkawy, T. Y. (1977). Neural control of oesophageal peristalsis—a conceptional analysis. *Gastroenterology*, **72**, 546

Dilwari, J. B. and Misiewicz, J. J. (1973). Action of metoclorpramide on the gastro-oesophageal junction in man. *Gut*, **14**, 380

Dilwari, J. B., Newman, A., Poleo, J. and Misiewicz, J. J. (1973). The effect of prostaglandins and of anti-inflammatory drugs on the oesophagus and the cardiac sphincter in man. *Gut*, **14**, 822

DiMarino, A. J. and Cohen, S. (1973). The adrenergic control of lower oesophageal sphincter function. *J. Clin. Invest.*, **52**, 2264-2271

Dobson, A. (1959). Active transport through the epithelium of the reticulo-rumen sac. *J. Physiol., Lond.*, **146**, 235-251

Dodds, W. J., Hogan, W. J. and Miller, W. N. (1976). Reflux oesophagitis. *Am. J. Dig. Dis.*, **21**, 49

Dodds, W. J., Hogan, W. J., Miller, W. N., Barreras, R. F., Arndorfer, R. C. and Stef, J. J. (1975a). Relationship between serum gastrin concentration and lower oesophageal sphincter pressure. *Am. J. Dig. Dis.*, **20**, 201-207

Dodds, W. J., Hogan, W. J., Miller, W. N., Stef, J. J., Arndorfer, R. C. and Lydon, S. B. (1975b). Effect of increased intra-abdominal pressure on lower oesophageal sphincter pressure. *Am. J. Dig. Dis.*, **20**, 298-307

Dodds, W. J., Hogan, W. J., Stef, J. J., Miller, W. N., Lydon, S. B. and Arndorfer, R. C. (1975c). A rapid pull-through technique for measuring lower oesophageal sphincter pressure. *Gastroenterology*, **68**, 437-443

Donne, A. (1834). Recherches sur quelques unes des proprietes chimiques des secretions et sur les courants electriques qui existent dans les corps organises. *Ann. Chim. Phys.*, **57**, 398

Donner, M. W., Silbiger, M. L., Hookman, P. and Hendrix, T. R. (1966). Acid barium swallows in the radiographic evaluation of clinical oesophagitis. *Radiology*, **87**, 220-225

Earlam, R. J. (1972). Further experience using the epigastric pain reproduction test in duodenal ulceration. *Br. Med. J.*, **1**, 683-685

Eastwood, G. L., Castell, D. O. and Higgs, R. (1975). Experimental oesophagitis in cats impairs lower oesophageal sphincter pressure. *Gastroenterology*, **69**, 146-153

Farrell, R. L., Castell, D. O. and McGuigan, J. E. (1974). Measurements and comparisons of lower oesophageal sphincter pressure and serum gastrin levels in patients with gastro-oesophageal reflux. *Gastroenterology*, **67**, 415-422

Farrell, R. L., Roling, G. T. and Castell, D. O. (1973). Stimulation of the incompetent lower oesophageal sphincter. A possible advance in the therapy of heartburn. *Am. J. Dig. Dis.*, **18**, 646

Fisher, R. S., Malmud, L. S., Roberts, G. S. and Lobis, I. F. (1976). Gastro-oesophageal scintiscanning to detect and quantitate gastro-oesophageal reflux. *Gastroenterology*, **70**, 301

Fisher, R. S., Malmud, L. S., Roberts, G. S. and Lobis, I. F. (1977). The lower oesophageal sphincter as a barrier to gastro-oesophageal reflux. *Gastroenterology*, **72**, 19-22

Freeland, G. R., Higgs, R. H. and Castell, D. O. (1977). Lower oesophageal sphincter responses to oral administration of cimetidine in normal subjects. *Gastroenterology*, **72**, 28-30

Fyke, F. E., Code, C. F. and Schlegel, J. F. (1956). The gastro-oesophageal sphincter in healthy human beings. *Gastroenterologie (Basel)*, **86**, 135

Garrett, J. M. and Goodwin, D. H. (1969). Gastro-oesophageal hypercontracting sphincter. *J. Am. Med. Assoc.*, **208**, 992-998

Geall, M. G., Code, C. F., McIlrath, D. C. and Summerskill, W. H. J. (1970). Measurement of gastrointestinal transmural electric potential difference in man. *Gut*, **11**, 34-37

Gibbs, D. (1976). Endoscopy in the assessment of reflux oesophagitis. In *Clinics in Gastroenterology. Disorders of Oesophageal Motility* (ed. Michael Atkinson), January, 1976

Giles, G. R., Mason, M. C., Humphries, C. and Clark, C. G. (1969). Action of gastrin on lower oesophageal sphincter in man. *Gut*, **10**, 730-734

Goodal, R. J. R., Hay, D. J. and Temple, J. G. (1980). Assessment of the rapid pullthrough technique in oesophageal manometry. *Gut*, **21**, 169-173

Goyal, R. K. and McGuigan, J. E. (1975). Failure of gastrin antiserum to influence lower oesophago-sphincter pressure: a double blind controlled study. *Gastroenterology*, **68**, 951

Goyal, R. K. and Rattan, S. (1975). Nature of the vagal inhibitory innervation of the lower oesophageal sphincter. *J. Clin. Invest.*, **55**, 1119-1126

Goyal, R. K. and Rattan, S. (1978). Neurohumural, hormonal and drug receptors for the lower oesophageal sphincter. *Gastroenterology*, **74**, 598-619

Grantham, R. N., Code, C. F. and Schlegel, J. F. (1970). Reference electrode sites in determination of potential differences across the gastro-oesophageal muscular junction. *Mayo Clin. Proc.*, **45**, 265-274

Grossman, M. I. (1973). What is physiological? *Gastroenterology*, **65**, 994

Habibulla, K. S. (1972). The diaphragm as an anti-reflux barrier. A manometric, oesophagoscopic and transmucosal potential study. *Thorax*, **27**, 692-702

Harris, L. D., Winans, C. S. and Pope, C. II (1966). Determination of yield pressures: a method for measuring anal sphincter competence. *Gastroenterology*, **50**, 754-760

Harrison, G. K. (1969). Oesophageal muscle changes in achalasia. *Lancet*, **i**, 530

Helm, W. J., Schlegel, J. F., Code, C. F. and Summerskill, W. H. J. (1965). Identification of the gastro-oesophageal mucosal junction by transmucosal potential in healthy subjects and patients with hiata hernia. *Gastroenterology*, **48**, 23-25

Higgs, R. H., Smith, R. D. and Castell, D. O. (1974). Gastric alkalinisation. Effect on lower oesophageal sphincter pressure and serum gastrin. *New Engl. J. Med.*, **291**, 486-490

Hogben, C. A. M. (1955). Active transport of chloride by isolated frog gastric epithelium: origin of the gastric mucosal potential. *Am. J. Physiol.*, **180**, 641-649

Hollis, J. B. and Castell, D. O. (1972). Amplitude of oesophageal peristalsis as determined by rapid infusion. *Gastroenterology*, **63**, 417-422

Holly, E. (1977). Pressure pH measurement in the human gastro-oesophageal sphincter: A computer analysis. Ph.D. Thesis, University of London

Humphries, T. J. and Castell, D. O. (1977). Pressure profile of oesophageal peristalsis in normal humans as measured by direct intra-oesophageal transducers. *Am. J. Dig. Dis.*, **22**, 641

Ingelfinger, F. J. (1958). Oesophageal motility. *Phys. Rev.*, **38**, 533-584

Itoh, Z., Honda, R., Aizawa, I., Takeuchi, S., Hiwatashi, K. and Couch, E. F. (1978). Interdigestive motor activity of the lower oesophageal sphincter in the conscious dog. *Am. J. Dig. Dis.*, **23**, 239-247

Jennewein, H. M., Waldeck, F., Siewert, R., Weiser, F. and Thimm, R. (1973). The interaction of glucagon and pentagastrin on the lower oesophageal sphincter in man and dog. *Gut*, **14**, 861-864

Jensen, D. M., McCallum, R. W. and Walsh, J. H. (1977a). Human lower oesophageal sphincter response to submaximal and maximal effective doses of synthetic human gastrin 1 (G17) is not inhibited by atropine. *Gastroenterology*, **A-15**, Abstract 58

Jensen, D. M., McCallum, R. W. and Walsh, J. H. (1977b). Human lower oesophageal sphincter response to submaximal and maximal effective doses of synthetic human big gastrin (G34) and gastrin (G17). *Gastroenterology*, **A-61**, Abstract 244

Johnson, L. F. and Demester, T. R. (1974). Advantages of distal oesophageal 24 hour pH monitoring over other tests for gastro-oesophageal reflux. *Gastroenterology*, **66**, 716

Johnson, L. F., Demester, T. R. and Haggitt, R. G. (1974). Oesophageal histology correlated to objective measurements of gastro-oesophageal reflux. *Gastroenterology*, **66**, 717

Kantrowitz, P. A., Siegel, C. I. and Hendrix, T. R. (1966). Differences in motility of the upper and lower oesophagus in man and its alteration of atropine. *Bull. Johns Hopkins Hosp.*, **118**, 476

Kaye, M. D. and Showalter, J. P. (1971). Manometric configuration of the lower oesophageal sphincter in normal human subjects. *Gastroenterology*, **61**, 213

Kaye, M. D. and Showalter, J. P. (1974). Measurement of pressure in lower oesophageal sphincter—the influence of catheter diameter. *Am. J. Dig. Dis.*, **19**, 860-863

Kline, M. M., McCallum, R. W., Curry, N. and Sturdevant, R. A. L. (1975). Effect of gastric alkalinisation on lower oesophageal sphincter pressure on serum gastrin. *Gastroenterology*, **68**, 1137-1139

Koelz, H. R., Hollinger, A. P., Sauberli, H., Largiader, F., Siewart, R. and Blum, A. L. (1978). Effect of gastric antrum on regulation of lower oesophageal sphincter pressure in the dog. *Am. J. Physiol.*, **234** (2), E157-E161

Krawitz, J. J., Snape, W. J. Jr. and Cohen, S. (1977). Role of histaminergic receptors in the control of lower oesophageal function. *Gastroenterology*, **A59**, Abstract 237

Lind, J. F., Cotton, D. J., Blanchard, R., Crispin, J. S. and Dimopolo, S. (1969). Effect of thoracic displacement and vagotomy on the canine gastro-oesophageal junction. *Gastroenterology*, **56**, 1078-1085

Lind, J. F., Warrian, W. G. and Wankling, W. J. (1966). Responses of the gastro-oesophageal junctional zone to increases in abdominal pressure. *Can. J. Surg.*, **9**, 32-38

Lipshutz, W. and Cohen, S. (1971). Physiological determinants of lower oesophageal sphincter function. *Gastroenterology*, **61**, 16-24

Lipshutz, W., Hughes, W. and Cohen, S. (1972). The genesis of the lower oesophageal sphincter pressure; its identification through the use of gastrin antiserum. *J. Clin. Invest.*, **51**, 522-529

Lipshutz, W., Tuch, A. F. and Cohen, S. (1971). A comparison of the site of action of gastrin 1 on lower oesophageal sphincter and antral circular smooth muscle. *Gastroenterology*, **61**, 454-460

Lyndon, S. B., Dodds, W. J., Hogan, W. J. and Arndorfer, R. C. (1975). The effect of manometric assembly diameter on intraluminal oesophageal pressure recording. *Am. J. Dig. Dis.*, **20**, 968-970

Mann, C. V., Greenwood, R. K. and Ellis, F.H. Jr. (1964). The oesophago-gastric junction. *Surg., Gynec. Obst.*, **118**, 853-862

Mann, C. V. and Shorter, R. G. (1964). Structure of the canine oesophagus and its sphincter. *J. Surg. Res.*, **IV**, 160-163

Meckeler, K. J. and Ingelfinger, F. J. (1967). Correlation of electric surface potentials, intraluminal pressure and nature of tissue in the gastro-oesophageal junction of man. *Gastroenterology*, **52**, 966-971

Mei, N., Salducci, J. and Monges, H. (1972). Afferent vagal impulses from the lower oesophageal sphincter of the cat. *Rend. Gastroenterol.*, **4**, 65-68

Meltzer, S. J. (1899). On the causes of the orderly progress of the peristaltic movements in the oesophagus. *Am. J. Physiol.*, **2**, 266-272

Miller, W. N., Graneshapper, W. J., Dodds, W. J., Hogan, W. J., Arndorfer, R. C. and Stef, J. J. (1974). Preliminary report on Millhon–Crites intra-oesophageal motility probe. *Am. J. Dig. Dis.*, **13**, 929–933

Millhon, W. A., Hoffman, D. E. and Jarvis, P. (1968). Preliminary report on Millhon–Crites intraoesophageal motility probe. *Am. J. Dig. Dis.*, **13**, 929-933

Miolan, J. P. and Roman, C. (1973). Activity of vagal efferent fibres innervating the dog's cardia. *J. Physiol. (Paris)*, **66**, 171-198

Nebel, O. T. and Castell, D. O. (1972). Lower oesophageal sphincter pressure changes after food ingestion. *Gastroenterology*, **63**, 778

Olsen, A. M. and Schlegel, J. F. (1965). Motility disturbances caused by oesophagitis. *J. Thorac. Cardiovasc. Surg.*, **50**, 607-612

Pope, C. E. II (1967). A dynamic test of sphincter strength: its application to the lower oesophageal sphincter. *Gastroenterology*, **52**, 779-786

Pope, C. E. II (1976). Pathophysiology and diagnosis of reflux oesophagitis. *Gastroenterology*, **70**, 445

Price, S. and Castell, D. O. (1978). Oesophageal mythology. *J. Am. Med. Assoc.*, **240**, 44

Rattan, S. and Goyal, R. K. (1974). Neural control of lower oesophageal sphincter: influence of vagus nerves. *J. Clin. Invest.*, **54**, 899-906

Rattan, S. and Goyal, R. K. (1976). Effect of dopamine on the oesopnageal smooth muscle in vivo: evidence of excitatory and inhibitory dopamine receptors. *Gastroenterology*, **70**, 377-381

Rehm, W. S. (1946). Evidence that the major portion of the gastric potential originates between the submucosa and mucosa. *Am. J. Physiol.*, **147**, 69

Resin, H., Stern, D. H., Sturdevant, R. A. C. and Isenberg, J. I. (1973). Effect of C-terminal octapeptide of CCK on lower oesophageal sphincter pressure in man. *Gastroenterology*, **64**, 946-949

Siegel, C. I. and Hendricks, J. R. (1963). Oesophageal motor abnormalities induced by acid perfusion in patients with heartburn. *J. Clin. Invest.*, **42**, 686-695

Siewart, R., Weiser, F. and Jennewein, H. M. (1974). Clinical and manometric investigation of the lower oesophageal sphincter and its reactivity to pentagastrin in patients with hiatus hernia. *Digestion*, **10**, 287-297

Smith, B. (1970). The neurological tension in achalasia of the cardia. *Gut*, **11**, 388-391

Stanciu, C. and Bennett, J. R. (1972). The effect of smoking on gastro-oesophageal reflux. *Gut*, **13**, 318

Stanciu, C. and Bennett, J. R. (1973). Metoclorpramide in gastro-oesophageal reflux. *Gut*, **14**, 275

Stef, J. J., Dodds, W. J., Hogan, W. I., Linehan, H. J. and Stewart, E. T. (1974). Intraluminal oesophageal manometry. An analysis of variables affecting recording fidelity of peristaltic pressures. *Gastroenterology*, **67**, 227-230

Thomas, P. A. (1977). The action of some gastrointestinal polypeptide hormones on the isolated perfused canine gastro-oesophageal sphincter. M.S. Thesis, University of London

Thompson, H. (1976). Pathology of reflux oesophagitis. In *Clinics in Gastroenterology. Diseases of Oesophageal Motility* (ed. Michael Atkinson), January 1976

Tuch, A. and Cohen, S. (1973). Lower oesophageal sphincter relaxation: studies on the neurogenic inhibitory mechanism. *J. Clin. Invest.*, **52**, 14-20

Tumen, H. J., Stein, G. N. and Shlansky, F. (1960). X-Ray and clinical features of hiatal hernia—significance of hiatal hernia of minimal degree. *Gastroenterology*, **38**, 873

Tuttle, S. G., Betarello, A. and Grossman, M. I. (1960). Oesophageal acid perfusion test and a gastro-oesophageal reflux test in patients with oesophagitis. *Gastroenterology*, **38**, 861

Tuttle, S. G., Betarello, A. and Grossman, M. I. (1961). Gastro-oesophageal regurgitation. *J. Am. Med. Assoc.*, **176**, 498-500

Tuttle, S. G. and Grossman, M. I. (1958). Detection of gastro-oesophageal reflux by simultaneous measurement of intraluminal pressure and pH. *Proc. Soc. Expl Biol. Med.*, **98**, 225

Wankling, W. J., Warrian, W. G. and Lind, J. F. (1965). The gastro-oesophageal sphincter in hiatus hernia. *Can. J. Surg.*, **8**, 61-67

Winans, C. (1977). Manometric asymmetry of lower oesophageal high pressure zone. *Am. J. Dig. Dis.*, **22**, 348

Winans, C. S. and Harris, L. D. (1967). Quantitation of lower oesophageal sphincter competence. *Gastroenterology*, **52**, 773-778

Wingate, D. L. (1976). The eupeptide system: a general theory of gastrointestinal hormones. *Lancet*, i, 529

Wright, L. F., Slaughter, R. L., Gibson, R. G. and Hirschowitz, B. I. (1975). Correlation of lower oesophageal sphincter pressure and serum gastrin levels in man. *Am. J. Dig. Dis.*, **20**, 603-606

Zboralske, F. F. and Dodds, W. J. (1969). Roentgenographic diagnosis of primary disorders of oesophageal motility. *Radiol. Clin. North Am.*, **7**, 147-162

5
The Pylorus

Alan G. Johnson

'It is as if always small amounts of the contents of the stomach pass over into the intestine and, so to speak, close the door behind them.'

(S. Moritz, 1901)

The word 'pylorus' means 'door-keeper' and this quotation describes accurately, if rather fancifully, the two main functions of the pylorus: to limit the amount of chyme that passes into the duodenum at any one time and to prevent reflux of the duodenal contents back into the stomach.

ANATOMY

Unlike the lower oesophageal sphincter, the pylorus is a clearly identifiable structure, with the prepyloric vein of Mayo marking its distal limit on the serosal surface, where a thickened ring of circular muscle is easily palpable. However, this ring of muscle is on the gastric side of the mucosal change that marks the gastroduodenal junction and it is a graduated thickening from its proximal to its distal end (figure 5.1). It is broken up into fasciculi of different sizes by strands of connective tissue. The narrowed orifice just before the duodenum is due to the greatest thickening and is best called the pyloric ring, for reasons that will become apparent. The mean length of the ring is 6.7 mm, measured radiologically (Edwards, 1961b), whereas the whole of the thickened terminal antral muscle is 2.5–3.0 cm long in the adult. Torgersen (1942) laid special stress on the loop arrangements of the muscle fibres, believing that these were responsible for the change of shape

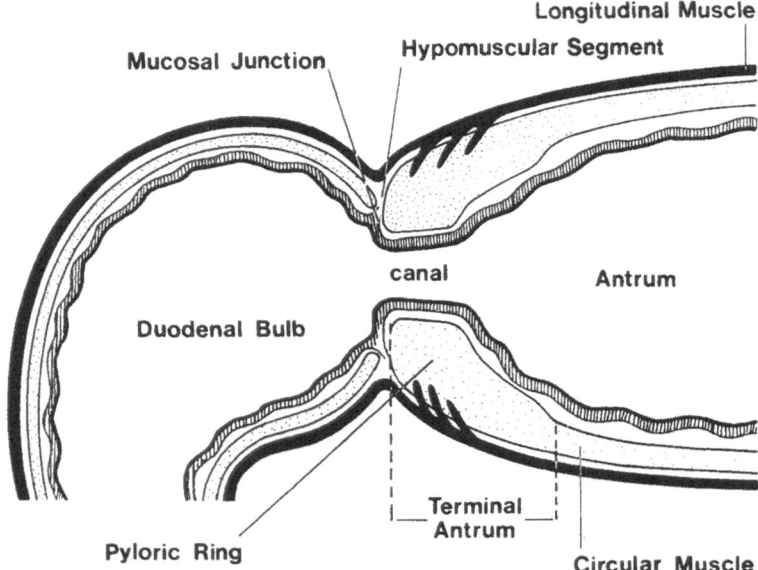

Figure 5.1   **Diagram** of anatomy of gastroduodenal junction.

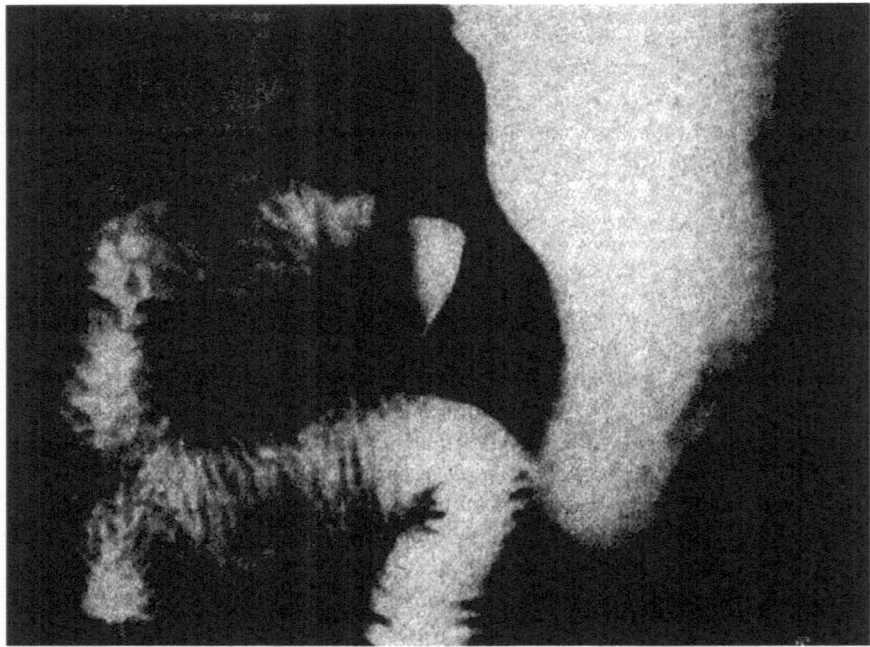

Figure 5.2   Air-contrast barium meal examination showing normal terminal antrum, pyloric canal and duodenal cap.

of the terminal antrum. Figure 5.2 shows the anatomy of the region as demonstrated by radiology.

Just beyond the pyloric ring is the hypomuscular segment, which may be identified from the serosal aspect as a circular groove. The circular muscle of the stomach is not continuous with the duodenal circular muscle across this junction and usually only a few superficial longitudinal fibres pass across, most of the deeper fibres dipping into the circular muscle (Horton, 1928). Torgersen (1942) describes a duodenal part of the pyloric sphincter belonging to the bulb and contracting with it. This is the most proximal ring of the duodenal circular muscle and may be important in pyloric closure (see below). A caricature of the antral circular muscle thickening is seen in hypertrophic pyloric stenosis in infants, where the abrupt change to the thin muscle wall of the duodenum is very obvious and can easily be opened by mistake in Ramstedt's operation of pyloromyotomy. Figure 5.3 is a radiograph of the rare adult form of hypertrophic pyloric stenosis, showing the long narrowing of the pyloric canal extending the full length of the thickened pyloric muscle. The neural elements in the myenteric plexus pass across the junction, which is important in the co-ordination of the gastric

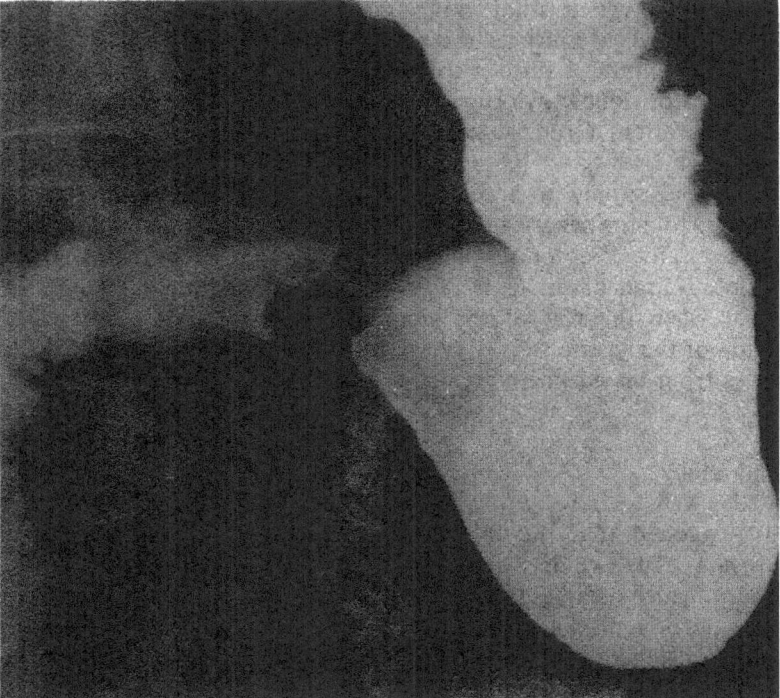

Figure 5.3 Barium meal showing adult hypertrophic pyloric stenosis. Note the longer, narrower pyloric canal compared with figure 5.2.

and duodenal contractions (see page 108). The subserosal plexus also continues through to the duodenum with the outer longitudinal muscle fibres, but it is not clear whether the submucous plexus is interrupted or continuous. There is almost a complete block in the submucous lymphatics, but the subserosal lymphatics pass across the junction. This may be significant in the spread of carcinoma of the stomach.

The junction between gastric and duodenal mucosa occurs at the hypomuscular segment, where the mucosa is tethered to the underlying connective tissue between the circular muscle of the stomach and duodenum. This junction can be defined by a potential difference electrode, because the transmucosal potential difference of the stomach is 27 mV more negative than that of the duodenum. The gastric mucosa, which is very mobile over the antrum, usually pouts into the duodenum to a varying extent—rather like the cervix into the vagina. This mucosal plug may be a factor in preventing reflux but, if excessive, may give rise to symptoms—the prolapsing mucous membrane syndrome.

Occasionally at endoscopy we have observed prolapsing of the less mobile duodenal mucosa back into the stomach through the pyloric ring while reflux is occurring. The most proximal duodenum in man is dilated into a duodenal bulb which is not so prominent in many other species.

A congenital atresia near the pylorus is a rare anomaly and may be a prepyloric septum, a fibrous cord or discontinuous blind ends. Although most cases of double pylorus are really gastroduodenal fistulae following peptic ulceration, a true congenital double pylorus does occur (Sufian *et al.*, 1977).

The vagal supply to the gastroduodenal junction is via the pyloric branches from the hepatic branch of the anterior vagus, and one of the aims behind selective vagotomy in man was to leave the hepatic branch with its pyloric sub-branches intact in the hope that pyloric function would remain normal when the rest of the stomach was extrinsically denervated by division of the gastric vagal fibres. The sympathetic nerve supply is via the arteries from the coeliac plexus.

Terminology

It is suggested that the following terminology be adopted to prevent confusion. The whole structure should be called the *gastroduodenal junction,* which includes the following parts. The *antrum* is usually taken to be the portion of the stomach distal to the incisura, although the true histological junction is not detectable macroscopically. The gradual distal thickening of the circular muscle should be designated the *terminal antrum,* and the most terminal ring of thickened muscle, the *pyloric ring* or *pyloric canal* (on radiology). Beyond this is a very thin *hypomuscular segment* before the dilated *duodenal bulb*. The term *pyloric sphincter* is best avoided, because it may imply certain physiological characteristics of a sphincter which are not true of the pylorus (see under 'Physiology').

Conclusion

Forsell in 1913 concluded: 'We can, on account of its anatomic structure, consider, with good grounds, the sphincter pylorus as a complete sphincter; a muscular diaphragm built up around a connective tissue septum, with radial and circular muscle bundles which, like an iris, can diminish the lumen of the tube-shaped canal in different degrees and which in the human body, with a finely differentiated organisation, is only excelled by the sphincter of the iris.' It remains to be seen whether subsequent study of the physiology supports this deduction.

PHYSIOLOGY

As the pyloric canal and ring are composed of gastric circular muscle, it would be expected to contract and relax in association with the stomach. Some of the first observations of the motility of this area were made by Cannon in 1898 in cats by fluorography recorded by rapid drawings on long rolls of paper. He observed: 'If the pylorus does not relax, it is evident that a wave approaching it pushes the food into a blind elastic pouch, the only exit from which is through the advancing constricted ring. The constrictions are deeper near the end of the antrum, and the rings are small; consequently the food is squirted back through them with considerable violence ... over and over again the process is repeated till the sphincter at last opens and allows the more fluid parts to pass.' He therefore concluded that the main function of the pylorus was to regulate the flow between stomach and duodenum by being closed most of the time and opening occasionally.

Crider and Thomas in 1937 tested the effect on gastric emptying in dogs of keeping the pylorus open with a metal tube. They found no alteration in the rate of gastric emptying and noted much bile in the stomach. From this and other studies (Wheelon and Thomas, 1920, 1922; Thomas *et al.,* 1934) they concluded that antral contractions, not the pylorus, regulate gastric emptying and that the main function of the pylorus was to prevent regurgitation. Louckes *et al.* (1960), using the inductograph method for studying the pylorus in dogs, found that the pyloric ring was completely closed during 5 per cent of each antral cycle, completely open during 35 per cent, and either closing or opening during 60 per cent while providing some obstruction to flow of contents. They, like Thomas and colleagues, argued that the true functions of the pylorus were to prevent reflux and act as a sieve to prevent evacuation of large particles.

In 1966 Carlson *et al.* used cineradiography to study the gastroduodenal junction in dogs. They observed that, during gastric emptying, the whole terminal antrum, including the pyloric ring, contracted almost simultaneously. Before this event a small amount of barium had been propelled into the duodenum, but the passage of the rest of the barium was halted so that it was 'retropelled' back into the body of the stomach as it came up against the closed pylorus. They also noted that the duodenal contractions occurred just after the pyloric ring had closed. The closure of the pyloric ring, therefore, both cut short the flow of gastric contents into the duodenum and prevented reflux back into the stomach by being closed while the duodenum contracted. This sequence is summarised in figure 5.4.

The ring of contraction becomes narrower as it passes down towards the antrum and is only completely closed off when it is nearly at the pylorus.

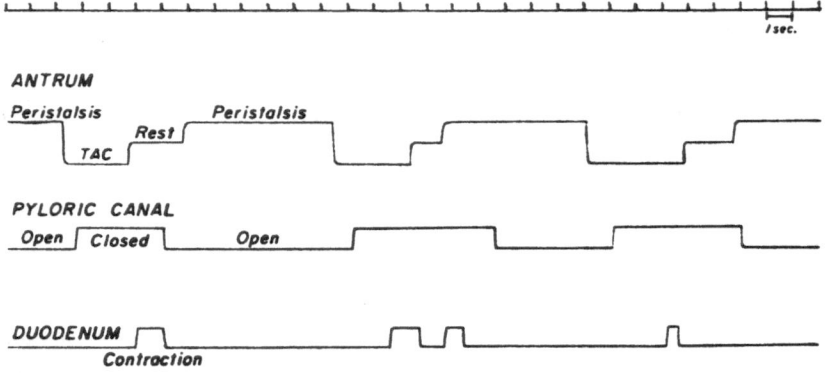

Figure 5.4 Sequence of antral, pyloric and duodenal contractions in dogs, studied by cineradiography (after Carlson *et al.*, 1966).

This is why only a small volume of chyme passes into the duodenum with each contraction. It must be stressed that this study was with dogs and during vigorous gastric emptying; but it confirmed again the important concept that the pylorus is *open* most of the time, closing at the end of the gastric contraction, unlike the lower oesophageal sphincter, which is closed most of the time and only relaxes just before a bolus of food reaches it. The fact that the pylorus rests in an open position has been repeatedly demonstrated in man by direct vision at endoscopy (when anticholinergics have not been given).

Mechanisms of Control of Gastroduodenal Contractions

Gastric contractions are controlled by an electrical pacemaker situated near the greater curve of the stomach at the junction of body and fundus. This pacemaker, although not identifiable structurally, is the area from which a regular slow electrical wave—the pace-setter potential (PP), basic electrical rhythm (BER) or electrical control activity (ECA)—arises and spreads distally and around the stomach, travelling towards the pylorus (figure 5.5).

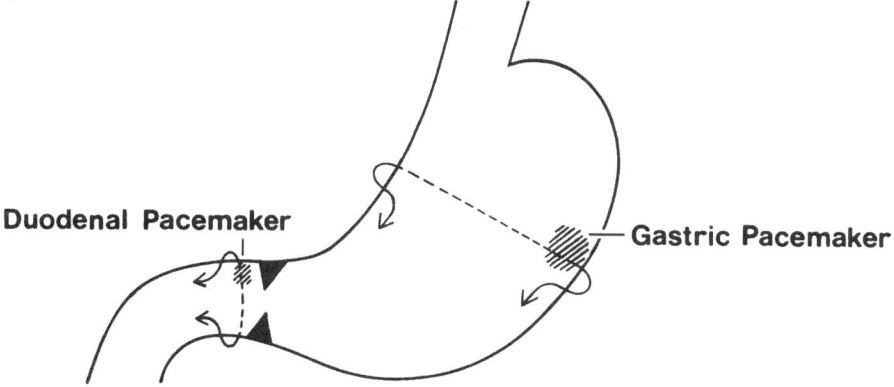

Duodenal Pacemaker   **Gastric Pacemaker**

Figure 5.5   Diagram of the pacemakers of stomach and duodenum.

The rate of conductivity of the PP down the stomach becomes more rapid as it progresses towards the pylorus, so that the contractions of the pyloric canal and the pyloric ring are almost synchronous (figure 5.6). In the dog this PP discharges at 5 cycles per minute and in man at 3 cycles per minute. By itself it does not necessarily give rise to contraction. Contractions are associated with fast electrical activity, 'spike' potentials or electrical response activity following the PP. It is the added influence of vagal tone or hormones that turns the PP into an actual contraction. Vagotomy or sympathectomy does not alter the PP rate but reduces the strength and co-ordination of contractions as well as their even propagation along the stomach. During the phase of fast gastric emptying, contractions occur at nearly maximum rate—that is, the majority of PPs turn into a contraction (figure 5.6). In one study only 13 per cent of the PPs turned into contractions in the fasting state but after feeding 71 per cent produced contractions (Edwards and Rowlands, 1968).

The duodenum also has a pacemaker or several pacemakers. In the dog it is situated less than 1 cm distal to the pyloric ring in the very first part of the duodenum (Hermon-Taylor and Code, 1971) (figure 5.5). There is probably another pacemaker near the opening of the bile duct. The intrinsic PP rate

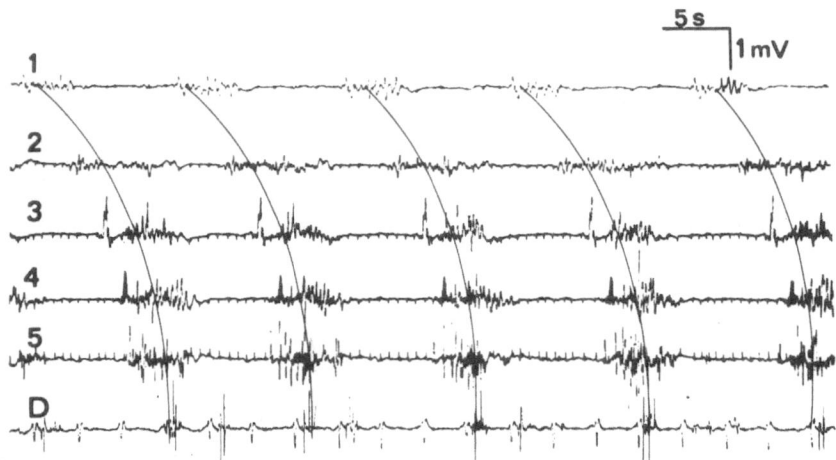

Figure 5.6   Recording of electrical activity of stomach and duodenum. Electrodes 1–5 are placed progressively down the antrum and electrode D is on the first part of the duodenum. Each antral PP shows spike (fast) activity but the more rapid duodenal PP only shows spikes when the antral fast activity reaches it.

of the duodenum is 16–18 cycles per minute in the dog and 11–12 cycles per minute in man and is normally conducted only caudally (Bass *et al.*, 1961). Again by no means all the slow waves turn into spike potentials all the time but, as in the antrum, the proportion is increased by feeding. The intrinsic rates of the pacemaker of the small intestine decrease progressively from the pylorus to the ileocaecal valve.

Gastroduodenal Co-ordination or Linkage

The different intrinsic rates of the PP of the stomach and duodenum present a problem. Unless there is some co-ordination, the antral contents would frequently be propelled into an already contracted duodenal cap, instead of the cap contracting just afterwards to propel the contents onwards. During gastric emptying the great majority of duodenal cap contractions—whether observed on cineradiography or electrically—occur following a terminal antral contraction. How is it achieved? As seen in figure 5.6, the duodenal PP only produces the rapid electrical activity of a contraction when an antral contraction reaches it, despite there being a marked interruption of the muscle layers at the hypomuscular segment. Code has shown that the gastroduodenal PPs are not linked either during fasting or after a meal. There are three possible mechanisms for linkage of contractions.

(1) Electrical transmission via the few longitudinal muscle fibres that traverse the junction.

(2) Electrical transmission via the nerve plexuses.

(3) The bolus of chyme reaching the duodenum stimulates a contraction of the cap.

Bedi and Code (1972) transected the gastroduodenal junction and only resutured the mucosa. They found that linkage was not restored across the junction even though the stomach was emptying chyme normally. This makes the third suggestion, that it is due to the chyme, unlikely.

Electron and light microscopic studies after excision and resuture of the pyloric ring in the cat (Barrett, 1976) have shown return of co-ordinated gastroduodenal activity after 3 weeks when the nerve plexus has regenerated and its disappearance again when the regenerating nerve fibres became enmeshed in fibrous tissue. So it seems likely that the transmission of electrical impulses across the gastroduodenal junction is by the nerve plexus. This adds anatomical support to the conclusion of Atanassova (1969) that the pathway is neurological.

The Resting Tone of the Pylorus

The sequence of events during gastric emptying is fairly clear. The question, however, that causes not a little controversy is the state of the pylorus when it is not contracting and in the interdigestive phase when the stomach is not emptying. Cineradiological studies have already suggested that the pylorus is open much of the time, and Atkinson et al. (1957) studied the pyloric resting pressure in man by withdrawing pressure-sensitive balloons from the duodenum to the antrum. The balloons were 7 mm in diameter and were pulled through when there was little antral activity. No rise in pressure was recorded at the pyloric ring. When the balloons were enlarged to 10, 12, 15 and 20 mm in diameter, the 10 mm balloon occasionally produced a rise in pressure and the larger balloons recorded a rise more frequently. Sometimes it was impossible to pull through the 15 and 20 mm balloons (Edwards, 1961a). Andersson and Grossman (1965) similarly found no consistent rise in pressure on pulling through a 5 or 10 mm diameter, water-filled balloon in supine human subjects. These results suggest that the pyloric ring, most of the time, offers little or no resistance to being stretched to 7–12 mm diameter.

It was all the more surprising, therefore, when Fisher and Cohen (1973a), using a collection of perfused catheters with a total outside diameter of 5.4 mm, found a consistent zone of high pressure (mean 5.3 mmHg and 1.5 cm long) in the pylorus of healthy humans. The subjects were lying in the right lateral position. Kaye *et al.* (1976), however, using a circumferentially sensitive miniature transducer assembly (2 mm in diameter) and a 5.4 mm diameter perfused catheter assembly, failed to reveal a zone of high pressure in eight healthy, fasting subjects, and suggested that Fisher and Cohen's findings were due to the sharp angulation at the gastroduodenal junction produced by the subject lying on his side. Similarly, a water-filled tube (1.2 mm outside diameter) did not register a rise in pressure when drawn through the healthy gastroduodenal junction, but a 5 mm balloon sometimes did (Code, 1970).

We have recently looked at the problem by two different techniques. In the first we used the Honeywell motility probe (Model 31, external diameter 5 mm) with miniature distal transducers, pulling it through with synchronous linked radiological screening. Both the pressure recordings and the X-ray pictures are synchronised via a split screen unit onto the same videotape. Figure 5.7 shows the rise in pressure starting as the transducer is drawn through the pyloric ring in a non-ulcer subject. We found a variation in pull-through pressures within the same individual at different times, but in patients with Type I gastric ulcer (lesser curve without duodenal disease) it was common to find no rise in pressure, which suggests that the pylorus was more dilated. A rise in pressure was only registered, if at all, as the transducer passed through the pyloric ring itself. The second technique was

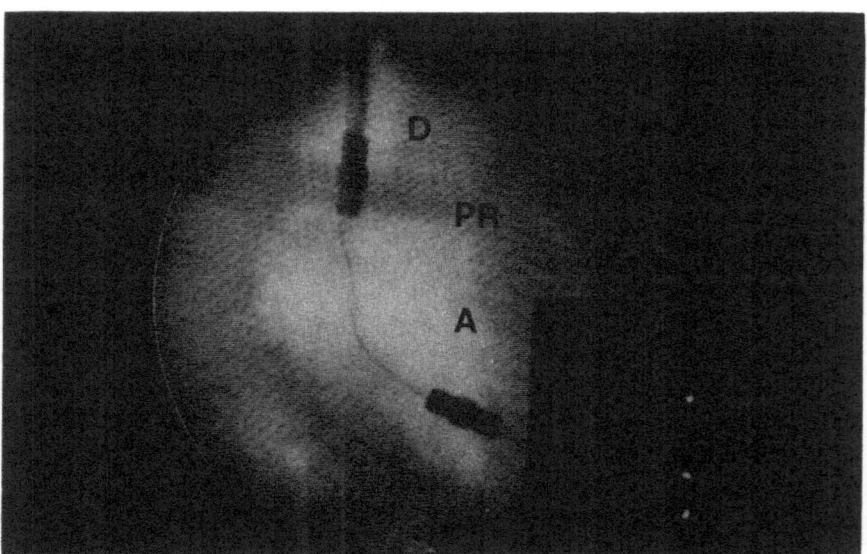

Figure 5.7 Synchronous radiology and pull-through studies using Honeywell (Model 31) motility probe (external diameter 5.0 mm). Notice rise in pressure of lowermost trace as distal transducer is pulled back through the pyloric ring. A = antrum; D = duodenal cap; PR = pyloric ring.

to record the pyloric diameter and pull-through pressure under direct vision at endoscopy. The patient was given just a small amount of diazepam with no other drug and a balloon catheter was passed down the biopsy channel of the endoscope and inflated in the duodenum, and the balloon (maximum diameter 11–13 mm) was connected to a transducer. Rings drawn on the balloon at intervals were used to measure the diameter before the pull-through pressure was increased.

The mean (± 2 SD) pyloric diameter of normal subjects (three measurements in each) was 12.8 ± 3.3 mm, in gastric ulcer patients 16.0 ± 2.6 mm and in duodenal ulcer patients 6.4 ± 3.7 mm. The diameter of gastric ulcer patients was significantly greater than that of duodenal ulcer patients. Measurements were made between antral contractions while the pylorus relaxed fully, and only if normal rhythmic antral contractions were present (Munk et al., 1977). To interpret any pull-through measurements meaningfully, one must know the phase of antral contraction during which the observation was made, as the pylorus is only fully open during 35 per cent of the antral cycle (Louckes et al., 1960). It is possible that pull-through pressures are different when the stomach is full, but Edwards (1961a), using the 7 mm balloons, did not find any rise in pressure in five normal subjects with a full stomach.

From all these different methods of studying resting pyloric diameter some general conclusions can be reached. When the normal subject is supine, the pylorus does not give a high-pressure zone and remains open with a resting diameter of between 8 and 15 mm. It is only when the measuring devices are of this range of diameter that a pressure rise will be consistently recorded. There is no doubt, however, that during an antral contraction the pressure in the pyloric ring can be very high (40–50 mmHg).

Some of the discrepancies between external and internal measurements of pyloric function may be explained by a recent observation that (in dogs) the external part of the circular muscle of the pyloric ring behaves like terminal antrum but the internal part responds differently to various stimuli, and has spontaneous activity and a strong inhibitory innervation (Golenhofen et al., 1979). This supports the following observations that it can contract independently of terminal antral contraction.

Can the Pylorus Contract Independently of the Antrum?

In terms of static tone, this seems to be true. Fisher and Cohen (1973a) found an increase in pull-through pressure with duodenal acidification in normal subjects, but the length of the high-pressure zone was 2.5 cm, which is nearly the whole length of the terminal antrum, not just the pyloric ring. Moreover, the change of mucosal potential difference occurred half-way along the high-pressure zone, which suggests that some of the pressure rise was from muscle covered by duodenal mucosa. Intraduodenal olive oil and exogenous secretin (1 u kg⁻¹ h⁻¹) and CCK (Karolinska 2.0 Ivy-dog units kg⁻¹ h⁻¹) also produced a rise in pull-through pressure.

In endoscopic studies performed in our department a bolus injection of CCK (Karolinska 1.0 Ivy-dog units kg⁻¹ h⁻¹) within 2 min inhibited all antral contractions and narrowed the pyloric ring, sometimes closing it completely (figure 5.8). Clearly, tonic contraction of the ring can occur in the absence of antral activity and independently of tonic contraction of the terminal antrum and pyloric canal. *In vitro* experiments show opossum pyloric circular muscle to be more sensitive to CCK than the adjacent antrum and duodenum (Fisher *et al.*, 1973).

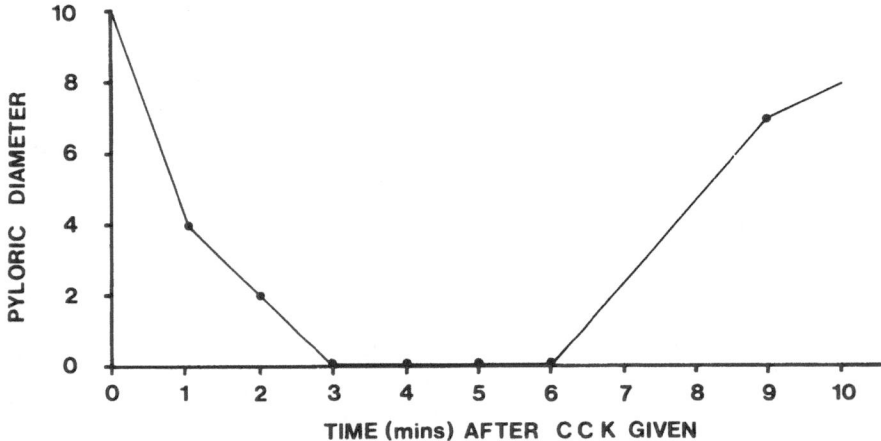

Figure 5.8   Response of pyloric ring to CCK (1 u kg⁻¹ GIH Karolinska) in a normal subject.

Does it Matter Whether There is a High-pressure Zone at the Pylorus?

If the pyloric ring is open a few millimetres, it will still allow of reflux of contents during a duodenal contraction, and even a pressure of 10 mmHg may not resist duodenal contractions of the order of 50–70 mmHg. What is important in the dual function of preventing reflux and limiting the flow of chyme is the timing of the pyloric closure. If the pylorus closes prematurely, then flow of chyme into the duodenum will be reduced. On the other hand, if it closes too late after a duodenal contraction has occurred or alternatively too soon while the duodenal cap is still contracting, there will be reflux.

What is the Significance of the Resting Diameter of the Pylorus?

The actual resting diameter of the pyloric ring has several important effects. If it is narrow, only a small amount of chyme will pass at any one time. In hypertrophic pyloric stenosis of children the very narrow canal only allows minute amounts to pass through before it closes. On the other hand, if it is very wide, more will pass through with each contraction but it may not close completely (see under 'Mechanisms of reflux', page 123). Probably the most important function of the diameter is in selection of particle size. It seems that the pyloric ring acts as a barrier to the passage of particles over a particular diameter. If these particles are food, they are returned to the body of the stomach for further trituration. If the particle is a foreign body, it will not pass and therefore impaction lower down the gastrointestinal tract is prevented. In addition, the strong retropulsive action of the antral contractions ensures that the foreign body is repeatedly returned to the body or fundus of the stomach and does not become impacted and obstruct gastric emptying.

Particle size selection by the pylorus was originally observed in 1898 by Cannon, using pellets of bismuth and starch. It has more recently been well demonstrated in dogs by Schlegel and colleagues (1966), using solid spheres 1.0 and 1.5 cm in diameter, some complaint and some incompressible, mixed in a liquid. The liquid emptied fastest but 1.0 cm spheres, both compliant and incompressible, also left the stomach in due course. Of the 1.5 cm spheres, only the compliant ones left the stomach. Thus, the pylorus selected size and consistency. This also implies that the pylorus cannot be passively stretched to allow a large particle to pass, probably because it is starting to contract at the time the sphere reaches it. Similar studies have been done in man, using compliant rubber balloons inflated to different sizes and swallowed on the end of a tube together with a regular meal (Salessiotis, 1972). In no subject did the 2.0 cm or 2.5 cm balloon pass through the pylorus, but in four the 1.9 cm balloon passed and in nine the 1.8 cm. 1.9 cm, then, seems to be the maximum diameter that the normal adult human pylorus will allow to pass. Using a balloon catheter down the endoscope, we have found that the mean resting diameter of normal subjects (without atropine) under these conditions was 12.8 mm and, although a larger balloon could be pulled through, it registered a rise in pressure in the process, showing that there was a muscular tone resisting the passage of the balloon.

Extrinsic Nervous Control of the Pylorus

The classical concept of a sphincter was linked with the idea of 'reciprocal innervation'—i.e. the sphincter relaxed with parasympathetic stimulation and contracted with sympathetic stimulation, whereas the neighbouring intestine did the reverse. It is not quite so simple with the pylorus. As we have seen, it behaves as part of the terminal antrum, and atropine both inhibits antral contractions and relaxes the pylorus. The isolated perfused gastric preparation of the dog has been particularly useful in sorting out the various controlling factors. Vagal stimulation increased antral motility but inhibited the gastroduodenal junction at pulse widths greater than 2.0 ms (Hardcastle and Aylward, 1969). Acetylcholine increased the pressures in both antrum and pylorus—which suggests that there are some non-cholinergic vagal inhibitory fibres. This is further confirmed by studies in the anaesthetised dog, where, after atropine, there is significant spontaneous contractile activity and an inhibition–relaxation response is produced by electrical vagal stimulation (Telford *et al.*, 1979). Recently a non-cholinergic, non-adrenergic, inhibitory innervation has been found in muscle strips of the pyloric muscle from cat, dog, opossum and man, that is unaffected by hormones (Anuras *et al.*, 1974). Little is known about the sympathetic innervation to the pylorus itself, although after thoracolumbar sympathectomy there is no disturbance of gastric emptying. There are both α- and β-adrenergic receptors in stomach and duodenum. In the stomach both are inhibitory, but in the duodenum and the rest of the small intestine, β-adrenergic drugs may initiate spike potentials, whereas α-adrenergic drugs still inhibit spike potentials (Daniel, 1965). Neither vagotomy nor sympathectomy alters the gastric PP, but vagotomy does affect the co-ordination and propagation of contractions (see page 127). The pylorus normally reacts to nervous stimuli like the rest of the antrum but it may well have a nervous inhibitory or even stimulating mechanism of its own which enables it to react differently from the neighbouring stomach and duodenum.

Hormonal Control of the Pylorus

Cholecystokinin/pancreozymin is probably the most important digestive hormone and there is increasing evidence that it contracts the pyloric ring while inhibiting the antrum. Isenberg and Csendes (1972) found that the canine pylorus responded by tonic contraction to an infusion of octapeptide of CCK ($0.25–1.0$ μg kg^{-1} h^{-1}). Fisher and Cohen (1973a), using the technique described above, found that a combination of cholecystokinin and secretin had the same effect in man. We have repeatedly observed the contraction of the pyloric ring in response to a bolus injection of CCK (see figure 5.8). Both CCK and secretin inhibit antral contractions in the intact animal (Johnson *et al.*, 1966; Kelly *et al.*, 1969). As the hormones are linked to the acetylcholine system (the CCK effect on the antrum is inhibited by atropine, whereas the effect on the gall bladder is not), it is important to know whether studies have been done *in vivo* or *in vitro*, as removal of the extrinsic nerve supply may affect the response. In the isolated perfused canine stomach CCK stimulates the antrum and in the intact dog giving an anaesthetic changes the effect of an infusion of CCK from inhibition to stimulation (Denton and Gershbein, 1967). Inhibition of gastric emptying is probably a physiological effect of CCK (Debas *et al.*, 1975).

Gastrin and pentagastrin stimulate antral activity but have little effect on the pyloric ring (Anuras *et al.*, 1974; Lipshutz and Cohen, 1972), but there is evidence that they antagonise the effect of CCK and secretin (Fisher *et al.*, 1973). In the isolated perfused preparation gastrin has the same effect; it may also have a trophic effect on pyloric muscle. However, preliminary work in our department in man suggests that pentagastrin tonically contracts the pyloric ring while stimulating antral contraction. Motilin potentiates the effect of acetylcholine on rabbit pyloric muscle *in vitro* (Domschke *et al.*, 1976) and also causes contraction of the antrum and duodenum; it produces changes similar to the interdigestive myoelectric complex of the antrum, pylorus and duodenum. When interpreting results, it must be remembered that Boots pancreozymin contains both secretin and motilin. In addition, intraduodenal acid, used in a number of studies, releases all three hormones. Table 5.1 summarises the probable effects of these hormones in man, but the work has been done on a variety of animals, sometimes *in vivo* and sometimes *in vitro*; sometimes with the whole hormone molecules and sometimes with fragments (such as octapeptide or pentagastrin). It is therefore impossible to be sure of the true picture. In addition, these hormones also affect the neighbouring antrum and duodenum, and so the overall effect on gastric emptying is not determined solely by the response of the pyloric muscle.

Table 5.1 Summary of hormone effects on pyloric ring

Gastrin	? no effect (but many inhibit CCK)
CCK	contracts
Secretin	contracts
Motilin	contracts

Prostaglandins

The role of the prostaglandins in local modification of activity is not yet clear but may be of considerable importance. The antrum of human stomach contains both PGE and PGF in varying proportions (Bennett *et al.*, 1977). Indomethacin (an inhibitor of prostaglandin synthesis) increased both rhythmic activity and contractions to acetylcholine (ACh) in circular gastric muscle strips. PGE_2 (50–110 ng ml^{-1}) reduced rhythmic activity and inhibited ACh-induced contractions (Stockley and Bennett, 1975). It had no overall effect on nerve-mediated responses (Stockley, 1977). In studies on the canine pylorus, oral aspirin (but not indomethacin, phenylbutazone or systemic aspirin) reduced sphincter pressure and increased reflux. This may be a local effect rather than mediated through prostaglandins (Pantoja *et al.*, 1979).

The Pylorus as a Pump

Edwards and Rowlands (1968) conceived of the pyloric ring as part of the antral pump, squirting chyme either forwards or backwards. This concept was based on the evidence available at that time—namely, that the pyloric ring always behaves in the same way as the terminal antrum. More recent work on the hormones and inhibitory innervation has made the situation not quite so simple. Most of the time, during gastric emptying, the pylorus is acting as part of a pump but in this case it probably controls the amount of chyme pumped out and ensures that, normally, none returns. At other times it may be more independent.

The Pylorus as an Iris Diaphragm

The physiology of the pylorus is still confusing but the picture that is emerging is that of the internal part of the pyloric ring acting as an iris diaphragm of variable aperture like the iris of the eye. Continually under hormonal and nervous influence, the diameter is adjusted, to allow less or more of the gastric contents and smaller or larger particles to pass through. At certain times, mainly during terminal antral contraction, it closes completely, whatever its resting diameter had been, and prevents flow of contents in either direction. Whether or not the pyloric ring can contract in response to an isolated duodenal cap contraction will be discussed later.

INVESTIGATIVE TECHNIQUES IN MAN

Much of the physiology of this region has been worked out in dogs and cats. It is most important that the human pylorus be studied and that clinical abnormalities be detected easily in order to be valuable in the management of patients. Many of the techniques measure the result of pyloric malfunction—particularly duodenogastric reflux—rather than the malfunction itself.

Radiology

The limiting factor in the use of radiology is the length of time that particularly a normal subject can be exposed to irradiation. Although image-intensification has reduced the radiation, probably 5 min is the longest justifiable exposure of a volunteer with conventional machines. Duodenogastric reflux can be detected by the patient swallowing a small amount of barium sulphate, turning prone to fill the duodenum and then supine again, leaving the antrum filled with air. As events occur rapidly, continuous screening is required if reflux is to be detected. Grossly delayed gastric emptying can be detected on conventional barium meal. Structural abnormalities of the pylorus can be detected whether there be muscle hypertrophy, scarring from peptic ulceration, or deformity due to carcinoma. The diagnosis of 'pylorospasm' usually means the failure of barium to enter the duodenum, but there is no way of knowing what is happening in the duodenum and the delay may be due to absence or weakness of antral contractions. This term should only be used for a tonic contraction of the pylorus in the absence of antral and duodenal contractions—as observed after intravenous CCK (see figure 5.8). The disadvantages in using barium to study gastric emptying are that barium has a high specific gravity and does not behave like food. If mixed with food, it may separate out.

Pyloric Regurgitation Tests

A more reliable radiological method for detecting reflux is that devised by Capper et al. (1966) in which a mercury-weighted fine tube is allowed to pass into the duodenum, after which barium sulphate is introduced into the duodenum only down the tube, the stomach being left empty. However, such a method involves a tube *traversing* the pylorus. An alternative method is to use patients with a T-tube in the common bile duct after surgery. The duodenum can be filled with contrast medium via the bile duct, but the significance of the findings is open to doubt with a tube in the bile duct diverting the bile while the medium is hypertonic, and the immediate post-operative period is not a 'normal' situation. It does not seem justified in man to insert gastrostomy and duodenostomy tubes at surgery to investigate the flow of fluids across the pylorus in both directions.

Isotope Studies

Reflux can be assessed approximately by measuring bile pigment or bile salts in gastric juice. Rhodes et al. (1969) used radioactive bile salts to study reflux in man. This needed a tube in the stomach to sample the contents after a standard liquid meal, but no tube in the duodenum. Hobsley (Whitfield and Hobsley, 1977), on the other hand, believes that the amount of duodenogastric reflux can be calculated from the sodium content of gastric juice. Possibly this may be so for the normal subject, but if there is an inflamed gastric mucosa with back-diffusion of hydrogen ions and exchange for other cations, it is probably unreliable. This is not the place to review techniques for measuring gastric emptying, but isotopes are particularly useful, as the labelled substance can be dispersed evenly around the normal meal. When isotopes are used, the two most important points of technique are to measure liquid and solid phases separately and to start the measurements immediately after the meal is taken, because the initial emptying pattern may be more important than the overall emptying time, particularly after operations (see below). Sheiner (1975) has reviewed the available techniques for studying gastric emptying.

Pull-through Techniques

These may be performed with perfused open-tip catheters, small balloons or miniature transducers. It is important to know what is happening either side of the pylorus—by either synchronous radiology or further recording channels. The position of the patient, the relationship to meals and the fact that the pull-through cannot be straight, as in the inferior oesophageal sphincter, because of the curvature of the stomach, all make the interpretation difficult. In addition, care must be taken to avoid any drugs that might affect motility.

In view of the different modes of action of the pylorus compared with the inferior oesophageal sphincter, pull-through studies by themselves are unlikely to be of much use in clinical diagnosis except in extreme situations such as pyloric stenosis and the wide patulous pylorus. However, these can be detected by simpler means.

Telemetron Capsules

Although useful in avoiding tubes in the stomach, the difficulty with these capsules is their failure to remain in one place, as they tend to be moved about with the contents. They are much more suitable for measuring caecal or lower ileal activity.

Electromyography

In animals much useful information has come from chronically implanted electrodes on the serosal surface of the stomach, pylorus and duodenum. It is possible to do this in man at operation (with informed consent), leading the wires out through a drainage wound (Duthie *et al.*, 1971). After a few days they can be pulled out with the surgical drains. This is not very useful for diagnostic purposes, as information and recordings can only be taken in the first few post-operative days.

More promising is the use of suction electrodes on the mucosal surface (Monges and Salducci, 1970; Waterfall *et al.*, 1973). This technique is still being developed but could be useful in detecting unco-ordinated gastric motility in patients with delayed gastric emptying. There is some evidence that ulcers or small carcinomas may produce ectopic sites of PP, but there is a problem in keeping the electrodes on the mucosa and positioning them precisely. It may be possible to record the gastric electrical activity with electrodes on the skin (Sarna *et al.*, 1973).

Endoscopy

Fibre optic endoscopy provides a good opportunity for direct observation of the pylorus. Gross abnormalities in pyloric size and shape can be assessed visually. The very small pylorus that fails to relax with atropine probably is affected by scarring from the duodenum, as is the deformed or irregular pylorus. Conversely, the large patulous pylorus is obvious because the wide-diameter endoscope passes through it with ease. The condition of sedation must be carefully standardised but videotapes can be taken for future analysis. We have used a combination of direct vision of the antrum and pylorus with pressure recordings from a fine balloon catheter passed into the duodenum down the biopsy channel of the gastroscope. These are then synchronised on the same videotape, and so the motility of antrum, pylorus and duodenum can be observed. This has the advantage that there is no limit on study time, as when radiology is used. Some endoscopists set great store by the amount of bile in the stomach. Gross difference may be significant, but often reflux results from the patient being given atropine beforehand, retching a little as the endoscope is passed or coughing, which may produce reflux through a resting, open pylorus.

Other Methods

One of the most ingenious ways of studying the *timing* of pyloric closure was to put a small light into the duodenum with a photoelectrical cell in the stomach—the whole assembly being passed orally: whenever the pylorus was completely closed, no light shone through on to the cell. It proved too cumbersome and uncomfortable for routine investigation of patients.

Summary

In detecting functional abnormalities of the pylorus the resting, empty stomach is not ideal, because, as we have seen, the hormones released by a meal are important. Responses to standard hormones and to drugs may be an important part of the assessment. Fat, which is so often associated with bilious regurgitation and dyspeptic symptoms, is probably the most useful single stimulus of pyloric activity. In studies with a modified pyloric regurgitation test, when the *timing* of pyloric ring closure may be the measure of its proper function, more sophisticated recording methods are required with multiple channel assemblies. It is generally agreed that pressure studies by themselves do not give enough information but should be combined with observations on the movement of gastric and duodenal contents and ideally with electromyographical recordings as well.

Finally, when the results of recordings are being interpreted, it is important to remember that the different phases of the interdigestive migrating myoelectrical complexes are associated with different degrees of activity in the stomach and duodenum.

The following scheme of investigation in man is suggested.

(1) *Radiological:* Structural deformity.
Gross delay in gastric emptying—effect of drugs?
Repeated pyloric reflux.

(2) *Endoscopic:* Using a balloon catheter to measure pyloric size and events in the duodenum with direct observation of antrum. Instillation of acid or fat in the duodenum and of exogenous hormones and drugs (e.g. atropine) can be used to study the pyloric response. By this method the tight pylorus due to scarring is distinguished from the pylorus in spasm, and the wide-open pylorus which can respond normally to CCK (for example) distinguished from the patulous pylorus that is unresponsive (see below).

To study reasons for abnormalities, two other techniques can be used:

(3) *Pressure-sensitive devices* in antrum, pyloric ring and duodenal cap to study co-ordination of contractions in association with flow of barium across the pylorus.

(4) *Electromyography*—with mucosal suction electrodes. This could be particularly useful clinically in the patient with marked delay in emptying after truncal vagotomy. It may be possible to 'pace' the stomach to start co-ordinated contractions again, as Kelly and La Force (1972) have demonstrated in dogs with implanted electrodes.

MEDICAL AND SURGICAL THERAPEUTIC IMPLICATIONS IN DISEASE

Structural and Functional Abnormalities of the Pylorus

Well-known examples of structural abnormalities include the muscle hypertrophy of the whole pyloric canal seen in pyloric stenosis of infancy and the rare purely muscle hypertrophy in adults. The pressures during a pyloric contraction in the adult disease may be very high (> 100 mmHg). Fibrosis due to chronic duodenal ulcer may produce a fixed, irregular pylorus that does not vary its diameter. This may lead to severely delayed gastric emptying in the late stages and marked reflux in the early stages because the pylorus cannot close. Infiltration by carcinoma may produce the same effect. A pyloric canal ulcer may delay gastric emptying by inducing oedema and possibly spasm (see below).

There are also functional abnormalities of the pylorus. The word functional' does not mean psychological but a disorder of function in the absence of an obvious structural lesion. The most important example is gastric ulcer.

Gastric Ulcer and Duodenogastric Reflux

From radiological, isotope and chemical data (Capper, 1967; Rhodes et al., 1969; Johnson and McDermott, 1974; Duplessis, 1965), there is good evidence that gastric ulcer patients regurgitate through the pylorus before and after meals more than healthy subjects. Patients with gallstone dyspepsia before and after cholecystectomy show a similar tendency (Johnson, 1975). Beneventano and Schein (1970) argued that pyloric regurgitation is a physiological variant but their study was in patients soon after exploration of their bile ducts with a T-tube in position—far from normal conditions in a group of patients with a known high incidence of regurgitation. Studies in healthy control subjects have shown minimal regurgitation (Capper, 1967). When a gastric ulcer heals, reflux persists (Black et al., 1971; Cocking and Grech, 1973), which suggests that it is a primary defect rather than secondary to the presence of the ulcer. It may also explain the high recurrence rate of gastric ulcer. Indeed, those celebrated investigators John Hunter (Owen, 1861) and Beaumont (1833) both concluded many years ago that bile did not normally appear in the stomach of a healthy person.

What, then, is the physiological defect that allows of regurgitation through an apparently normal pylorus? There are four possibilities.

Absence of Pressure Barrier?   Fisher and Cohen (1973b) found a similar resting pyloric pressure in gastric ulcer patients as in normal subjects, whereas Valenzuela and Defilippi (1976) found a significantly lower pressure in gastric ulcer and a higher pressure in duodenal ulcer patients; both groups were using a series of open-tipped perfused catheters. Munk *et al.* (1977) found at endoscopy a significantly larger diameter pyloric ring in gastric ulcer patients than in duodenal ulcer patients, with the normal subjects in the intermediate position—the exact corollary in terms of diameter of the pressure rises found by Valenzuela.

Failure of Response to Hormones?   Fisher and Cohen (1973b) found that in gastric ulcer patients the pylorus did not respond to CCK and secretin or to duodenal acidification, whereas the normal subjects did respond. Valenzuela and Defilippi reported a similar failure of response to duodenal acidification. Wormsley (1972) observed an increase in the already present regurgitation in gastric ulcer subjects after administration of CCK and secretin but no change in normal subjects. Munk *et al.* (1977), on the other hand, found at endoscopy a dramatic contraction of the pyloric ring in gastric ulcer patients in response to intravenous CCK (Karolinska 1 u kg^{-1} i.v.), but the effect of a single bolus lasted only 10 min (figure 5.9).

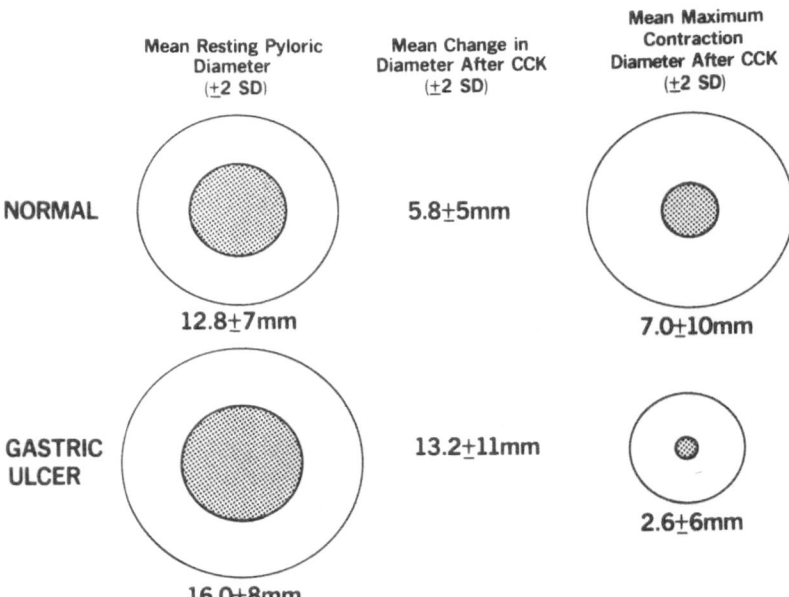

Figure 5.9   Comparison of response of pyloric diameter to CCK (1 u kg^{-1}) in five normal subjects and nine subjects with active gastric ulceration (the hatched circle represents the mean diameter and the open circles 2 SD).

It is possible that the higher bolus dose overcame some inhibitory mechanism which prevented the lower infusion dose of Fisher and Cohen causing a contraction. Indeed, Fisher and Boden (1975) found that they could reverse the dysfunction in gastric ulcer patients by acidifying the antrum. It is tempting to suggest that the high fasting gastrin levels in the gastric ulcer patient inhibited the effect of CCK, although the serum gastrin concentration (measured by radioimmunoassay) did not decrease during antral acidification. Rovelstad (1976) points out that hypergastrinaemia remains an attractive explanation for gastric ulcer. None of these explanations of reflux is entirely satisfactory unless the pylorus is *incapable of closing tightly during a duodenal cap contraction*. This can only be discovered by measuring the pressure in the pyloric ring at this time.

The Timing of Pyloric Closure?   Careful analysis of videotape recordings with synchronous pressure recordings (Johnson *et al.*, 1973) have led us to conclude that there are three motility patterns leading to reflux:

(1) Occasionally when the pylorus is so patulous that it fails to close completely when an antral contraction passes over it. In this case the regurgitation occurs at the time of a normal emptying contraction.

(2) When a true retroperistaltic wave occurs in the second part of the duodenum in the absence of an antral contraction. The contents of the duodenum are then pushed back ahead of the contraction ring—which only reaches the duodenal side of the pylorus after the contents have gone into the stomach. There is therefore no mechanism for closing the pylorus before the contents reach it, unless there happens to be an antral contraction. This situation has been reproduced in dogs by Kelly and Code (1977) by pacing the distal duodenum. They produced consistent retroperistaltic waves and reflux. Capper (1967) observed in gastric ulcer patients that duodenal activity, including retroperistaltic contractions, was particularly vigorous.

(3) When a duodenal cap contraction originates in the distal part of the cap and propels contents in both directions in the absence of an antral contraction to close the pylorus, again the bolus is retropelled *ahead* of the contraction ring, which appears to bisect the duodenal cap. These patterns are illustrated in figure 5.10. It is possible that the stimulating effect of β-adrenergic receptors in the duodenum, with their inhibitory effect on the antrum, could lead to this situation (see page 114).

Can the Pylorus Close in Response to an Isolated Duodenal Contraction?   This is the really important question, for, if it cannot, we would all reflux each time a duodenal cap contraction occurred out of phase with the antrum. As we have seen, during the height of gastric emptying

NO REFLUX

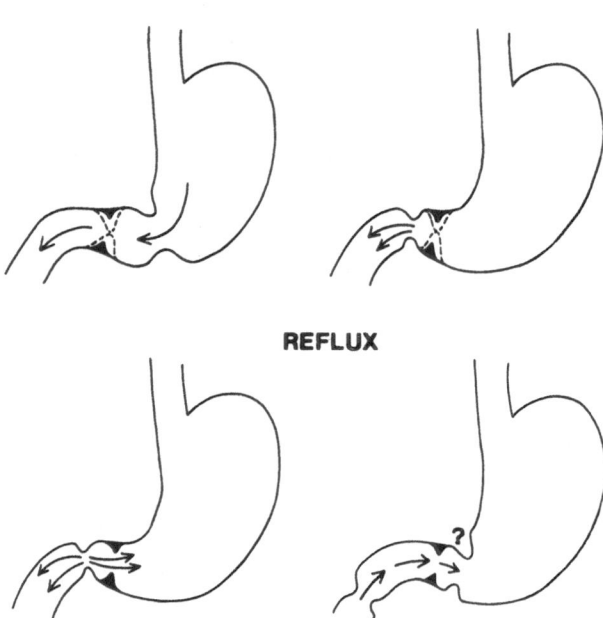

REFLUX

Figure 5.10 Diagram showing antroduodenal motility patterns that prevent and cause reflux. Reflux is prevented by a progressive antroduodenal contraction and a duodenal contraction starting close to pylorus. Reflux can occur with a duodenal contraction starting further distally in the cap or with a retroperistaltic wave from the second or third part of the duodenum.

most but not all of the cap contractions occur in phase with an antral contraction, but during the interdigestive phase this is not so. Our studies suggest that whereas gastric ulcer and non-ulcer dyspepsia subjects *do* regurgitate with an isolated duodenal cap contraction, the symptomless subject does not (Johnson *et al.*, 1973). Perhaps, after all, the *duodenum* is the key to reflux, and if the dominant pacemaker is just beyond the pylorus, a contraction first closes the pylorus before sweeping distally down the duodenum. If a dominant pacemaker arises more distally, the pylorus does not close in the same way. This concept at present still requires final proof but it is a plausible theory. There is some evidence from the isolated perfused canine preparation that the duodenal end of the pyloric canal can close with a duodenal contraction (Hardcastle *et al.*, 1970), and Torgensen (1942) suggested that a proximal duodenal circular muscle contraction could close the pylorus. In patients we have observed on several occasions, endoscopically, the pylorus closing with a duodenal contraction in the absence of an antral contraction. The most important factor in reflux, whether or not the resting pylorus is narrowed or dilated, may be the site of origin of the duodenal contraction.

Pylorospasm

'Pylorospasm' is a term used by radiologists when barium stays in the antrum and will not leave the stomach despite changes in posture. The trouble with a diagnosis of spasm is that (a) the defect may be absent antral contractions, and (b) the duodenum may be contracting rapidly and strongly but it cannot be observed, as no barium has yet filled it. At endoscopy one has occasionally observed a tightly closed pylorus, in the absence of antral contractions, which relaxes with atropine. It may well be that a tonically contracted pyloric ring is due to a temporarily high circulating level of CCK or other hormone, or to nervous factors.

The Pylorus and Ulcer Surgery

Until recently operations for peptic ulcer involved cutting across, excising or by-passing the pylorus. It is not surprising that there were some side-effects; in fact, it is surprising that they were so few.

Particle Size

A rare but well-known complication of Polya partial gastrectomy was intestinal obstruction due to orange pith or other undigested solid that had passed through the large stoma and obstructed lower down the intestine. The other side of the coin is the *dumping syndrome,* where (particularly the liquid) contents rush out of the stomach into the small intestine. These problems have led some authors (e.g. Salessiotis, 1972) to advocate a stoma no larger than the normal pylorus. The problem here is that there are no powerful antral contractions to propel the contents through such a small stoma. An alternative approach has been the pylorus-preserving gastrectomy, in which the antrum is removed up to about 1–2 cm from the pyloric ring (Maki *et al.,* 1967). Emptying studies suggest that some function of the pylorus is preserved in this way (Liavag *et al.,* 1972), giving further weight to the suggestion that the pylorus can function independently of the antrum; but the actual anatomical line of division, and thus the amount of terminal antral muscle preserved, may vary from patient to patient.

Reflux

By-passing or dividing the pylorus also produces the problem of bile reflux. This is universal after Polya gastrectomy or gastroenterostomy but not after a Roux-en-Y reconstruction (Lawson, 1964). After pyloroplasty it is also present but it may not be as bad. A pyloroplasty usually makes the pylorus incapable of closing by altering its diameter and shape. Figure 5.11 shows the free reflux of barium put into the duodenum of a patient with a pyloroplasty.

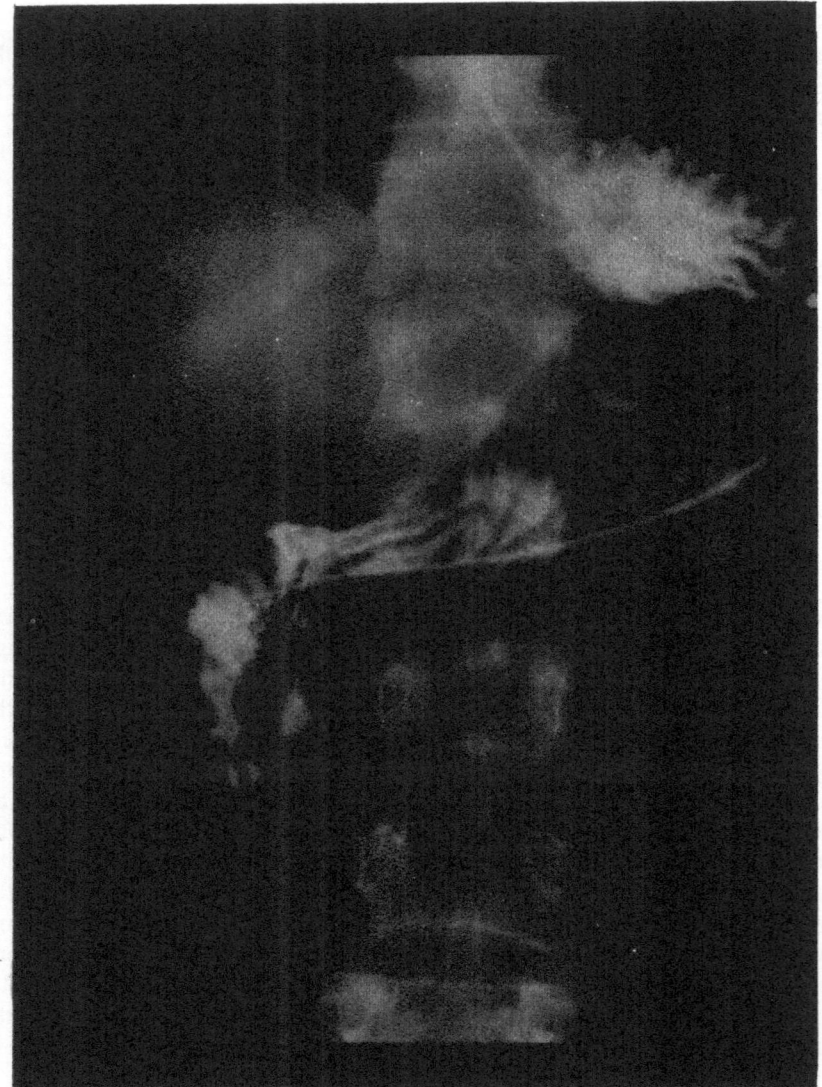

Figure 5.11   Radiograph showing free reflux after wide pyloroplasty. The barium has been introduced directly into the duodenum by a fine catheter.

Vagotomy

Pyloroplasty was advocated as an addition to truncal vagotomy because of the delayed emptying produced by the vagotomy. However, many of the early patients had very severe disease and moderate pyloric stenosis. How does vagotomy affect gastroduodenal motility? Using mucosal electrodes in man, Stoddard *et al.* (1975) found that after truncal vagotomy and pyloroplasty (TV & P) and proximal gastric vagotomy (PGV) there is no change in the frequency of the pace-setter potential (PP). Five days after TV & P the triphasic form of the PP became sinusoidal and there were few action potentials, whereas after PGV the PP was normal and there was only slightly less motor activity than before operation. The only change with passage of time after operation was an increase in percentage of activity. Moreover, in dogs gastroduodenal co-ordination was retained after PGV but not after other forms of vagotomy.

Gastric emptying studies indicate that gastric emptying is more normal in both speed and form after PGV than other vagotomies, but all types of vagotomy denervate the fundus, which leads to impairment of receptive and reflex relaxation and more rapid initial emptying of fluids (Wilbur and Kelly, 1973).

There is, therefore, every indication, both theoretical and practical, to preserve the gastroduodenal junction during gastric surgery. However, a badly scarred pylorus that is malfunctioning needs widening or by-passing. No satisfactory studies have been done on pyloric reflux after PGV. Theoretically there should be no difference from before operation.

Surgical Reconstruction of a Pyloric Sphincter

At the lower oesophageal sphincter a Nissen fundoplication—encircling the lower oesophagus with the fundus of the stomach—reproduces and strengthens some of the actions of the sphincter. It is not nearly so easy to correct, surgically, an incompetent pylorus. The creation of a non-return valve involves the distal end of the stomach protruding into and being completely surrounded by the duodenal cap, so that a cap contraction would also occlude the gastric opening. A similar idea has been applied to the intestine, but so far no surgical reconstruction of the pyloric mechanism has been effective (Grier *et al.,* 1971). A Roux-en-Y reconstruction is the only satisfactory way of diverting duodenal contents from the stomach, but it requires a covering vagotomy and such a major procedure is hardly justified even if the reflux gastritis is severe.

Other Diseases and Pyloric Function

There is some evidence that patients with chronic bronchitis reflux through the pylorus more than others. Certainly in the absence of antral and duodenal contractions with the pylorus resting open, coughing can produce reflux, as can be observed at endoscopy. There is also evidence that cigarette smoking increases pyloric reflux, and heavy cigarette smokers have a higher incidence of gastritis and gastric ulcer (Read and Grech, 1973). Valenzuela and Defilippi (1976) found a decrease in basal pyloric pressure when the patient smoked one cigarette.

Drugs and the Pylorus

Many of the common drugs prescribed in clinical practice for dyspepsia contain a combination of antacid and atropine or related substance. As every endoscopist knows, the atropine-like substances relax the pylorus while at the same time inhibiting antral and duodenal contractions. This leads to delayed gastric emptying but not necessarily to pyloric reflux, as there are no duodenal contractions. Atropine has also been found to block the rise in pyloric pressure produced by acid infusion of the duodenum. Cholinergic stimulant drugs stimulate antral and duodenal contractions (and acid secretion) and adrenergic stimulants abolish contractions (Daniel, 1965).

Of particular interest is the drug metoclopramide, which speeds gastric emptying but does not affect gastric secretion. It does so by a number of actions. It increases the strength of gastric contractions, turning them into progressive waves that sweep through the pylorus into the duodenum. It also improves co-ordination of the linkage between antral and duodenal contractions and delays the terminal antral contraction that cuts short the flow of chyme (Kelly, 1973). In summary, it switches on the gastric emptying motility pattern while overcoming the antral brake mechanism. It has also been found to increase the resting pressure of the pyloric ring (Valenzuela and Defilippi, 1976). The drug does not alter the gastric pacemaker rate but turns more pace-setter potentials into actual contractions, and it therefore has little effect on a stomach that is already emptying at maximum rate. The mode of action is not clear, but it is thought to enhance the effect of acetylcholine on muscle, probably by increasing acetylcholine release from the post-ganglionic nerve endings (Hay, 1977), and its effects are antagonised by atropine. It may also block dopamine inhibition, which may have relevance to the pyloric ring itself.

Metoclopramide has been found to prevent recurrence of duodenal ulcers (Moshal, 1973), but it seems to reverse the abnormalities of motility associated with gastric ulcer (Miller *et al.*, 1979). Newer dopamine inhibitors, such as domperidone, will need to be studied in this region.

POSSIBLE FUTURE ADVANCES

It has been established that in certain abnormalities, notably gastric ulcer, there is a malfunction of the pylorus, but why this occurs is still not known. There are several areas of research that need to be followed.

The Duodenal Control of Pyloric Closure

This will need careful correlation of electrical and mechanical activity, especially looking for ectopic duodenal pacemakers that may affect the direction of transmission of impulses and contractions.

Polypeptide Hormones and the Pylorus

The upper GI hormones are secreted together after a meal. Although the effect of individual hormones on the pylorus gives some information, the balance between agonists and antagonists can only be studied by measuring all the hormones at one time. This work must await reliable assays of important hormones such as CCK and also the assurance that radioimmunoassay measurements relate to biological activity.

The Prostaglandins

The modulating effect of the prostaglandins on the responses to other hormones may be crucial to motility disorders of the region. Recent work suggests that prostaglandins synthesised in the gastric mucosa protect it against damage by chemical irritants (Robert *et al.*, 1979), and inhibition of prostaglandin synthesis such as indomethacin and aspirin may also alter motility.

Psychological Factors

There is evidence that psychological stress is related to peptic ulcer disease and it is also known that stress will alter gastric and duodenal motility (Johnson, 1971).

The pathways are probably nervous but the effects on motility may be influenced by hormones. So much functional dyspepsia is related to stress that this area needs thorough investigation by workers from different disciplines and possibly with new techniques.

Techniques

It is still often impossible to compare two pieces of work, because different techniques have been used. Sometimes the outside diameter of an apparatus being pulled through the pylorus is not even stated. We need standardisation of techniques or, more accurately, a clear knowledge of exactly what parameter of motility each piece of apparatus is measuring. It is important that the studies be done on intact man. Extrapolation from the behaviour of a strip of opossum muscle is not always justified.

Therapy

As our understanding of control mechanisms is developing, drugs should be developed which are increasingly selective in their influence on motility. This will be particularly important if the existence of non-adrenergic, non-cholinergic inhibitory nervous pathways is established. Metoclopramide is a useful start but we need further drugs of that kind.

The function and control of the gastroduodenal junction will turn out to be far more complex than anyone had thought. There is at present no justification for entrenched and overdogmatic views! Every new piece of evidence must be carefully scrutinised and, if authentic, accepted, even if it cannot be fitted into an existing hypothesis.

The picture that is emerging is of a mechanism so delicate and complex that it should deter all but the most insensitive surgeon from destroying it with one sweep of the knife, unless it is irreparably damaged or the patient's life is at stake. Perhaps the gastroenterologist should give the pylorus the same respect that the ophthalmologist accords to the iris of the eye?

ACKNOWLEDGEMENTS

I am grateful to Mr M. Munk for help in the preparation of the chapter, to Mr Ganley and Medical Illustration Department of Charing Cross Hospital for the illustrations and to Miss Heather Wright for secretarial assistance. Figure 5.6 was kindly supplied by Professor J. Salducci, Hopital Nord, Marseille, France.

REFERENCES

Andersson, S. and Grossman, M. I. (1964). Profile of pH, pressure and potential difference at gastroduodenal junction in man. *Gastroenterology*, **49**, 364

Anuras, S., Cooke, A. R. and Christensen, J. (1974). An inhibitory innervation of gastroduodenal junction. *J. Clin. Invest.*, **54**, 529

Atanassova, E. (1969). The role of the intramural nervous system in correlating the spike activity between the stomach and the duodenum. *Dokl. Bolg. Akad. Nauk*, **22**, 1337

Atkinson, M., Edwards, D. A. W., Honour, A. and Rowlands, E. N. (1957). Comparison of cardiac and pyloric sphincters: a manometric study. *Lancet*, **ii**, 918

Barret, G. S. (1976). Arnott Demonstrations, Royal College of Surgeons of England

Bass, P., Code, C. F. and Lambert, E. H. (1961). Motor and electrical activity of the duodenum. *Am. J. Physiol.*, **201**, 287

Beaumont, W. (1883). *Experiments and Observations on the Gastric Juice and the Physiology of Digestion*, Allen, Plattsburgh, p. 153

Bedi, B. S. and Code, C. F. (1972). Pathway of co-ordination of post-prandial, antral and duodenal action potentials. *Am. J. Physiol.* **222** (5), 1295

Beneventano, T. C. and Schein, C. J. (1970). Pyloric sphincter incompetence in man: a physiological variant. *Gastroenterology*, **59**, 518

Bennett, A., Stamford, I. F. and Stockley, H. L. (1977). Estimation and characterisation of prostaglandins in the human gastrointestinal tract. *Br. J. Pharmacol.*, **61**, 579 P

Black, R. B., Roberts, G. and Rhodes, J. (1971). The effect of healing on bile reflux in gastric ulcer. *Gut*, **12**, 552

Brown, B. H., Smallwood, R., Duthie, H. L. and Stoddard, C. J. (1975). Intestinal smooth muscle potentials recorded from surface electrodes. *Med. Biol. Eng.*, 97

Cannon, W. B. (1898). The movements of the stomach studied by means of Röntgen rays. *Am. J. Physiol.*, **1**, 359

Capper, W. M. (1967). Factors in the pathogenesis of gastric ulcer. *Ann. R. Coll. Surg. Engl.*, **40**, 21

Capper, W. M., Airth, G. R. and Kilby, J. O. (1966). A test for pyloric regurgitation. *Lancet*, **ii**, 621

Carlson, H. C., Code, C. F. and Nelson, R. A. (1966). Motor action of the canine gastroduodenal junction: a cineradiographic, pressure and electric study. *Am. J. Dig. Dis.*, *(NS)*, **11**, 155

Cocking, J. B. and Greech, P. (1973). Pyloric reflux and the healing of gastric ulcers. *Gut*, **14**, 555

Code, C. F. (1970). The mystique of the gastroduodenal junction. *Rend. Gastroenterol.*, **2**, 20

Crider, J. O. and Thomas, J. E. (1937). A study of gastric emptying with the pylorus open. *Am. J. Dig. Dis.*, **4**, 295

Daniel, E. E. (1965). The electrical and contractile activity of the pyloric region in dogs and the effects of drugs. *Gastroenterology*, **49**, 403

Debas, H., Farooq, O. and Grossman, M. I. (1975). Inhibition of gastric emptying is a physiological action of cholecystokinin. *Gastroenterology*, **68**, 1211

Denton, R. W. and Gershbein, L. L. (1967). *In vivo* contractility of smooth muscle by cholecystokinin concentrates. *Arch. Int. Pharmacodyn.*, **166**, 473

Domschke, N., Strunz, U., Mitzregg, P., Domschke, S., Wünsch, E. and Demling, L. (1976). Motilin and motilin analogues: mode of action. *Scand. J. Gastroenterol.*, **11**, Suppl. 39, 25

Duplessis, D. J. (1965). Pathogenesis of gastric ulceration. *Lancet*, **i**, 974

Duthie, H. L., Kwong, N. K., Brown, B. H. and Whittaker, G. E. (1971). Pacesetter potential of the human gastroduodenal junction. *Gut*, **12**, 250

Edwards, D. A. W. (1961a). Physiological concepta of the pylorus. *Proc. R. Soc. Med.*, **54**, 930

Edwards, David (1961b). Some radiological aspects of pyloric disease. *Proc. R. Soc. Med.*, **54**, 933

Edwards, D. A. W. and Rowlands, E. N. (1968). Physiology of the gastroduodenal junction. In *Handbook of Physiology* (Section 6), Am. Physiological Society, Washington, D.C., p. 1985

Fisher, R. S. and Boden, G. (1975). Reversibility of pyloric sphincter dysfunction in gastric ulcer. *Gastroenterology*, **69**, 591

Fisher, R. and Cohen, S. (1973a). Physiological characteristics of the human pyloric sphincter. *Gastroenterology*, **64**, 67

Fisher, R. S. and Cohen, S. (1973b). Pyloric sphincter dysfunction in patients with gastric ulcer. *New Engl. J. Med.*, **288**, 273

Fisher, R. S., Lipshutz, W. and Cohen, S. (1973). The hormonal regulation of pyloric sphincter function. *J. Clin. Invest.*, **52**, 1289

Forsell, G. (1913). Quoted from Horton, B. T. (1928). Pyloric muscle tone with special reference to pyloric block. *Am. J. Anat.*, **41**, 197–225

Golenhofen, K., Ludtke, F. E., Milenov, K. and Siewert, R. (1979). Excitatory and inhibitory effects on canine pyloric musculature. In *Proceedings 7th International Symposium on Gastrointestinal Motility, Iowa, 1979* (in press)

Grier, R. L., Nelson, A. W. and Lumb, W. V. (1971). Experimental sphincter for short bowel syndrome. *Arch. Surg.*, **102**, 203

Hardcastle, J. D. and Aylward, M. (1969). A study of gastric emptying and the associated mechanical electrical activity of the gastroduodenal junction. In *Proc. 2nd Int. Symposium GI Motility, Rome, 1969, Rend. Gastroenterol.*, 1, Suppl 2, 137

Hardcastle, J. D., Green, W. E. R. and Ritchie, H. D. (1970). A study of the motility of the gastroduodenal junction in the isolated perfused canine stomach [Abstract]. In *Proc. 4th World Congress Gastroenterology, Copenhagen, 1970*, p. 83

Hay, A. M. (1977). Pharmacological analysis of the effects of metoclopramide on the guinea pig isolated stomach. *Gastroenterology*, 72, 864

Hermon-Taylor, J. J. and Code, C. F. (1971). Localisation of the duodenal pacemaker and its role in the organisation of duodenal myoelectric activity. *Gut*, 12, 40

Horton, B. T. (1928). Pyloric musculature, with special reference to pyloric block. *Am. J. Anat.*, 41, 197

Isenberg, J. I. and Csendes, A. (1972). Effect of octapeptide of cholecystokinin on canine pyloric pressure. *Am. J. Physiol.*, 222, 428

Johnson, A. G. (1971). The action of metoclopramide on human gastroduodenal motility. *Gut*, 12, 421

Johnson, A. G. (1975). Cholecystectomy and gallstone dyspepsia. *Ann. R. Coll. Surg. Engl.*, 56, 69

Johnson, A. G., March, Catherine and Kirk, C. J. C. (1973). Does pyloric competence depend on antro-duodenal co-ordination? In *Proc. 4th Int. Symposium GI Motility, Vancouver, 1973*, p. 505

Johnson, L. P., Brown, J. C. and Magee, D. C. (1966). Effect of secretin and cholecystokinin-pancreozymin extracts on gastric motility in man. *Gut*, 7, 52

Kaye, M. D., Mehta, S. J. and Showalter, J. P. (1976). Manometric studies of the human pylorus. *Gastroenterology*, 70, 477

Kelly, J. M. (1973). Metoclopramide in the vagotomised stomach. Part II—in dog. *Postgrad. Med. J.*, 49, Suppl. 4, 83

Kelly, K. A. and Code, C. F. (1977). Duodenal-gastric reflux and slowed gastric emptying by electrical pacing of the canine duodenal pacesetter potential. *Gastroenterology*, 72, 429

Kelly, K. A. and La Force, R. C. (1972). Pacing the canine stomach with electrical stimulation. *Am. J. Physiol.*, 222, 588

Kelly, K. A., Woodward, E. R. and Code, C. F. (1969). Effect of secretin and cholecystokinin on canine gastric electrical activity. *Proc. Soc. Expl Biol. Med.*, 130, 1060

Lawson, H. H. (1964). Effects of duodenal contents on gastric mucosa under experimental conditions. *Lancet*, i, 469

Liavag, I., Roland, M. and Broch, A. (1972). Gastric function after pylorus-preserving resection for gastric ulcer. *Acta Chir. Scand.* 138, 775

Lipshutz, W. and Cohen, S. (1972). Interaction of gastrin I and secretin on gastrointestinal circular muscle. *Am. J. Physiol.*, 222, 775

Louckes, H. S., Quigley, J. P. and Kersey, J. (1960). Inductograph method for recording muscle activity, especially pyloric sphincter physiology. *Am. J. Physiol.* 199 (2), 301

Maki, T., Shiratori, T., Hatafuku, T. and Sugawara, K. (1967). Pylorus-preserving gastrectomy as an improved operation for gastric ulcer. *Surgery*, 61, 838

Miller, L. J., Longstreth, G. F., Go, V. L. W. and Malagelada, J.-R. (1979). Dysfunction of the stomach with gastric ulceration: correction by metoclopramide. *Gastroenterology*, 76, 1204

Monges, H. and Salducci, J. (1970). A method of recording the gastric electrical activity in man. *Am. J. Dig. Dis.*, 15, 271

Moritz, S. (1901). Studien uber die motorische thatigkeit des magens. *Z. Biol.*, 42, 565

Moshal, M. G. (1973). Trials with metoclopramide in duodenal ulceration. *Postgrad. Med. J.*, 49, Suppl. 4, 100

Munk, J., Gannaway, R. M., Hoare, Mary and Johnson, A. G. (1977). The direct measurement of pyloric diameter and tone in man and their response to cholecystokinin. In *Gastrointestinal Motility in Health and Disease*, MTP Press, p. 349

Owen, R. (1861). *Essays and Observations* (ed. John Hunter), J. van Voorst, London, p. 156

Pantoja, J. L., Defilippi, C., Valenzuela, J. E. and Csendes, A. (1979). Nonsteroidal anti-inflammatory drugs: effect on pyloric sphincter and duodenogastric reflux. *Dig. Dis. Sci.*, 24, 217

Read, N. W. and Grech, P. (1973). Effect of cigarette smoking on competence of the pylorus:

preliminary study. *Br. Med. J.*, **3**, 313

Rhodes, J., Barnardo, D. E., Phillips, S. F., Rovelstad, R. A. and Hofman, A. F. (1969). Increased reflux of bile into the stomach in patients with gastric ulcer. *Gastroenterology*, **57**, 241

Robert, A., Nezamis, J. E., Lancaster, C. *et al.* (1979). Cytoprotection by prostaglandins in rats: prevention of gastric necrosis produced by alcohol, HCl, NaOH, hypertonic NaCl and thermal injury. *Gastroenterology*, **77**, 433

Rovelstad, R. A. (1976). The incompetent pyloric sphincter: bile and mucosal ulceration. *Am. J. Dig. Dis.*, **21**, 165

Salessiotis, N. (1972). Measurement of the diameter of the pylorus in man. *Am. J. Surg.*, **124**, 331

Sarna, S. K., Bowes, K. L. and Daniel, E. E. (1973). Post operative gastric electrical control activity in man. In *Proc. 4th Int. Symposium GI Motility, Vancouver, 1973*, p. 7

Schlegel, J. F., Coburn, W. M. Jr. and Code, C. F. (1966). Gastric emptying of solid and compliant spheres in dogs [Abstract]. *Physiologist*, **9**, 283

Sheiner, H. J. (1975). Gastric emptying tests in man [progress report]. *Gut*, **16**, 235

Stockley, H. L. (1977). Personal communication

Stockley, H. L. and Bennett, A. (1975). Modulation of activity by prostaglandins in human gastrointestinal muscle. In *Proc. 5th Int. Symposium GI Motility, Leuven, Belgium, 1975*

Stoddard, C. J., Smallwood, R., Brown, B. H. and Duthie, H. L. (1975). The immediate and delayed effects of different types of vagotomy on human myoelectrical activity. *Gut*, **16**, 165

Sufian, S., Ominsky, S. and Matsumoto, T. (1977). Congenital double pylorus. *Gastroenterology*, **73**, 154

Telford, G. L., Mir, S. S., Mason, G. R. and Ormsbee, H. S. III (1979). Neural control of the canine pylorus. *Am. J. Surg.*, **137**, 92

Thomas, J. E., Crider, J. O. and Mogan, C. J. (1934). A study of reflexes involving the pyloric sphincter and antrum and their role in gastric evacuation. *Am. J. Physiol.*, **108**, 683

Torgersen, J. (1942). The muscular build and movements of the stomach and duodenal bulb especially with regard to the problem of the segmental divisions of the stomach in the light of comparative anatomy and embryology. *Acta Radiol. (Stockholm)*, Suppl. 45

Valenzuela, J. E. and Defilippi, C. (1976). Pyloric sphincter studies in peptic ulcer patients. *Am. J. Dig. Dis.*, **21** (3), 229

Waterfall, W. E., Duthie, H. L. and Brown, B. H. (1973). The electrical and motor actions of gastrointestinal hormones on the duodenum in man. *Gut*, **14**, 689

Wheelon, H. and Thomas, J. E. (1920). Observations on the motility of the antrum and the relation of rhythmic activity of the pyloric sphincter to that of the antrum. *J. Lab. Clin. Med.*, **6**, 124

Wheelon, H. and Thomas, J. E. (1922). Observations on the motility of the duodenum and the relation of duodenal activity to that of the pars pylorica. *Am. J. Physiol.*, **59**, 72

Whitfield, P. F. and Hobsley, M. (1977). Failure to detect back diffusion in human gastric aspirate. *Gut*, **18**, A947

Wilbur, B. G. and Kelly, K. A. (1973). Effect of proximal gastric, complete gastric and truncal vagotomy on canine gastric electric activity, motility and emptying. *Ann. Surg.*, **178**, 295

Wormsley, K. G. (1972). Aspects of duodeno-gastric reflux in man. *Gut*, **13**, 243–250

6
The Biliary Sphincter

A. L. G. Peel and H. H. Thompson

INTRODUCTION

In 1543 Vesalius demonstrated that the common bile duct enters the duodenum and not the stomach, as had previously been supposed. Glisson (1654) made the first description of a sphincter surrounding the termination of the bile duct, and he suggested that its function was to prevent the reflux of chyme into the bile duct. Luschka (1869) failed to identify a distinct sphincter and suggested that duodenal muscle alone exerted a sphincteric action. The papilla, onto which the bile duct opens, and not the ampulla formed by the joining of the bile duct and duct of Wirsung, was described by Vater in 1720. In 1887 Rugero Oddi published his studies on the sphincter which has since borne his name. He demonstrated it in several species of animals, concluded that it was anatomically and functionally distinct from the duodenum, and measured its resistance. He even suggested that its dysfunction may give rise to 'morbid affections' of the biliary tract (Hand, 1963).

Since Oddi's publication the sphincter has been intensively studied, but many aspects of its anatomy and physiology, including its degree of independence from the duodenum, remain controversial. The advent of endoscopic retrograde cholangiography has increased clinical interest in the choledochal sphincter, attention being directed to its possible role in biliary disease. The sphincter can now be divided not only surgically, but also endoscopically; the indications for these procedures are at present under evaluation.

ANATOMY

Comparative Anatomy

The anatomy of the choledochoduodenal junction and its relationship to the termination of the pancreatic ducts show considerable species variation. Mann and his associates (1920) studied the relationship between the common bile duct and the pancreatic duct in 16 species. They divided them into three groups: (1) biliary and pancreatic ducts open separately into the duodenum (ox, pig, rabbit, guinea-pig, striped gopher); (2) ducts are distinct but share a common entrance into the duodenum (man, horse, dog, cat); (3) principal pancreatic duct and common bile duct join to provide a common channel that carries pancreatic juice and bile into the duodenum (goat, sheep, deer, mouse, rat, pocket gopher). Many animals, including man, have an additional pancreatic duct which opens into the duodenum, and in the dog this is the larger. The distance of the choledochoduodenal junction from the pylorus varies among different animals (Mann *et al.*, 1920; Hallenbeck, 1967). A choledochoduodenal junction close to the pylorus usually has a well-developed sphincter, and it has been suggested that this may be to prevent reflux of duodenal contents up into the bile duct (Germain *et al.*, 1977). Most vertebrates have a gall bladder; however, why some (e.g. deer, rat, horse) do not is not known. Animals without a gall bladder have been found to have a poorly developed sphincter (Boyden, 1965) which requires less pressure to overcome its resistance than that in animals which possess a gall bladder (Mann, 1919). Why such variation exists in these aspects of the anatomy of the biliary tract is not understood.

Human Anatomy

The distal part of the common bile duct in man runs in a groove on the dorsal surface of the pancreas, where it is intimately related to the duodenum, with no intervening tissue for a distance of 8–22 mm (Klune, 1964). Thereafter it pierces the duodenal muscle and runs a variable distance in the submucosa before turning towards the lumen to open onto the papilla of Vater. The course through the duodenal wall is therefore S-shaped. The site of the papilla varies, the distance from the pylorus ranging from 44 to 142 mm (Sterling, 1953). The incidence at different sites is shown in figure 6.1 (Lurje, 1937). There is also considerable variation in the manner in which the pancreatic and common bile ducts terminate. In 85 per cent of people there is a common channel; there are separate openings onto the papilla in 13 per cent; and there is an atretic duct of Wirsung in 2 per cent (Hand, 1963). The portion of duct distal to the point where the

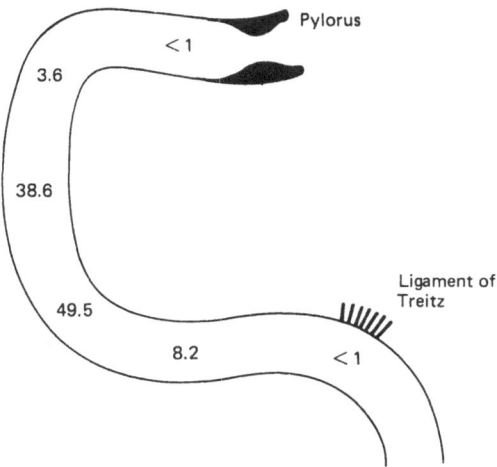

Figure 6.1   The site of the papilla in 194 cadaveric dissections (percentages) (after Lurje, 1937).

common bile duct and pancreatic duct join is called the ampulla of Vater. However, a dilatation of this part of the duct to form an ampulla is the exception rather than the rule—a fact mentioned by Vater.

Existence of an Anatomical Sphincter

The major controversy surrounding the anatomy of the choledochal sphincter concerns whether or not it is separate from the duodenal musculature through which the terminal bile duct passes (Ivy, 1934; Michels, 1955). Oddi (1887), Hendrickson (1898) and Nuboer (1931) considered the sphincter to consist of intrinsic muscle distinct from that of the duodenum, a view opposed by Porsio (1929, 1933) and Schreiber (1944). The most extensive investigation of this problem has been made by E. A. Boyden and his colleagues at the University of Washington in Seattle. They studied macerated specimens of the sphincter of Oddi in several species (Boyden and Schwegler, 1936; Boyden, 1937, 1955, 1957 a,b, and 1966; Eickhorn and Boyden, 1955), and although finding considerable variation in the arrangement of the muscular bundles of the sphincter between species, concluded that there was an intrinsic sphincter. However, Boyden also suggests that the extrinsic duodenal muscle may affect resistance at the choledochoduodenal junction by virtue of the arrangement of its muscle fibres around the terminal portion of the common bile duct and the oblique course of the duct through the duodenal wall (Eickhorn and Boyden, 1955; Boyden, 1965). This latter view is shared by others (Sandblom *et al.*, 1935; Hallenbeck, 1967; Persson, 1972).

Embryology

The common bile duct and the proximal part of the duct of Wirsung are derived embryologically from the ventral duodenal diverticulum, while the accessory pancreatic duct is formed from the dorsal duodenal diverticulum (Hamilton *et al.*, 1964). A detailed study of the embryology of the sphincter was made by Schwegler and Boyden (1937a–c) and has been used to support the concept of an intrinsic sphincter. In the first month of intrauterine life, the bile duct and the pancreatic duct unite just before they pass through the window in the duodenal muscle. The first sphincter muscle fibres develop at the choledochal window from mesenchyme surrounding the ducts at about the tenth week, 4 weeks after the appearance of the intestinal muscle, which suggests that the sphincter is a separate entity. The mesenchymal septum between the two ducts advances towards the papilla, separating the two ducts and decreasing the size of the common channel. If it reaches the summit of the papilla, the two ducts will open separately into the duodenum. Intrinsic sphincter muscle differentiates from mesenchyme in a direction from the choledochal window to the papilla.

Microscopic Anatomy

The sphincter can be divided into the choledochal sphincter, the pancreatic sphincter, the sphincter ampullae and the sphincter papillae (figure 6.2). The choledochal sphincter is the most prominent, extending for a distance of 2–3 mm outside the duodenal wall (Hand, 1963); it has been further divided into a pars superior and a pars inferior (Kreilkamp and Boyden, 1940). The sphincter ampullae is well-developed in only one in six individuals, as is the sphincter papillae. The pancreatic sphincter surrounds the terminal portion of the pancreatic duct before it joins the common bile duct. Associated with the pars superior of the choledochal sphincter are bundles of extrinsic duodenal muscle. These auxiliary bands have been divided into three types (Kreilkamp and Boyden, 1940): (1) reinforcing fibres that strengthen the margins of the window; (2) connecting fibres that hold the ducts to the intestine; (3) longitudinal fibres that shorten and erect the papilla. Boyden (1965) believes that contraction of the pars superior forces bile back up into the common bile duct and that contraction of the pars inferior expels bile into the duodenum. In spite of these studies the existence of an intrinsic sphincter of Oddi is still disputed (Floquet *et al.*, 1977).

The oblique course of the bile duct through the duodenal wall may be an anti-reflux mechanism (Germain *et al.*, 1977). When the duodenal muscle contracts, it may occlude the intramural portion of the duct directly or the rise in intraduodenal pressure may occlude the submucosal part of the duct.

The mucosa of the terminal portion of the common bile duct and the

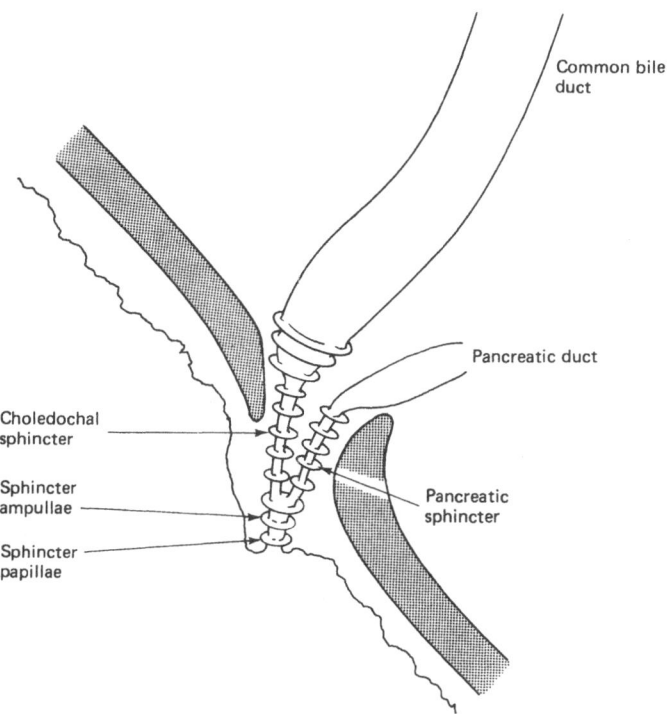

Figure 6.2 Diagrammatic representation of the choledochoduodenal junction in man.

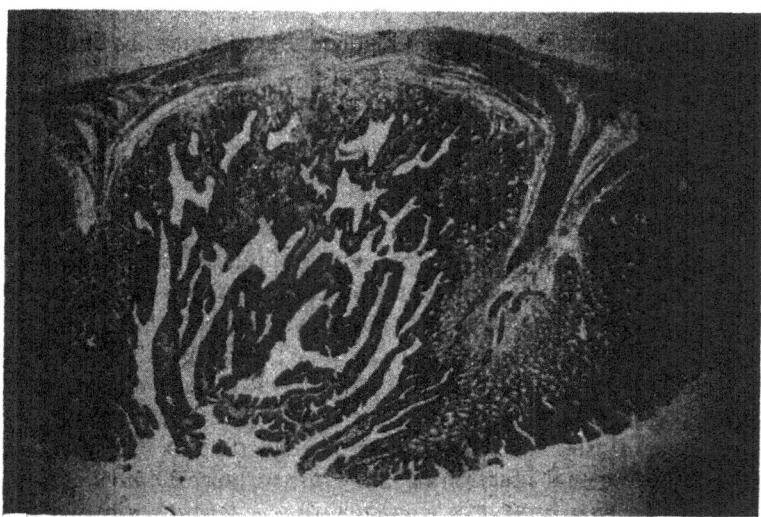

Figure 6.3 Section of the ampulla of the rabbit showing the arrangement of mucosal folds within the lumen ('Venetian blind system').

common channel is thickened, narrowing the lumen to produce an X-ray appearance of the choledochoduodenal junction (Fernandez-Cruz and Pera, 1977). The mucosa sends many projections into the lumen and these may cross the entire lumen of the duct. This has been called the Venetian blind system (Giermann and Holle, 1961) and has been suggested to be an anti-reflux mechanism (figure 6.3). With increasing age the thickness of these intraluminal projections increases, which makes them polypoid (Fernandez-Cruz and Pera, 1977). The submucosa contains dilated thin-walled blood vessels which have been referred to as the 'plexus papillaris' (Fernandez-Cruz and Pera, 1977). It has been suggested that filling of this plexus may cause erection of the papilla.

Extrahepatic Bile Ducts

Relevant to an understanding of the physiology of the sphincter region is a discussion of the anatomy of the extrahepatic bile ducts. Peristaltic waves in the common bile duct have been observed in the common bull head (Higgins, 1928) and opossum (Dubois and Hunt, 1932); however, the existence of such activity in higher mammals, including man, is disputed (Burnett and Shields, 1958; Hauge and Mark, 1965; Watts and Dunphy, 1966). The consensus is that the amount of muscle in the duct wall is minimal and that common bile duct peristalsis does not occur (Csendes *et al.*, 1979). Mirizzi (1939) described a sphincter in the wall of the common hepatic duct, but this view has not been substantiated either anatomically or functionally (Negri, 1941). Lutkens (1926) described a sphincter at the origin of the cystic duct from the gall bladder. Its existence has been denied (Nuboer, 1931); but more recently (Øster *et al.*, 1980) a high-pressure zone has been found at this site.

PHYSIOLOGY

The finding that intracholedochal pressure is higher than intraduodenal pressure implies an area of resistance to bile flow, located at the choledochoduodenal junction. Withdrawal pressure profile studies demonstrate a zone of elevated pressure which corresponds anatomically with the sphincter region (Hauge and Mark, 1965; Bourke and Ritchie, 1970). The pressure within the sphincter zone is higher in living subjects than in cadavers (Øster *et al.*, 1980), which suggests that the resistance at the choledochoduodenal junction is partly due to muscle activity, and not solely due to the structural characteristics of the termination of the bile duct. As the anatomy of the choledochoduodenal junction shows much species variation, it seems likely that its physiology does likewise. This should be borne in mind in interpreting results of studies using different species and extrapolating them to man (Boyden, 1965).

Methods Used to Study the Choledochal Sphincter

A number of methods have been used to investigate the function of the sphincter, but few record activity of the muscle directly.

Measurement of Yield Pressure

Elman and McMaster (1926) recorded the pressure, as measured by a saline column, required to attain flow into the common bile duct and hence through the sphincter region. Since then various terms have been used, including 'perfusion pressure', 'filling pressure', 'resistance pressure', 'opening pressure', 'passage pressure' and 'yield pressure', to describe this sphincteric resistance. The value of pressures measured in this way is questionable. It has been shown that the onset of flow frequently represents filling of the common bile duct rather than flow into the duodenum. The extent of such filling depends upon the elasticity of the bile duct, which itself can be affected by inflammation and fibrosis. Furthermore, Berci and Johnson (1965) have shown that flow into the duodenum may occur before the plateau or yield pressure is reached. They also found that the musculature around the lower end of the bile duct was easily fatigued by repeated testing. Nevertheless, with this technique several facts have emerged. The yield pressure is higher in animals with a gall bladder than in those without (Mann, 1919). Elman and McMaster (1926) demonstrated that feeding, or just showing, food to dogs reduced the yield pressure. More recently it has been advocated as a useful adjunct to cholangiography in deciding whether to explore the common bile duct at operation (Daniel, 1972; White *et al.*, 1972) or as an indication for direct surgery on the papilla (Daniel, 1972; Hunter, 1972).

Pull-through Pressure Profile

Pressure recording catheters have been passed into the lumen of the terminal bile duct to measure sphincter activity (Hauge and Mark, 1965). More recently, with perfused catheters passed into the sphincteric region during endoscopic retrograde cholangiography, the method has been extended to man (Nebel, 1975; Csendes *et al.*, 1979). The technique has demonstrated a high-pressure zone in the sphincteric region (figure 6.4), and the sphincter has been shown to exhibit phasic activity (see below)

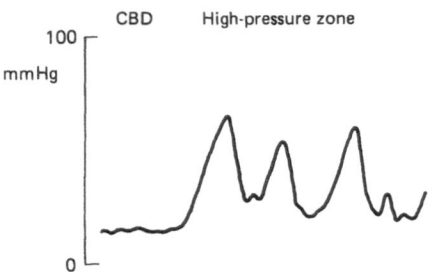

Figure 6.4   Pull-through study in man showing phasic contractions in the high-pressure zone.

which is independent of duodenal activity. The disadvantage of the method is that it is not known to what extent the presence of a catheter within the lumen of the sphincter region affects the activity of the sphincter muscle.

Choledochal Perfusion Techniques

Perfusion of the choledochoduodenal junction through a catheter placed in the common bile duct has been a technique widely used to assess the effect of hormones and various other substances on the sphincter. Either the bile duct is perfused at a constant pressure and flow into it recorded (Lueth, 1931; Bergh and Layne, 1940; Hedner and Rossman, 1969), or the bile duct is perfused at a constant rate and changes of pressure in it recorded (Lin and Spray, 1971; Persson, 1972). Whichever technique is used, and assuming that the common bile duct is a passive conducting tube with little inherent activity, any change in rate of flow or common bile duct pressure, respectively, will be due to changes in resistance at the choledochoduodenal junction. Common bile duct pressure is also determined in part by the rate of bile secretion by the liver and the presence of a gall bladder; therefore, the bile duct has to be divided below the origin of the cystic duct if the recordings are to accurately reflect sphincter activity. Such a procedure has been criticised as being unphysiological (Shore *et al.*, 1971).

Other Techniques

Other methods have been used to look at the activity of the sphincter more directly. Shore *et al.* (1971) avoided any instrumentation of the bile duct by inserting a duodenal cannula opposite the papilla in dogs and observing directly the flow of bile into the duodenum under various conditions. The sphincteric muscle has been studied *in vitro* (Toouli and Watts, 1972), and cinecholangiography has been used to observe the passage of contrast medium through the sphincter region. Recordings of the electrical activity of the sphincter (Ishioka, 1959; Sarles *et al.*, 1974; Toouli *et al.*, 1980b) have provided some information on the function of the sphincter.

Characteristics of the Choledochoduodenal Junction

Several factors affect bile duct pressure, including the rate of secretion of bile by the liver and the presence and activity of the gall bladder, but the most important is the choledochal sphincter. It controls the flow of bile into the duodenum, prevents reflux of duodenal contents into the bile duct (Csendes *et al.*, 1979) and is responsible for gall bladder filling. It has been shown by several workers that if an indwelling cannula is positioned in the sphincteric region, the gall bladder does not fill (Copher *et al.*, 1926; Whitaker, 1926). Perhaps the two most frequent questions asked concerning the physiology of the choledochal sphincter are: to what extent is the sphincter independent of the activity of the surrounding duodenum? and what pattern of sphincter activity determines flow of bile into the intestine?

Duodenal Influence

The degree to which the activity of the sphincter is distinct from that of the surrounding duodenal muscle has not yet been ascertained. Lueth (1931) measured simultaneously resistance at the choledochoduodenal junction and intraduodenal pressure, and found that sphincter activity was 'intimately co-ordinated with peristalsis and tone, but may function independently of the duodenum'. A similar conclusion was arrived at by Sandblom *et al.* (1935). The techniques used to record duodenal activity in most studies designed to investigate this problem do not accurately reflect contraction of the duodenal longitudinal muscle through which the bile duct passes, nor do they localise contraction to the sphincter region. To assess the effect of duodenal activity on the choledochoduodenal junction, Persson and Ekman (1972) devised the ingenious technique, using the cat, of passing lengths of femoral vein through the duodenal wall at various distances from the choledochoduodenal junction. They measured resistance at the choledochoduodenal junction by a perfusion technique and simultaneously recorded duodenal activity by perfusing the pieces of vein in a similar manner. The conclusion of the work was that sphincter activity was independent from the activity of duodenal muscle a short distance away from the choledochoduodenal junction, but that the duodenal muscle immediately surrounding the choledochal sphincter behaved like the sphincter and not like the rest of the duodenum—i.e. it responded to cholecystokinin by relaxation, while the rest of the duodenum responded by contraction.

Ono *et al.* (1968) used a combination of cinecholangiography and electrical recordings of the sphincter and adjacent duodenum as a means of assessing sphincter independence. They found that spike discharge of the sphincter was coincident with an arrest of the flow of contrast medium from the bile duct into the duodenum, while duodenal spike discharge did not always coincide with cessation of flow. Several other reports of simultaneous recordings of sphincter and duodenal electrical activity are available, but they do not all agree that the sphincter acts independently of the duodenum. Results from the surgical clinic of Hirosaki University (Ishioka, 1959; Kasai, 1960; Maki, 1961) and from France (Sarles *et al.*, 1974), using the rabbit, support the concept of sphincter independence, as do Nana *et al.* (1963), using the dog. However, other Japanese workers (Taniku, 1960; Hayashi, 1963; Tanaka, 1965) find electrical discharge from the sphincter essentially the same as from the duodenum. Such differences in results cannot solely be attributed to species differences, since Nana, Taniku and Hayashi all used dogs. The overall impression is that the sphincter can exhibit activity independent of the duodenum, but to what extent bile flow is influenced by duodenal activity is unclear.

Phasic Activity

The pattern of sphincter contraction is likely to reflect its role in the control of bile transit from the bile duct into the duodenum. Higgins (1927) suggested that, in the guinea-pig, bile was 'milked' into the intestine by simultaneous closure of the superior part of the sphincter and ampullary peristaltic waves forcing bile out into the duodenum. In the opossum (Dubois and Hunt, 1932) peristaltic waves pass down the common bile duct, and following each wave the ampulla becomes more and more distended. After several such contractions a larger peristaltic wave progresses across the ampulla, expelling bile into the intestine. Boyden (1965) believes that the sphincteric region acts as a pump in those animals—e.g. guinea-pig and rabbit—who have poor gall bladder function and put out large quantities of dilute bile. The sphincter of several other species, including man, has been shown to exhibit intermittent or phasic contractions (figure 6.4) (Bergh and Layne, 1940; Persson, 1972), but the function of these is disputed.

In the dog the sphincter undergoes intermittent contractions about every 5 s (Hauge and Mark, 1965; Crispin *et al.*, 1970). Csendes *et al.* (1979) recorded a frequency in man of 7.5 per minute, whereas Gennen *et al.* (1980) recorded a frequency of 4 per minute. Persson (1971) found that tetrodotoxin (a blocker of nerve conduction) increased the frequency of spontaneous contractions and concluded that it was an inherent myogenic phenomenon which could be modified by non-cholinergic, non-adrenergic nerves.

The function of the phasic activity of the sphincter is debated. Watts and co-workers (Watts and Dunphy, 1966; Toouli and Watts, 1972) studied the canine sphincter both *in situ* and *in vitro*, recorded phasic activity, and suggested that the sphincter may act as a pump to ejaculate bile into the duodenum. Cinecholangiogram studies (Torsoli *et al.*, 1973) have shown that contraction in the sphincter zone starts in the middle and spreads proximally and distally. The superior (retention) sphincter pushes bile up into the common bile duct, while the sphincter ampullae expels bile into the duodenum. *In vitro* studies performed by Toouli and Watts (1972) demonstrated that cholecystokinin (CCK) increased phasic activity of the sphincter muscle. They concluded that as bile flow into the duodenum is promoted by CCK, bile must be actively 'milked' into the duodenum by the intermittent sphincter activity. On the other hand, in man Gennen *et al.* (1980) found that CCK depressed the phasic activity. Persson (1972a) strongly opposes the view that bile is actively transported through the sphincter region and considers the sphincter to be a gate which simply opens to allow bile to pass through.

Most studies have used perfusion techniques to assess bile flow. Cessation of flow into the common bile duct or an increase in duct pressure marks a resistance to flow across the sphincter. However, if the sphincter region acts as a pump, the superior part of the sphincter would close while the distal part is pushing bile into the duodenum. If the sphincteric region is considered to be a gate, a resistance to flow through the sphincter would prevent the passage of bile into the duodenum. The interpretation of the results obtained with perfusion techniques depends entirely on which concept of choledochal sphincter function one supports. In a similar way, it is unclear whether duodenal peristalsis inhibits or actively transports bile through the choledochoduodenal junction. What is needed to help solve these problems is a method of correlating entry of bile into the duodenum with phasic contractions of the choledochal sphincter.

Factors Influencing the Choledochal Sphincter

In 1917 Meltzer proposed that the gall bladder and choledochal sphincter were under nervous control. He suggested a 'Law of Contrary Innervation' to explain the reciprocal response of the gall bladder and sphincter. However, this was soon followed by the work of Ivy with cholecystokinin (CCK), and since then it has been supposed that the muscle of the biliary tract is mainly under hormonal control.

Hormones

Potter and Mann (1926) demonstrated that feeding causes synchronous contraction of the gall bladder and relaxation of the choledochal sphincter. This finding was followed by the observation that the denervated gall bladder also contracts in response to food (Whitaker, 1926) and in 1928 by the extraction of CCK from the intestinal mucosa of the pig by Ivy and Oldberg. Carotid-to-carotid cross-circulation experiments by Ivy and

Oldberg and the vivi-perfused gall bladder preparation of Houssay and Rubio (1932) confirmed the hormonal status of CCK. In man, Sandblom (1933) produced contraction of the gall bladder by a transfusion of blood from donors digesting egg yolks, whereas blood from a fasting donor had no effect. Thus, it was established that the muscle of the biliary tract was under hormonal control.

In 1935 Sandblom et al. produced relaxation of the choledochal sphincter by an injection of CCK. Since then this observation has been confirmed by many other workers using purified preparations of CCK or its carboxyl-terminal octapeptide (Crema et al., 1962; Lin and Spray, 1969, 1971; Persson, 1972). Caerulein, a decapeptide, isolated from the skin of an Australian frog, is structurally related to CCK and has similar effects to it on both the gall bladder and the choledochal sphincter (Lin and Spray, 1969). The choledochal sphincter is more sensitive to CCK than the gall bladder or the liver, on which CCK has a choleretic action (Lin and Spray, 1971). It has therefore been concluded (Lin, 1975) that the action of CCK on the choledochal sphincter is physiological rather than pharmacological. The action of this hormone on the sphincter is not affected by atropine, propranolol, phenoxybenzamine or pentolinium, which suggests that neither adrenergic nor cholinergic nerves are involved in its action on the sphincter. Persson (1972) believes that CCK mediates its response on the gall bladder and sphincter of Oddi by affecting tissue levels of cyclic AMP (cAMP). CCK reduced the level of gall bladder cAMP and increased sphincter cAMP.

The phasic activity of the sphincter was depressed by CCK in a study in man (Gennen et al., 1980), yet an in vitro study using the dog (Toouli and Watts, 1972) showed it generally to increase phasic activity. It would be inappropriate to suggest that CCK, released by food, contracted the gall bladder and the choledochal sphincter; however, referring back to the previous section on phasic activity, if such activity increases flow through the sphincteric region, then CCK might be expected to increase activity of the sphincter.

The effect of the other gastrointestinal hormones on the choledochal junction is less well documented. Most reports find that gastrin and its analogues relax the sphincter (Lin and Spray, 1969; Agosti et al., 1971; Lin, 1971). Lin (1975) considers this action to be pharmacological rather than physiological. However, in vitro studies (Toouli and Watts, 1972) have shown that gastrin increases activity of the circular muscle of the sphincter, and a human study showed gastrin to increase pressure within the lumen of the sphincter (Nebel, 1975). Secretin has been found to decrease choledochal resistance in the conscious dog (Lin and Spray, 1971). Lin (1975) suggests that physiologically it does not affect the sphincter independently but may potentiate the action of cholecystokinin. However, Nebel (1975) found secretin to increase sphincter pressure. Glucagon has been found to relax the sphincter by most workers (Lin and Spray, 1969; Andersson *et al.*, 1972; Nebel, 1975), but Csendes *et al.* (1979) found no effect using a dose sufficient to inhibit duodenal activity.

Nerves

Perception of food causes reduction of resistance to bile flow at the choledochoduodenal junction (Potter and Mann, 1926; Elman and McMaster, 1926), which suggests a nervous mechanism influencing the choledochal sphincter. Acetylcholine causes contraction of both the gall bladder and the sphincter of Oddi (Persson, 1971); contraction of the sphincter also occurs with stimulation of the vagus nerves (Crema *et al.*, 1964). Persson (1972) found α-adrenergic receptors mediating contraction, and β-adrenergic receptors mediating relaxation, in the sphincter of Oddi. Intestinal muscle contains α- and β-receptors which both mediate relaxation (Ahlquist and Levy, 1959). The splanchnic nerves provide the sympathetic supply to the biliary tract, and Baumgarten and Lange (1969), using a fluorescence technique, have demonstrated adrenergic nerves in the choledochal sphincter of the cat. Stimulation of the right splanchnic nerve causes contraction of the sphincter and relaxation of the gall bladder (Persson, 1972). The physiological importance of nervous regulation of the biliary tract is unclear, but it has been suggested that adrenergic effects operate in the interprandial phase, promoting gall bladder filling.

Morphine

Morphine has been known for a long time to cause increased resistance to bile flow (Reach, 1912) and thus has been contraindicated in the treatment of biliary pain. Many studies have confirmed this effect (Butsch *et al.*, 1936; Gaensler and McGowan, 1950; Persson, 1971). However, morphine is also known to cause an increase in duodenal tonus, and this alone could increase resistance at the choledochoduodenal junction. Persson's studies (1972) indicate that morphine does have a direct action on the sphincter as well as its action on the surrounding intestinal muscle.

Miscellaneous Substances

The action of various other substances on the sphincter have been studied. Prostaglandin E_2 shares with CCK the dual effects on biliary muscle, contracting the gall bladder and relaxing the choledochal sphincter (Andersson *et al.*, 1972). Magnesium sulphate given intraduodenally also contracts the gall bladder and relaxes the sphincter (Boyden *et al.*, 1943), possibly by causing the release of CCK. Menguy *et al.* (1958) found that alcohol given intraduodenally increased choledochal and pancreatic duct pressures by causing a rise in sphincteric resistance, and Nossell and Efron (1955) found, in man, that whisky increased choledochal pressure. Such observations have led to speculation about the role of alcohol in the aetiology of pancreatitis. Amyl nitrite has consistently been found to relax the sphincter (Bergh, 1942).

Much information concerning the physiology of Oddi's sphincter has been acquired but several questions have only been partially answered. Newer techniques are required to identify the mechanisms whereby bile is transported through the sphincter region and also the role of duodenal motility, if any, in the passage of bile through the intestinal wall.

INFLAMMATORY LESIONS OF THE SPHINCTER OF ODDI

Benign pathological changes in the papilla and sphincter were described by Del Valle from Buenos Aires in 1926 in a paper entitled 'Chronic retractile sclerous odditis' (Del Valle *et al.*, 1965). In this article the author reported a patient who developed abdominal pain and jaundice some years after cholecystectomy. At operation the common bile duct was dilated and the lower end indurated. A transduodenal 'papillosphincterotomy' was made, but no calculi were found in the bile ducts. A wedge biopsy of the papilla subsequently showed fibrous replacement of the intrinsic sphincter fibres. The patient died of bronchopneumonia, and autopsy revealed that fibrosis involved not only the papilla and Oddi's sphincter, but also the terminal part of the pancreatic duct. The changes of chronic pancreatitis were not present.

Del Valle *et al.* (1965), Zinny (1965) and Ahualli (1966) have described the sequence of pathological changes thought to take place at the distal end of the common bile duct: chronic infection, initially localised to the mucosa and then infiltrating the fibres of Oddi's sphincter with subsequent fibrosis. These changes may remain localised or may spread to involve not only a long segment of the distal bile duct, but also the pancreatic duct in up to 63 per cent of cases (Del Valle *et al.*, 1965). Secondary changes in the bile ducts and liver result from long-standing obstruction and infection in the biliary tree, ultimately leading to biliary cirrhosis.

Calame (1957) in Geneva considered the histological changes to include adenomatosis, microadenomata, inflamed adenofibromata or sclerosis. He found acute inflammatory change to be rare, unlike the South American authors, and considered papillitis an incorrect term. Subsequently, authors have used a profusion of descriptive terms, with the result that a satisfactory pathological classification of the stages of 'odditis' has not really been achieved. In the French literature Hepp (1966a,b) simply refers to odditis (*l'oddité*), and this simplification has much to recommend it, provided that the author produces evidence to substantiate the diagnosis (see below). Others refer to *l'oddité stenosante* (Leonard and Massion, 1965), *l'oddité sclereuse* (Stalport, 1965) or *la maladi du sphincter d'Oddi* (Mallet-Guy *et al.*, 1950). The Spanish surgeon Pi-Figueras (1966) grouped the stenosing process into *papille ictergene* (Salembier, 1970, subsequently defined this as an isolated stenosis limited to the papilla only), *papillo-oddité hyperplaseque ou oedemateuse, oddité fibreuse ou sclero-oddité,* and reported 20 cases. In the same year Sciacca (1966) from Rome described the microscopic appearances of the papilla, which may be oedematous, hypertrophic or atrophic and retracted, but usually has granulation tissue at the tip. The essential microscopic changes should include glandular and mucosal hyperplasia, inflammatory cell infiltrate (variable in degree), and fibrosis with replacement of the intrinsic muscle fibres, with the process on occasions extending to involve a long segment of the common bile duct and the terminal portion of the pancreatic duct.

Classification of Types of Odditis

Sciacca (1966) has classified 'papillitis', 'papillo-odditis' and 'odditis' according to their aetiology into primary, secondary (associated with calculi in common bile duct or gall bladder) and residual (following previous surgical intervention). In 1970 Salembier from Lille published a review of 207 cases of *stenose oddienne* (table 6.1); only three cases fulfilled the criteria of primary stenosis (*papillites icterienne*). The rarity of this syndrome is stressed by Hepp (1966) in Paris, and Stalport (1965) in Belgium, who found an incidence of less than 1 per cent on review of 177 patients undergoing common duct exploration. Most cases are associated

Table 6.1   Odditis—classification and incidence (from Salembier, 1970)

	No. of cases	
Primary (*papillites icterienne*)	3	
Secondary	3	
odditis and cholecystitis		
(i) acalculous	12	
(ii) calculous	85	(5% of all cases of cholelithiasis confined to gall bladder)
odditis and choledocholithiasis	88	(9% of all cases of common bile duct stones)
odditis and chronic pancreatitis	5	
Residual		
(post-cholecystectomy)	13*	

*Including two patients with chronic pancreatitis.

either with multiple small gallstones apparently confined to the gall bladder or with detectable common bile duct stones, although in the context of acute pancreatitis it is now well recognised that stones may pass into the common bile duct and through the papilla.

Criteria for the Diagnosis of Odditis

The criteria for diagnosis of odditis or benign stenosis of the sphincter of Oddi as laid down by Hepp (1966a,b) and Salembier (1970) include:

(1) *Clinical.* Episodic biliary type pain. Del Valle *et al.* and other South American authors leave the reader in little doubt that chronic fibrosing retracting odditis will lead to biliary hypertension causing a characteristic pattern of pain (Del Valle *et al.*, 1965), with acute spasms alternating with long periods of chronic discomfort similar to that occurring in patients with primary or recurrent common duct stones. Jaundice, however, was considered to be less common.

(2) *Radiological.* Intravenous cholangiography showing stenosis, unresponsive to amyl nitrate or other antispasmodics, dilation of the bile ducts and either delayed or no flow of contrast media into the duodenum. Similar findings are found during per-operative cholangiography.

(3) *Operative instrumentation.* Difficulty in negotiating instruments through the papilla—e.g. No. 3 Bakes dilator (Schein and Beneventano, 1968).

(4) *Pathological.* Fibrosis and the changes previously described.

(5) *Manometric.* The existence of biliary hypertension (elevated intracholedochal pressure) has been considered fundamental to making a diagnosis of stenosing odditis by many authors (Mallet-Guy, 1950, 1952; Mester *et al.*, 1952; Stalport, 1964; Pi-Figueras, 1966; Sciacca, 1966; Salembier, 1970). During perfusion studies intracholedochal pressure is normally less than 15 cm; higher levels are suggestive of obstruction and in stenosing odditis yield pressures well in excess of 30 cm water are frequently found (Daniel, 1972; Hunter, 1972). The nature of the obstruction is revealed more clearly when radiology is performed synchronously—i.e. to differentiate calculus obstruction from stenosis. Stalport (1964) has emphasised the value of antispasmodics (succinyl choline): in the absence of an impacted calculus, stenosis is likely if an elevated perfusion pressure does not fall within the normal range (10–18 cm water), thus helping to exclude temporary spasm of Oddi's sphincter.

Investigation of the Patient with Suspected Odditis

As has been described in previous chapters, certain sphincters can be investigated with a high degree of accuracy pre-operatively. Thus, the gastro-oesophageal junction can be studied radiologically, endoscopically, manometrically obtaining withdrawal pressure profiles, supplemented by recordings of pH and the mucosal potential difference. Unfortunately, this is less readily achieved in the case of the biliary sphincter.

Estimation of hepatic enzymes—in particular, elevation of the alkaline phosphatase—may be a helpful indicator of obstruction to bile flow in the anicteric patient; it is not completely reliable and unless combined with electrophoresis gives no information as to the cause (Leading Article, 1977; Warnes et al., 1977). Similarly, estimation of the time of arrival in duodenal juice of a marker, BSP, known to be secreted in bile following its intravenous injection may be helpful (Caroli and Tanasoglu, 1953), and a time prolonged beyond 16 min in a patient who has undergone surgical or autocholecystectomy signifies obstruction. The test is, however, extravagant in manpower and requires duodenal intubation.

Oral cholecystography supplemented with cholecystokinin or morphine has been used by Leonard and Massion (1965). These Belgian workers claim that when both pain and dilation of the common bile duct are recorded, the test is positive and indicates pathology at the lower end of the bile duct. Intravenous cholangiography, combined with tomography, can be expected to provide more detail, but may be inapplicable, since its use is restricted to the anicteric or mildly icteric patient. In a satisfactory examination a diagnosis of papillitis, hypertonia or stenosis of Oddi's sphincter is suggested by delay in the opacification of the biliary tree, dilation of the bile ducts, delayed entry of contrast media into the duodenum, a deformed choledochoduodenal junction and persistent opacification of the common bile duct 3 h after intravenous injection.

Leonard and Massion (1965) have classified the cholangiographic signs of odditis. Indirect ones included delay in the appearance of contrast media (10 min after injection), delay in obtaining the peak concentration (60 min) and delay in evacuation of the dye into the duodenum (180 min). They also regarded total or segmental dilatation of the common bile duct of more than 14 mm as significant. Direct signs were grouped into abnormalities of the sphincter zone and abnormalities in the zone immediately proximal to the sphincter. In odditis the sphincteric zone appears hooked and elongated, dye may pool in the duct of Wirsung, and morphine produces either no visible response or an exaggerated contraction. The suprasphincteric zone may be either clubbed or bulbous, or it may be irregular, tortuous and narrowed.

In the jaundiced patient either percutaneous transhepatic cholangiography with the Chiba or Okuda needle or endoscopic retrograde cholangiography is of value in delineating the bile ducts and sphincteric region. It is not always possible to draw definite conclusions, but these tests have a high yield of helpful information.

Endoscopic manometric studies of the distal common bile duct are now feasible (Rosch et al., 1976; Ribiero et al., 1977). Results are not always easy to interpret, owing to the lack of reproducibility of the ampullary zone pressure recordings. Intraductal pressure recordings are more reliable. Rosch *et al.* (1976) suggest a single lumen catheter with an end hole and perfused at 0.5 ml water per minute to be most satisfactory. The recording of a normal sphincteric zone, illustrated in figure 6.4, was taken during a withdrawal profile using a side hole catheter used at 0.2 ml min^{-1} (Ribiero, 1977). A zone of elevated pressure has been consistently found by some corresponding to the sphincter choledochus (Ribiero, 1977; Toouli *et al.*, 1980a). Others have not been able to verify this, although human, canine and porcine studies would suggest that failure to recognise the zone of elevated pressure was largely technical, as the region is very susceptible to trauma and readily fatigues during withdrawal pressure studies (Bourke and Ritchie, 1970; Peel, 1976). Rosch and co-workers found this technique to be a reliable method for confirming or refuting a diagnosis of papillary stenosis. The mean gradient between intracholedochal and intraduodenal pressures is normally 8.8 mmHg, but this rises to a mean of 17.8 mmHg in patients with papillary stenosis.

Delray *et al.* (1965) have found measurement of flow rates useful in establishing a diagnosis of stenosis. In patients with a normal choledochoduodenal junction 10 ml of saline can be expected to flow into the biliary system within 60 s at a pressure of 30 cm water, but in patients with obstruction including stenosis the rate is less (6 ml min^{-1} at 30 cm perfusion pressure) and is not improved with amyl nitrate inhalation.

THERAPEUTIC CONSIDERATIONS IN SPHINCTERIC DISORDERS

At the time of writing functional disorders of the sphincter of Oddi in patients who have not undergone previous biliary tract surgery remain to be categorised. These and strictures of the distal common bile duct due to chronic pancreatitis and malignant disease will not be discussed. Two groups of patients will be considered in detail: first, patients with benign biliary tract disease, including choledocholithiasis, with or without stenosis of the region of the sphincter of Oddi occurring primarily (very rare) or associated with gall bladder stone (Group 1); second, patients with a suspected abnormality of the choledochoduodenal region giving rise to symptoms after previous cholecystectomy (Group 2).

Group 1: Patients with Suspected Common Bile Duct Stones or Sphincteric Stenosis

Since most of these patients present with troublesome symptoms, including recurrent episodes of abdominal pain often accompanied by fever and jaundice, that tend to progress in severity in the course of time, investigation is nearly always indicated. This is usually followed by treatment of a surgical nature. Careful consideration, however, must be given to the patient's general state of health, and for the elderly debilitated patient suffering from transient attacks of pain and mild jaundice due to calculous disease no active intervention may be the correct decision. Alternatively, an attempt at medical dissolution in anicteric patients with non-opaque gallstones and a functioning gall bladder may be advisable, or where expert facilities exist endoscopic papillotomy or sphincterotomy with balloon or basket extraction of the calculi may relieve the jaundice. For the majority of patients a surgical approach is applicable.

Intra-operative Assessment

In the UK intra-operative pre-exploratory cholangiography, originally described by Mirizzi in Argentina in 1942, is now widely regarded as essential before any operative manoeuvre is carried out on the bile ducts. For the surgeon it has several advantages: it demonstrates the anatomy, detects calculi, avoids unnecessary bile duct surgery and assesses the lower end of the bile duct. Attention to technique is important (Le Quesne and Whiteside, 1960; Devlin et al., 1978) in order to achieve good results, and in this respect the addition of fluoroscopy has been found helpful (Shennan, 1974). Slow injection of contrast medium, rotation to move the bile duct away from the vertebral column and four or more radiographs taken after the injection of the appropriate volume of diluted dye have all been shown to improve the quality of this investigation. The precise number of duct stones, however, may not be accurately assessed on the radiographs (Burke, 1972).

Assessment of the distal common bile duct during intra-operative cholangiography may be difficult. The importance of free flow of contrast medium into the duodenum is well known (Le Quesne and Whiteside, 1960). A wide range of descriptive terms have been used to denote appearances considered to be associated with stenosing odditis, the most frequent being 'serpent's head' (Sciacca, 1966). In order to avoid unnecessary surgery in addition to the cholecystectomy, it is important to differentiate between spasm and stenosis at the lower end of the bile duct, and in this respect the value of antispasmodics is well documented (Mallet-Guy, 1952; Stalport, 1964; Ahualli, 1966).

Several authors have stressed the value of manometry in detecting obstruction at the lower end of the common bile duct (previously described) (Caroli, 1946; Mallet-Guy and Dudfield Rose, 1956), particularly when combined with radiology (Daniel, 1972; Hunter, 1972; White et al., 1972). Others are of the opinion that there is little correlation between intracholedochal pressures and pathological changes at the sphincter (Dahl-Iversen et al., 1957; Jacobsson, 1965).

Using synchronous radiology and manometry, Ribiero (1979) studied 76 patients undergoing cholecystectomy. Using a known rate of flow (maximum 5 ml min⁻¹), he recorded intracholedochal and intraduodenal pressures and the radiological image of the bile duct simultaneously on a screen. In 20 of these patients an abnormal record was obtained, in that intracholedochal pressure gradually rose to a high plateau level, and the flow of dye into the duodenum was delayed beyond 3 min or failed to occur. In 13 of these 20 patients, stones were present, but in 7 it is uncertain whether spasm or stenosis was the cause. Continuation of this study on a large scale may shed light on this difficult problem. Although theoretically sound, the practical results of withdrawal pressure pull-through studies have been inconclusive as yet.

Choledochoscopy, both flexible and rigid, has been shown to have a place in the detection and location of common duct stones (Shore and Shore, 1970; Shore et al., 1971; Ashby, 1976; Finnis and Rowntree, 1977). Recent studies confirm that it does not replace intra-operative pre-exploratory cholangiography in assessment of the bile duct (Kappas et al., 1979). Finnis and Rowntree (1977) found manipulation of the distal common bile duct and duodenum often necessary in order to obtain adequate visualisation: assessment of the function of the sphincteric region would thereby be limited. It is, however, likely to reduce residual calculi (Finnis and Rowntree, 1977; Kappas et al., 1979).

How Should the Common Bile Duct be Explored?

In the UK the standard approach to the common bile duct is via the supraduodenal route. Patency of the lower end of the common bile duct may be confirmed by blind instrumentation, and the inability to pass a No. 3 F.G. Bakes dilator through the papilla has been considered to indicate stenosis (Grage et al., 1960; Schein and Beneventano, 1968; Shingleton and Gamburg, 1970). The rigid bougie, however, may push the sphincter in front of it towards the duodenal lumen, thus appearing to pass through the papilla (Mahorner and Browne, 1955); it may cause a false passage, the most frequent being a site of entry into the duodenum proximal to the lower sphincter (see below), known as Barraya's transparency sign on cholangiograms (Fernandes-Cruz et al., 1975); and, finally, an iatrogenic fibrous stricture of the sphincteric region following overenthusiastic bouginage is well recognised (Zollinger et al., 1938; Reynolds, 1966). Although some surgeons favour primary closure of the bile duct (Collins, 1967; Wilkin, 1975; Ashby, 1978; Vassilakis et al., 1978), most insert a T-tube to temporarily decompress the biliary tree.

In patients with choledocholithiasis the aims of exploring the common bile duct are to remove all stones and to prevent further stone formation. On occasions the latter aim necessitates the establishment of adequate biliary drainage. Furthermore, it is mechanically unsound to aim to remove all calculous material from a tubular system by opening it half-way along its length and then closing it.

When is a drainage procedure needed? It is indicated for patients with grossly dilated ducts, ducts containing many small calculi or sand and mud, for a stone impacted in the sphincter (to aid removal and avoid the effects of a possible late stricture), for residual or recurrent stones and for stenosis at the lower end and in certain patients with hydatid disease or clonorchis infestation. The elderly patient with a grossly dilated bile duct forms a well-defined group (Leading Article, 1978), and it is interesting to speculate whether this is an atonic, 'baggy', duct perhaps secondary to an achalasia-like state. Further study of this group would be of great interest.

The types of procedures available include transduodenal papillotomy, sphincterotomy or sphincteroplasty, choledochoduodenostomy, endoscopic sphincterotomy and choledochojejunostomy Roux-en-Y. The first three procedures will now be considered in some detail. The fourth is favoured in France (Bismuth *et al.,* 1978), particularly in patients with residual or recurrent calculi. In the UK it is most widely indicated for certain long benign strictures of the extrahepatic duct system. Cholangitis, following this procedure, is usually related to overlooked calculi (usually intrahepatic associated with distorted intrahepatic ducts), and this has given rise to the high incidence (14 per cent) of late complications (Bismuth *et al.,* 1978). These authors reported only one case of anastomatic stenosis in 123 patients, but peptic ulceration occasionally occurred.

The transduodenal approach

The terms used to describe the different surgical operations carried out on the lower end of the common bile duct have led to confusion. Papillotomy divides the mucosa at the tip of the papilla, and the fibres of the sphincter papillae. Sphincterotomy divides, in addition, some of the fibres of the main biliary sphincter, the sphincter choledochus, in its intramural portion. When the mucosa of the bile duct and duodenum are then sutured, the term 'sphincteroplasty' may be applied. If such an incision divides all fibres of the biliary sphincter, and therefore extends proximally beyond the duodenal wall, suture of the cut edges is essential in order to avoid leakage of duodenal contents—this may be called a total sphincteroplasty.

The technique of sphincterotomy is described in detail elsewhere (Peel *et al.,* 1974). Adequate mobilisation of the duodenal loop and the head of the pancreas greatly facilitates the procedure, and identification of a 'flat stunted papilla' may be aided by the advancement of the ureteric catheter (used for cholangiography) inserted by way of the cystic duct. Before sphincterotomy is made it is particularly important to confirm that the probe or grooved dissector has passed into the papilla, and thence into the common bile duct, not the pancreatic duct. The tip of the probe should be seen to be in the supraduodenal portion of the common bile duct. The length of the incision should be sufficient to permit of insertion of instruments, and extraction of calculi, without difficulty.

Results of the transduodenal approach to common bile duct. An overall mortality of 5 per cent for 6291 cases collected from the literature has been reported. Comparative studies are few. Niederle (1967) of Czechoslovakia reported a 2.9 per cent mortality after biliary sphincterotomy, compared with 1.8 per cent after supraduodenal choledochotomy. In a retrospective study at the London Hospital, the mortality was least after the transduodenal approach (table 6.2) and the combined approach seemed most hazardous, although Aubrey and Edwards (1978) have found otherwise.

Table 6.2 Early post-operative complications after supraduodenal choledochotomy (SDC), transduodenal sphincterotomy (TDS) and combined SDC and TDS at the London Hospital (from Peel *et al.*, 1975)

	SDC (10 patients)	TDS (82 patients)	SDC and TDS (26 patients)
Mortality	4	2	2
Acute pancreatitis	1	0	1
Biliary peritonitis	1	0	2
Biliary fistula	1	0	1
Duodenal fistula	0	1	0
Duodenal obstruction	0	1	0
Cholangitis	5	0	3

Acute pancreatitis is a well-recognised hazard of biliary surgery, and certain authors have found that it is particularly frequent after the transduodenal approach (Walters *et al.*, 1961). It is a serious complication, with a mortality as high as 85 per cent (Hepp and Bismuth, 1966). In the London series it was infrequent (table 6.2), and this may be due to a combination of factors, including a low incidence of previous pancreatitis, avoiding intubation of the pancreatic duct, a transpapillary drain and trauma to the sphincter region as a result of blind instrumentation. Plasma amylase levels may be expected to rise during the first 48 h in about one-third of patients (Peel *et al.*, 1975), a similar proportion to that seen after supraduodenal choledochotomy (Keighley and Graham, 1973), and after ERCP (Liguory *et al.*, 1974). The late complications occurring in the London series are summarised in table 6.3.

Cholangitis. In seven of the ten patients after SDC and in one patient after TDS and two patients after the combined approach cholangitis was associated with residual calculi. In this series, therefore, it seemed that late

Table 6.3 Late post-operative complications after supraduodenal choledochotomy (SDC), transduodenal sphincterotomy (TDS) and combined SDC and TDS at the London Hospital (from Peel *et al.*, 1975)

	SDC (97 patients)	TDS (80 patients)	SDC and TDS (24 patients)
Cholangitis	10	1	2
Common bile duct stones			
necessitating re-operation	9	1	2
suspected clinically	3	0	0
Stenosis/Stricture	1	0	1
Pancreatitis	0	0	0

cholangitis was caused by obstruction to bile flow rather than the reflux of duodenal contents into the biliary tree, as previously suggested by Roux *et al.* (1965) and Moreaux and Teixeira (1966).

Residual or recurrent stone. One of the theoretical advantages of transduodenal sphincterotomy is that by allowing more complete removal of calculi and mud from the bile ducts and by providing permanent free drainage the incidence of residual or recurrent stone should be low. The figure of 1.3 per cent in the series is similar to that reported in the literature: 5 per cent (Wiechno, 1965); 4 per cent (Terquen, 1969); 0.4 per cent (Pi-Figueras, 1966). In the London series the combined approach did not improve the results. The routine use of intra-operative post-exploratory cholangiography can be expected to reduce the incidence of overlooked stone after both supraduodenal and transduodenal approaches, and choledochoscopy is also helpful in this respect (Ashby, 1978). It is of interest, however, that T-tube cholangiograms in four of the nine patients with further stones after SDC and one of the two patients after combined SDC and TDS were *normal*. In the three patients with residual stones who had had a sphincterotomy the stoma was widely patent, but the stones failed to pass, owing to their large size.

Stenosis or stricture. From experimental studies in dogs Eisman *et al.* (1959) and Webb *et al.* (1964) found that the sphincterotomy became stenosed, although more recent porcine studies (a model anatomically more similar to man) did not confirm this work (Peel, 1976). Niederle (1967) reported an incidence of less than 2 per cent in 345 patients. In the London series the patient who required re-operation for a terminal stricture of the bile duct 4 years after the original combined approach was found to have stenosis of the papilla, but the sphincter choledochus appeared intact—this may therefore represent an inadequate initial procedure.

Results of studies into certain long-term effects of biliary sphincterotomy Does subclinical stenosis occur? By modifying

Caroli's test the time of arrival in the duodenal aspirate of a marker BSP known to be excreted in bile following intravenous injection was recorded. The arrival time is defined as the time interval between the start of the intravenous injection and the first detection of BSP in the duodenal aspirate.

The normal arrival time for cholecystectomised patients is less than 16 min (table 6.4), and it is prolonged in patients with anicteric obstruction (and a non-functioning gall bladder). In 49 patients who had undergone cholecystectomy and transduodenal sphincterotomy up to 12 years previously the arrival time was prolonged in 2, which suggests a degree of subclinical stenosis.

Table 6.4   The time of arrival of BSP—duodenal aspirate in three groups of patients

Group of patients studied	No. of patients	Mean arrival time (AT)(min)	No. of patients with AT 16 min
After cholecystectomy	30	11.7 ± 2.3	−
Anicteric obstruction + NFGB	8	19.4 ± 1.2	8
After cholecystectomy and sphincterotomy	49	12.1 ± 4.4	2

Endoscopic examination of the stoma in eight patients 2–8 years after sphincterotomy revealed a widely patent non-rigid stoma in each. Endoscopic sphincterotomy would also appear to have a low incidence of stenosis (Koch *et al.*, 1977).

Does sphincterotomy lead to incompetence of the sphincter? The incidence of reflux during a standard barium meal has been quoted to be between 15 per cent and 43 per cent after sphincterotomy (Kourias *et al.*, 1966; Bohmig *et al.*, 1969; Jones and Smith, 1972). With a maximal stimulus, hypotonic duodenography, used to test sphincteric competence, reflux of barium into the common bile duct occurred in 20 of 51 patients up to 12 years after sphincterotomy (Peel *et al.*, 1975). Its occurrence was not related to the patients' age or the length of follow-up, but was more closely correlated with the length of the sphincterotomy incision. It was not associated with cholangitis or pancreatitis (barium was noted in the duct in six patients).

Is hepatic function impaired after sphincterotomy? In the London series routine liver function tests were obtained in 85 of 104 surviving patients after biliary sphincterotomy. BSP retention levels in plasma 45 min after injection were abnormal (Bodvall, 1973) in 14 of 49 sphincterotomised patients tested. Similar results have been reported following supraduodenal choledochotomy (Caroli *et al.*, 1950; Banki *et al.*, 1966; Lindenauer and Child, 1966; Aronsen, 1968). It seems likely that this abnormality reflects the original biliary pathology and is independent of the type of operation used to deal with it.

   Is sphincteric function abolished by sphincterotomy? In order to study this question, use has been made of morphine, a substance which is known to cause constriction of the lower end of the common bile duct (Jacobsson, 1965; Wiechno, 1965; Jones and Smith, 1972). In the London series the BSP arrival time was significantly prolonged by morphine in patients with an intact sphincter, and after sphincterotomy. Jones and Smith (1972) demonstrated that total sphincteroplasty ablated the pinch-cock action of musculature around the distal common bile duct. The results of duodenoscopic manometry of the bile duct and sphincteric region have been reported by Rosch *et al.* (1976) and Ribiero *et al.* (1977), using perfused single lumen end- or side-holed catheters. In patients with an intact sphincter, both groups of workers demonstrated a pressure gradient between bile duct and duodenum with an intervening high-pressure zone (range 18–45 mmHg, mean 31 mmHg). The mean pressure of the latter zone was much increased in patients with papillary stenosis, and reduced or abolished after surgical or endoscopic sphincterotomy. An example of tracings before and 2 months after surgical sphincterotomy is shown (figure 6.5). Further long-term results would prove interesting.

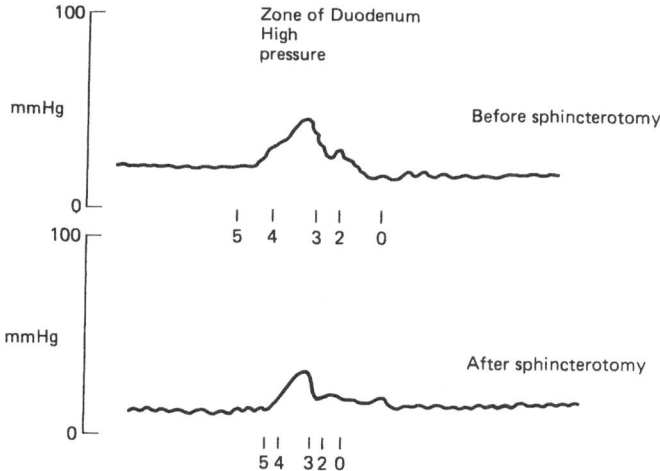

Figure 6.5 Endoscopic withdrawal pressure profiles in the same patient and 2 months after sphincterotomy (Ribiero, 1977).

It would seem that abolition of sphincteric activity is routinely achieved only after a total sphincteroplasty. In sphincterotomised patients the relative importance of the residual sphincteric fibres and the duodenal musculature has yet to be determined.

Choledochoduodenostomy

This operation can provide effective biliary drainage for patients with a grossly dilated common bile duct associated with calculous disease or stricture at the lower end of the duct (Johnson and Rains, 1972). It is particularly indicated in the elderly poor-risk patient (Madden *et al.*, 1970; Leading Article, 1978).

It has been criticised on account of the theoretical risks of allowing free reflux of duodenal contents into the biliary tree, giving rise to cholangitis, and of providing a blind sump which may give rise to infection, further stone formation or pancreatic inflammation. In the literature there is strong evidence to suggest that the incidence of cholangitis is low (0.4 per cent, Madden *et al.*, 1970; 3.7 per cent, Freund *et al.*, 1977), and that its occurrence signifies stenosis of the stoma—i.e. a descending cholangitis, and not an ascending cholangitis due to reflux (Schein and Beneventano, 1968; Madden *et al.*, 1970). Stenosis is unlikely to occur if a stoma of 25 mm or more is created (Capper, 1961; Schein and Beneventano, 1968; Johnson and Rains, 1972; Freund *et al.*, 1977). The importance of normal gastric acid secretion in preventing cholangitis has recently been reported (Cotton, 1979).

Problems from the blind sump seem infrequent (Madden *et al.*, 1970), although some authors do report the occurrence of stones (Freund *et al.*, 1977). The emptying of the common bile duct has been evaluated on post-operative barium meals—usually barium refluxes into the upper bile ducts and the sump, but the contrast rapidly empties back (Johnson and Rains, 1972), and none should be retained in the bile ducts 24 h after the study (Schein and Beneventano, 1968).

Liver function studies have not revealed impairment (Capper, 1961; Hadfield and Haziq ul Yaqin, 1970), and in this respect the results are similar to those found after transduodenal exploration.

When compared with transduodenal sphincterotomy, chole-dochoduodenostomy is similar in terms of mortality and morbidity (Thomas *et al.*, 1971) and it is a simpler procedure to perform (Madden *et al.*, 1970; Freund *et al.*, 1977), but the lower end of the bile duct is not directly visualised, which may lead to an inconclusive or incorrect diagnosis of a lump related to the choledochoduodenal area (Johnson and Rains, 1972).

Endoscopic papillotomy or sphincterotomy

Endoscopic electrosurgery can now offer treatment for certain cases of common bile duct obstruction. In a series of 267 patients (reported by Koch *et al.*, 1977) 222 had common bile duct stones, and in 192 the calculi were successfully removed. In 32 patients papillary stenosis was present, and the stricture was successfully divided, but in 2 re-stenosis has occurred, 1 of the cases subsequently proving to be malignant. These authors claimed that the complication rate was lower than for surgical sphincterotomy, although recognising that it is not always possible to be certain which sphincter had been divided and whether the cut had been confined to the intramural part of the duct.

Classen and Ossenberg (1977) have reported the results of 1107 endoscopic papillotomies performed in ten centres, mainly in Western Europe. In 63 per cent of patients stones passed spontaneously and in a further 26 per cent stones were extracted by means of a Dormia basket or balloon catheter: an 89 per cent success rate in stone removal. In this collected series serious complications such as pancreatitis, cholangitis, bleeding or perforation occurred in 94 patients (8.5 per cent), with a mortality of 1.08 per cent related to the papillotomy itself. Cholangitis was most likely to occur in patients with large common duct stones, owing to their impaction. The incidence of bleeding was correlated with the length of the papillotomy incision.

As with surgical sphincterotomy, the sphincter of Oddi is unavoidably and permanently damaged. Manometric studies have shown that the zone of high pressure is reduced or ablated (figure 6.5; Rosch *et al.*, 1976). Duodenal reflux is reported to occur in approximately 60 per cent of cases but does not appear to cause cholangitis (Classen and Ossenberg, 1977).

The indications for endoscopic papillotomy may be summarised:

(1) Overlooked or recurrent common bile duct stones in the older patient and probably in preference to re-operation in the younger patient. In the early post-operative period in a patient with a T-tube *in situ* either dissolution or extraction methods by this route may be preferred.

(2) Common bile duct stones with symptoms of obstruction in high-risk surgical patients who have not previously undergone cholecystectomy. This was the most frequent indication, according to Demling (1977).

(3) Isolated papillary stenosis, diagnostically confirmed by radiological and biochemical evidence of cholestasis, and manometric evidence of an increased choledochoduodenal pressure gradient. Demling (1977) regarded a gradient of more than 15 mmHg as indicating the presence of stenosis.

More recently Cotton (1980) has collated the results from 14 centres in Britain: a successful sphincterotomy was achieved in 87 per cent of 679 patients, with successful stone extraction or passage in 87 per cent. Complications, including pancreatitis, haemorrhage, perforation or cholangitis, occurred in 58 patients (8.5 per cent) and necessitated emergency surgery in 11 patients (1.6 per cent). Seven patients (1 per cent) died. These results compare favourably with surgical experience. Whereas the participants in this study would always choose endoscopic sphincterotomy in preference to surgery for the high-risk post-cholecystectomy patient with choledocholithiasis, they would rarely if ever consider this procedure for the low-risk young patient with a gall bladder *in situ*.

Although endoscopic division of a localised short segment papillary stenosis is a recognised procedure, it is not without risk—Seifert (1980) reported a complication rate of 23.8 per cent in 21 patients with short segment papillary stenosis, compared with 7.5 per cent in 171 patients undergoing papillotomy for choledocholithiasis. The corresponding mortality was 4.3 per cent for patients with stenosis, compared with 2.2 per cent for patients with common bile duct stones.

Recurrent stone and stenosis is reported as occurring in 0.8 per cent and 0.2 per cent, respectively, of patients after endoscopic sphincterotomy (Shapiro, 1980). Although short sphincterotomy has a low mortality and low early complication rate, it has a higher incidence of residual stone and recurrent cholangitis, compared with the results following a long incision. As yet the only clear guideline for the endoscopist about to undertake papillotomy is to limit the length of the incision according to the size of stone present and then to allow time for the spontaneous passage of the stones.

Group 2: Patients with a Suspected Abnormality of the Choledochoduodenal Region Giving Rise to Symptoms after Previous Cholecystectomy

The assessment of these patients must be comprehensive, and it is of importance to know the similarities and differences that exist between the original and current symptoms and signs. Details of the operative findings, including pre-operative cholangiography, should be reviewed. Details of the patients' socioeconomic status, with particular reference to alcohol consumption, are frequently relevant. Laboratory work-up must include the appropriate biochemical and immunological studies. Although useful information can be gained from intravenous cholangiography and ultrasonography, many patients require Chiba needle percutaneous transhepatic cholangiography or endoscopy and retrograde cholangiopancreatography (Blumgart *et al.*, 1977).

Two chief causes of post-cholecystectomy syndrome (PCS) have been considered in the literature (Bodvall, 1973):

(1) Organic causes related to the biliary and pancreatic systems, including common duct stone, benign or malignant stricture of the bile duct, pancreatic tumours, fibrous stenosis of the papilla, and a long cystic duct or gall bladder remnant. To these there must be added symptoms arising from other parts of the alimentary tract—e.g. hiatus hernia, peptic ulcer, etc.

(2) Functional causes, the so-called 'biliary dyskinesia'—the existence, diagnosis and treatment of which is ill understood.

What Are the Results of Investigating the Patients with PCS?

In patients presenting with jaundice after cholecystectomy, an organic cause may be expected and was demonstrated in all of 18 patients (the most frequent being retained stone, 67 per cent, but the ducts were normal on ERCP in 17 per cent) studied by Blumgart *et al.* (1977). These authors and others have noted the value of careful assessment in patients with right hypochondrial pain and mild recurrent jaundice, since some have abnormalities of bilirubin metabolism (Gilbert's or Dubin–Johnson syndrome), and may undergo unnecessary choledochotomy (Peel and Ritchie, 1974). In the non-jaundiced group of 21 patients with biliary colic and dyspepsia an abnormality is less frequently found and was detected in 62 per cent on ERCP (Blumgart *et al.,* 1977). In this group were included three patients with a stenosed or inflamed choledochoduodenostomy and debris and inspissated bile in the ducts, and four patients with stenosis of a sphincteroplasty stoma.

How Well-defined is the PCS?

After cholecystectomy mild attacks of pain may occur in nearly one in every four patients, but occasional attacks of severe pain (3 per cent), cholangitis (0.7 per cent) and continuous severe distress (1.7 per cent) are much less frequent (Bodvall, 1973a,b). The post-cholecystectomy syndromes were more frequent in women, in patients with gall bladders which contained stones rather than those affected by acalculous cholecystitis, in patients with a functioning as opposed to a non-functioning gall bladder at oral cholecystography, and in those with a longer preoperative history. The significance of the cystic duct stump is debated. In Gothenborg Bodvall (1973a,b), from a cholangiographic study of 500 PCS patients, found a significantly higher frequency of cystic duct remnant in patients with severe PCS (78 per cent), and residual stones (84 per cent), compared with asymptomatic or mildly dyspeptic patients (40 per cent). It can be seen that a cystic duct remnant *per se* has little clinical significance, but may give rise to symptoms by stone retention or formation, inflammation or possibly neuroma formation. Bodvall (1973a,b) reported that the width of the common bile duct is increased by age, by the presence of acute cholecystitis, and that in patients with severe distress after cholecystectomy a progressive dilatation is found—'in the absence of demonstrable calculi increasing CBD width is sound radiological evidence for the severe PCS distress'.

In the absence of organic obstruction at the choledochoduodenal junction, PCS symptoms could theoretically be due to achalasia, muscle hypertrophy, inco-ordination of the sphincters papillae, choledochus and pancreaticus, hypotonia, hypertonia or episodic spasms (Delmont, 1979).

How Can Patients with PCS be Treated?

After cholecystectomy consistent alterations of intracholedochal pressure have not been established (Jacobsson, 1957). This is in agreement with the view that vagotomy for hypertonic and splanchnic nerve resection for hypotonic states, as recommended by Mirizzi (1942), Hess (1961) and Mallet-Guy *et al.* (1970), are of limited long-term value (Bodvall, 1973a,b).

In a non-operative approach the value of choleretics and progestogens in both mild and severe distress has been reviewed (Bodvall, 1973a,b). Perhaps antispasmodics enjoy a wider usage and are certainly helpful in patients with episodic biliary type pain—so-called episodic post-cholecystectomy dyskinesia.

The place of surgery in the removal of residual calculi and repair of ductal stricture after cholecystectomy is not in dispute. For patients with spasm or stenosis at the sphincter both sphincterotomy or sphincteroplasty and choledochoduodenostomy are performed, but results are not always satisfactory. The presence of benign pancreatic disease, initially regarded as an acceptable indication for sphincterotomy (Doubilet and Mullholland, 1956), should lead to caution and this procedure should be restricted to some patients with relapsing acute pancreatitis, and a small number of patients with chronic pancreatitis with a short papillary stricture causing retention of pancreatic secretion (Warren, 1971; Dixon and Engler, 1971). Stenosis and inflammation of the stoma following choledochoduodenostomy performed when the biliary system is minimally dilated is well recognised (Blumgart *et al.*, 1977). Bodvall (1973a,b) has condemned both of these operations for patients with severe PCS distress on the grounds that the former carries a risk of pancreatitis, and the latter a risk of cholangitis and liver damage.

These patients present a challenge in management and it is to be hoped that more light will be shed as a result of dynamic studies, including endoscopic bile analysis, manometry and emptying patterns, biochemical provocation tests, and the use of isotopic scanning to obtain a dynamic picture.

REFERENCES

Agosti, A., Mantovani, P. and Mori, L. (1971). Actions of caerulein and related substances on the sphincter of Oddi. *Naunyn-Schmiedbergs Arch. Pharmakol.*, **208**, 114-118

Ahlquist, R. P. and Levy, B. (1959). Adrenergic receptive mechanism of canine ileum. *J. Pharmac. Exp. Ther.*, **127**, 146-149

Ahualli, A. (1966). Notre experimentation de la papillotomie. *Rev. Int. Hepat.*, **16**, 543-554

Andersson, K. E., Andersson, R. and Hedner, P. (1972). Effect of cholecystokinin on the level of cyclic AMP and on mechanical activity in the isolated sphincter of Oddi. *Life Sci.*, **11**, 723-732

Aronsen, K. F. (1968). Late effects of biliary stasis on the effective liver blood flow. *Acta Chir. Scand.*, **134**, 278-281

Ashby, B. S. (1976). Operative choledochoscopy using an experimental choledochoscope. *Gut*, **17**, 833

Ashby, B. S. (1978). Fibreoptic choledochoscopy in common bile duct surgery. *Ann. Coll. Surg. Eng.*, **60**, 399-403

Aubrey, D. A. and Edwards, J. L. (1978). The selective use of combined supraduodenal and trans-duodenal exploration of the common bile duct. *Br. J. Surg.*, **65**, 246-251

Banki, F., Stefanics, J., Maklary, L. and Nagy, L. (1966). Studies on intraduodenal excretion of BSP in surgically controlled partial biliary duct obstruction. *Deutsch. Vendan. Stoffweckselhr.*, **26**, 20-23

Baumgarten, H. G. and Lange, W. (1969). Extrinsic adrenergic innervation of the extrahepatic biliary system in guinea pigs, cats and rhesus monkeys. *Z. Zellforsch.*, **100**, 606-615

Berci, G. and Johnson, N. (1965). Functional studies of the extraheptic biliary system in the dog by use of a controlled biliary fistula. *Ann. Surg.*, **161**, 286-292

Bergh, G. S. (1942). The sphincter mechanism of common bile duct in human subjects: its reactions to certain types of stimulation. *Surgery*, **11**, 299-330

Bergh, G. S. and Layne, J. A. (1940). A demonstration of the independent construction of the sphincter of the common bile duct in human subjects. *Am. J. Physiol.*, **128**, 690-694

Bismuth, H., Franco, D., Corlette, M. B. and Hepp, J. (1978). Long term results of Roux en Y hepaticojejunostomy. *Surg., Gynec. Obstet.*, **142**, 161-167

Blumgart, L. H., Carachi, R., Imrie, C. W., Benjamin, I. S. and Duncan, J. G. (1977). Diagnosis and management of post-cholecystectomy symptoms: the place of endoscopy and retrograde choledochopancreatography. *Br. J. Surg.*, **64**, 809-816

Bodvall, B. (1973). The post-cholecystectomy syndrome. *Clin. Gastroenterol*, **2**, 103-126

Bohmig, H. J., Fritsch, A., Kux, M. and Stacher, G. (1969). Indikationein und ergetnisse der transduodenalen sphincterotomie. *Langenbecks Arch. Klin. Chir.*, **323**, 173-188

Bourke, J. B. and Ritchie, H. D. (1970). The pressure profile of the sphincter of Oddi in man and in the pig. *Rend. Gastroenterol.*, **2**, 160-161

Boyden, E. A. (1937). The sphincter of Oddi in man and certain representative mammals. *Surgery*, **1**, 25-37

Boyden, E. A. (1955). The choledocho and pancreatico-duodenal junction in the chimpanzee. *Surgery*, **37**, 918-927

Boyden, E. A. (1957a). The choledochoduodenal junction in the cat. *Surgery*, **41**, 773-781

Boyden, E. A. (1957b). The anatomy of the choledochoduodenal junction in man. *Surg., Gynec. Obstet.*, **104**, 641-652

Boyden, E. A. (1965). The comparative anatomy of the sphincter of Oddi in mammals, with special reference to the choledochoduodenal junction in man. In *The Biliary System* (A Symposium of the NATO Advanced Study Institute), Blackwell, Oxford, pp. 15-40

Boyden, E. A., Bergh, G. S. and Layne, J. A. (1943). An analysis of the reaction of the human gall bladder and sphincter of Oddi to magnesium sulphate. *Surgery*, **13**, 723-733

Boyden, E. A. and Schwegler, R. A. (1936). The sphincter of Oddi in the dog. *Am. J. Physiol.*, **116**, 14

Burke, M. (1972). Routine pre-operative cholangiography. *Br. J. Hosp. Med.*, **7**, 237-239

Burnett, W. and Shields, R. (1958). Movements of the common bile duct in man. *Lancet*, **ii**, 387-390

Butsch, W. L., McGowan, J. M. and Walters, W. (1936). Clinical studies on the influence of certain drugs in relation to biliary pain and to the variations in intrabiliary pressure. *Surg., Gynec. Obstet.*, **63**, 451-456

Calame, A. (1957). Pathologie et therapeutique chirurgicals de la stenose oddiennes. *Gastroenterologie*, **87**, 268–277

Capper, A. (1957). External choledochoduodenostomy. An evaluation of 125 cases. *Br. J. Surg.*, **49**, 292-300

Caroli, J. (1946). La radiomanometrie biliaire. *Sem. Hop. Paris*, **22**, 198-200

Caroli, J., Alliot, M. and Richard, H. (1950). Epreuve de la bromsulfonephtaleine. *Sem. Hop. Paris*, **24**, 1110-1122

Caroli, J. and Tanasoglu, Y. (1953). Le temps d'apparition de la bromesulfonephtalein dans la bile. *Sem. Hop. Paris*, **29**, 591-606

Classen, M. and Ossenberg, F. W. (1977). Non-surgical removal of common bile duct stones. *Gut*, **18**, 760-769

Collins, M. and Ossenberg, F. W. (1977). Non-surgical removal of common bile duct stones. *Gut*, **18**, 760-769

Collins, P. G. (1967). Primary closure of the common bile duct. *Br. J. Surg.*, **54**, 854-856

Copher, G. H. Kodama, S. and Graham, E. A. (1926). The filling and emptying of the gall bladder. *J. Exptl Med.*, **44**, 65-73

Cotton, P. B. (1979). Personal communication

Cotton, P. B. (1980). British experience with duodenoscopical sphincterotomy [Abstract], *International Biliary Association 2nd Annual Meeting*, 4 307-317

Crema, A., Berte, F., Bengi, G. and Frigo, E. M. (1964). The responses of the sphincteric areas of the extrahepatic biliary tract to the stimulation of sympathetic and parasympathetic nerves. *Acta Physiol. Lat. Am.*, **14**, 24-32

Crispin, J. S., Choi, Y. M., Wiseman, D. G. H., Gillespie, D. J. and Lind, J. F. (1970). A direct manometric study of the canine choledochoduodenal junction. *Arch. Surg.*, **101**, 215-218

Csendes, A., Kruse, A., Funch-Jensen, P., Øster, M. J., Ørnsholt, J. and Amdrup, E. (1979). Pressure measurements in the biliary and pancreatic duct systems in controls and in patients with gallstones, previous cholecystectomy or common bile duct stones. *Gastroenterology*, **77**, 1203-1210

Dahl-Iversen, E., Sørenson, and Westengaard, E. (1957). Pressure measurement in the biliary tract in patients after cholecystolithotomy and in patients with dyskinesia. *Acta Chir. Scand.*, **114**, 181-190

Daniel, O. (1972). The value of radiomanometry in bile duct surgery. *Ann. R. Coll. Surg. Eng.*, **51**, 357-372

Delmont, J. (1979). Personal communication

Delroy, C., Besancon, F., Pironneau, A. and Lopes-Macedo, L. (1965). Indication legitimes de la sphincterotomie oddienne sous conrole de la debrimetrie per-operatoire. *Rev. Int. Hepat.*, **15**, 985-997

Del Valle, D. Zinny, J. S. and Figueroa, M. (1965). Papillo-sphincterotomie. Indications et resultats. *Rev. Int. Hepat.*, **15**, 775-781

Demling, L. (1977). Endoscopic papillotomy and removal of gall stones. *J. R. Coll. Surg. Edin.*, **22**, 385-390

Devlin, H. B., Sahay, A. K., Tiwari, P. N., Galvin, P. B. and Peel, A. L. G. (1978). Cholecystectomy and a simple technique of operative cholangiography. *Br. J. Surg.*, **65**, 848-851

Dixon, J. A. and Engler, T. (1971). Growing role of early surgery in chronic pancreatitis: in a practical approach. *Gastroenterology*, **61**, 375-381

Doubilet, H. and Mulholland, J. H. (1956). An 8 year study of pancreatitis and sphincterotomy. *J. Am. Med. Assoc.*, **160**, 521-528

Dubois, F. S. and Hunt, E. A. (1932). Peristalsis of the common bile duct in the opossum. *Anat. Rec.*, **53**, 587-598

Eickhorn, E. P. and Boyden, E. A. (1955). The choledochoduodenal junction in the dog—a restudy of Oddi's sphincter. *Am. J. Anat.*, **97**, 431-451

Eisman, B., Brown, W. H., Virabutr, S. and Gottesfeld, S. (1959). Sphincterotomy: an evaluation of its physiologic rationale. *Arch. Surg.*, **79**, 294-297

Elman, R. and McMaster, P. D. (1926). The physiological variations in resistance to bile flow to the intestine. *J. Exptl Med.*, **44**, 151-171

Fernandez-Cruz, L. and Pera, C. (1977). A histological study of the sphincter of Oddi. In *The Sphincter of Oddi, Proc. 3rd Gastroenterol. Symp., Nice* (ed. J. Delmont), Karger, Basle, pp.13-20

Fernandez-Cruz, L., Pujol-Soler, R. and Pera, C. (1975). Dynamic morphology of the distal end of the common bile duct. *Chir. Gastroenterol.*, **9**, 379-384

Finnis, D. and Rowntree, T. (1977). Choledochoscope in exploration of the common bile duct. *Br. J. Surg.*, **64**, 661-664

Floquet, J., Laurent, J., Plenat, F. and Watrin, B. (1977). Is the sphincter of Oddi a reality in man? In *The Sphincter of Oddi, Proc. 3rd Gastroenterol. Symp., Nice* (ed. J. Delmont), Karger, Basle, pp. 21-24

Freund, H., Charuzi, I., Granit, G., Berlatzky, Y. and Eyal, J. (1977). Choledochoduodenostomy in the treatment of benign biliary tract disease. *Arch. Surg.*, **112**, 1032-1034

Gaensler, E. A. and McGowan, J. M. (1950). Activity of some newer spasmolytic agents on the biliary tract of man: a comparative study of isoprophyl-norepinephrine, actiphenine hydrochloride, methylamino-iso-octene and khellin. *J. Pharmacol. Exptl Therap.*, **99**, 304-311

Gennen, J. E., Hogan, W. J., Dodds, W. J., Stewart, E. T. and Arndorfer, R. C. (1980). Intraluminal pressure recording from the human sphincter of Oddi. *Gastroenterology*, **78**, 317-324

Germain, M., Martin, E. and Gremillet, C. (1977). Comparative anatomical study of the choledochoduodenal junction in man, pig, rabbit and rat. In *The Sphincter of Oddi, Proc. 3rd Gastroenterol. Symp., Nice* (ed. J. Delmont), Karger, Basle, pp. 6-12

Giermann, H. and Holle, G. (1961). Stereoskopische und mikroskopische intersuchungen zur pathologie des schleimhautre-liefs und klappenapparates de papilla vateri. *Acta Hepato-splenol.*, **8**, 189-205

Glisson, F. (1654). *Anatomia Hepatis*, 3rd edn, The Hague

Grage, T. B., Lober, P. H., Imamoglu, K. and Wangensteen, O. H. (1960). Stenosis of the sphincter of Oddi. A clinico-pathologic review of 50 cases. *Surgery*, **48**, 304-317

Hadfield, G. J. and Haziq ul Yaqin (1970). Obstruction to the lower end of the common bile duct. *Int. Surg.*, **54**, 142-152

Hallenbeck, G. A. (1967). Biliary and pancreatic intraductal pressures. In *Handbook of Physiology, Alimentary Canal*, Vol. 2 (ed. W. Heidel), Williams and Wilkins, Baltimore, pp.1007-1038

Hamilton, W. J., Boyd, J. D. and Mossman, H. W. (1964). *Human Embryology*, Heffer, pp.239-245

Hand, B. (1963). An anatomical study of the choledochoduodenal area. *Br. J. Surg.*, **50**, 486-494

Hauge, C. W. and Mark, J. B. D. (1965). Common bile duct motility and sphincter mechanism. I. Pressure measurements with multiple lumen catheter in dogs. *Ann. Surg.*, **162**, 1028-1038

Hayashi, A. (1963). Bioelectrographic study on the mechanism of bile discharge into the duodenum. *Fukuoka Acta Med.*, **54**, 307-329

Hedner, P. and Rossman, G. (1969). On the mechanism of action for the effect of cholecystokinin on the choledochoduodenal junction in the cat. *Acta Physiol. Scand.*, **76**, 248-254

Hendrickson, W. F. (1898). A study of the musculature of the entire extrahepatic biliary system, including that of the duodenal portion of the common bile duct and of the sphincter. *Bull. Johns Hopkins Hosp.*, **9**, 221-232

Hepp, J. (1966a). Oddites imaginaires et sphincterotomies abusives. *Ann-Chir.*, **20**, 343

Hepp, J. (1966b). Methodes d'exploration du sphincter d'oddi. *Ann-Chir.*, **20**, 372

Hepp, J. and Bismuth, H. (1966). Accidents et complications precoces de la sphincterotomie oddienne. *Rev. Int. Hepat.*, **16**, 497-519

Hess, W. (1961). *In Die erhrankungen der gallenwege unde des pankreas*, Georg Thieme, Stuttgart

Higgins, G. M. (1927). The extrahepatic biliary tract in the guinea pig. *Anat. Rec.*, **36**, 129-147

Higgins, G. M. (1928). Contraction of the gall bladder in the common bullhead (Amenorus nebulosus). *Arch. Surg.*, **16**, 1021-1038

Houssay, B. A. and Rubio, H. H. (1932). La function de la vesicula biliar injertoda y la hormona duodenocolec is loquinetica. *Rev. Soc. Argent. Biol.*, **8**, 369-378

Hunter, R. R. (1972). Choledochometry and transduodenal sphincterotomy. *Ann. R. Coll. Surg. Eng.*, **51**, 250-263

Ishioka, T. (1959). Electromyographic study of the choledochoduodenal junction and duodenal wall muscle. *Tohoku J. Exptl Med.*, **70**, 73-84

Ivy, A. C. (1934). The physiology of the gall bladder. *Physiol. Rev.*, **14**, 1-102

Ivy, A. C. and Oldberg, E. (1928). A hormone mechanism for gall bladder contraction and evacuation. *Am. J. Physiol.*, **86**, 599-613

Jacobsson, B. (1957). Determination of pressure in the common bile duct at and after operation. *Acta Chir. Scand.*, **113**, 483-488

Jacobsson, B. (1965). The morphology of the choledochoduodenal junction and the functional properties of the extrahepatic biliary ducts in cholecystectomised patients. *Rev. Int. Hepat.*, **15**, 939-952

Johnson, A. G. and Rains, A. J. H. (1972). Choledochoduodenostomy. A reappraisal of its indications based on a study of 64 patients. *Br. J. Surg.*, **59**, 277-280

Jones, S. A. and Smith, L. L. (1972). A reappraisal of sphincteroplasty (not sphincterotomy). *Surgery*, **71**, 565-575

Kappas, A., Alexander-Williams, J., Keighley, M. R. B. and Watts, G. T. (1979). Operative choledochoscopy. *Br. J. Surg.*, **66**, 177-179

Kasai, G. (1960). Electromyographic study on innervation of the choledochoduodenal junction. *Hirosaki Med. J.*, **11**, 293-299

Keighley, M. R. B. and Graham, N. G. (1973). The aetiology and prevention of pancreatitis following biliary tract operations. *Br. J. Surg.*, **60**, 149-152

Klune, G. A. (1964). Surgical anatomy of the common bile duct. *Arch. Surg.*, **89**, 995-1004

Koch, H., Rosch, W., Schaffner, D. and Demling, L. (1977). Endoscopic papillotomy. *Gastroenterology*, **73**, 1393-1396

Kourias, B., Tierris, E. and Papaevangelou, D. (1966). Resultats a distance de la sphincterotomie oddienne d'indication restreinte. *Rev. Int. Hepat.*, **16**, 581-585

Kreilkamp, B. L. and Boyden, E. A. (1940). Variability in the composition of the sphincter of Oddi: a possible factor in the pathologic physiology of the biliary tract. *Anat. Rec.*, **76**, 485-497

Leading Article (1977). *Br. Med. J.*, **3**, 75-76

Leading Article (1978). Bigger outlet for the bile duct? *Br. Med. J.*, **1**, 130-131

Leonard, P. and Massion, J. (1965). l'Apport pre-operatoire du medecin dans l'indication de la sphincterotomie. *Rev. Int. Hepat.*, **15**, 967-983

Le Quesne, L. P. and Whiteside, C. G. (1960). Discussion on cholangiography. *Proc. R. Soc. Med.*, **53**, 852-858

Liguory, C., Goverou, H., Chavy, A., Coffin, J. C. and Huguier, M. (1974). Endoscopic retrograde cholangiopancreatography. *Br. J. Surg.*, **61**, 359-367

Lin, T. M. (1971). Hepatic, cholecystokinetic and choldochal actions of cholecystokinin, secretin, caerulein and gastrin like peptides. *Proc. Int. Congr. Physiol. Sci.*, **9**, 1877

Lin, T. M. (1975). Actions of gastrointestinal hormones and related peptides on the motor function of the biliary tract. *Gastroenterology*, **69**, 1006-1022

Lin, T. M. and Spray, G. F. (1969). Effect of pentagastrin, cholecystokinin, caerulein and glucagon on the choledochal resistance and bile flow of dogs. *Gastroenterology*, **56**, 1178

Lin, T. M. and Spray, G. F. (1971). Choledochal, hepatic and cholecystokinetic actions of secretin, potentiation by cholecystokinin. *Gastroenterology*, **60**, 783

Lindenauer, S. M. and Child, C. G. (1966). Disturbances of liver functions in biliary tract disease. *Surg., Gynec. Obstet.*, **123**, 1205-1211

Lueth, H. C. (1931). Studies on the flow of bile into the duodenum and the existence of a sphincter of Oddi. *Am. J. Physiol.*, **99**, 237-252

Lurje, A. (1937). Topography of extrahepatic biliary passages with references to dangers of surgical technique. *Ann. Surg.*, **105**, 161-168

Luschka, H. (1869). Quoted by Hand (1963)

Lutkens, V. (1926). From Michels, N. A. (1955)

Madden, J. L., Chun, J. Y., Kandalaft, S. and Parekh, M. (1970). Choledochoduodenostomy. An unjustly maligned procedure? *Am. J. Surg.*, **119**, 45-52

Mahorner, H. and Browne, E. R. (1955). Results following transduodenal choledochampulotomy. *Am. J. Surg.*, **141**, 607-614

Maki, T. (1961). Functional independence of the muscle of Oddi from the duodenal wall muscle in bile flow mechanism. *Tohoku Igaku Zassi*, **63**, 36-48

Mallet-Guy, P. (1952). Value of pre-operative manometry and roentgenographic examination in the diagnosis of pathologic changes and functional disturbances in the biliary tract. *Surgery*, **94**, 385-393

Mallet-Guy, P. (1956). Die grandlager der peroperativen manometrie und cholangiographie. *Langenbecks Arch.*, **284**, 418-424

Mallet-Guy, P. and Dudfield Rose, J. (1956). Per operative manometry and radiology in biliary tract disorders. *Br. J. Surg.*, **44**, 55-68

Mallet-Guy, P., Feroldi, J. and Micek, F. (1950). Maladie du sphincter d'oddi. *Lyon-Chir.*, **45**, 181-199

Mallet-Guy, P., Kestens, P. J., Gignoux, M. and Murat, J. (1970). In *Syndrome Post-cholecystectomy*, Masson, Paris

Mann, F. C. (1919). A study of the tonicity of the sphincter at the duodenal end of the common bile duct (with special reference to animals without a gall bladder). *J. Lab. Clin. Med.*, **5**, 107-110

Mann, F. C., Foster, J. P. and Brimhall, S. D. (1920). The relation of the common bile duct to the pancreatic duct in common domestic and laboratory animals. *J. Lab. Clin. Med.*, **5**, 203-206

Meltzer, S. J. (1917). The disturbance of the Law of Contrary Innervation as a pathogenetic factor in diseases of the bile ducts and the gall bladder. *Am. J. Med. Sci.*, **153**, 469-476

Menguy, R. B., Hallenbeck, G. A., Bollman, J. L. and Grindlay, J. H. (1958). Intraductal pressures and sphincteric resistance in canine pancreatic and biliary ducts after various stimuli. *Surg., Gynec. Obstet.*, **106**, 306-320

Mester, Z., Vidra, G. and Dobos, I. (1952). Technique simplifie de la manometric biliaire per-operatoire. *J. Int. Chir.*, **12**, 20-31

Michels, N. A. (1955). *Blood Supply and Anatomy of Upper Abdominal Organs: with a Descriptive Atlas*, Lippincott, New York

Mirizzi, A. (1939). *Fisipatologia del Hepatocoledoco*, Buenos Aires

Mirizzi, A. (1942). Functional disturbances of the choledochus and hepatic bile ducts. *Surg., Gynec. Obstet.*, **74**, 306-318

Moreaux, J. and Teixeira, A. S. (1966). Les resultats eloignees de las sphincterotomie oddienne. *Ann. Chir.*, **20**, 340-342

Nana, A., Toader, C., Soltuz, V., Neumann, E. and Nana, M. (1963). The electrical biopotentials of the sphincter territories within the biliary pathway. *Gastroenterologia*, **100**, 182-198

Nebel, O. T. (1975). Effect of enteric hormones on the human sphincter of Oddi. *Gastroenterology*, **68**, 692

Negri, A. (1941). *La Histofisicopatología de la Vias Biliares*, Lopey, Buenos Aires

Niederle B. (1967). Sphincterotomy in biliary surgery. *J. R. Coll. Surg. Edin.*, **12**, 330-336

Nossel, H. L. and Efron, G. (1955). The effect of morphine on the serum and urinary amylase and the sphincter of Oddi: with some preliminary observations on the effect of alcohol on the serum amylase and the sphincter of Oddi. *Gastroenterology*, **29**, 409-416

Nuboer, J. F. (1931). Studien uber das extrahepatischen gallenwegessystem. *Erster Teil. Frankfurt Z. Path.*, **41**, 193-249

Oddi, R. (1887). D'une disposition a sphincter speciale de l'ouverture du canal choledoque. *Arch. Ital. Biol.*, **8**, 317-322

Ono, K., Watamabe, N., Suzuki, K., Tsuchida, H., Sugiyama, Y. and Abo, M. (1968). Bile flow mechanism in man. *Arch. Surg.*, **96**, 869-874

Øster, M. J., Csendes, A., Funch-Jensen, P. and Skjoldborg, H. (1980). Intraoperative pressure measurements of the choledochoduodenal junction, common bile duct, cysticocholedochal junction and gall bladder in humans. *Surg., Gynec. Obstet.*, **150**, 385-389

Peel, A. L. G. (1976). Thesis for Master of Surgery, University of Cambridge

Peel, A. L. G., Bourke, J. B., Hermon-Taylor, J., Maclean, A. D. W. M., Mann, C. V. and Ritchie, H. D. (1975). How should the common bile duct be explored? *Ann. R. Coll. Surg.*

Engl, **56,** 124-134

Peel, A. L. G., Hermon-Taylor, J. and Ritchie, H. D. (1974). Technique of transduodenal exploration of the common bile duct. *Ann. R. Coll. Surg. Engl,* **55,** 236-244

Peel, A. L. G. and Ritchie, H. D. (1974). Gilbert's syndrome in patients with gall bladder stones. *Ann. R. Coll. Surg. Engl,* **55,** 184-189

Persson, C. G. A. (1971). Excretory effect of tetrodotoxin on an isolated smooth muscle organ. *J. Pharm. Pharmacol.,* **23,** 986-987

Persson, C. G. A. (1972). Adrenergic, cholecystokinetic and morphine-induced effects on extra-hepatic biliary motility. *Acta Physiol. Scand., Suppl.,* **383,** 1-32

Persson, C. G. A. and Ekman, M. (1972). Effect of morphine, cholecystokinin and sympathomimetics on the sphincter of Oddi and intramural pressure in cat duodenum. *Scand. J. Gastroent.,* **7,** 345-351

Pi-Figueras, J. (1966). Indications et resultats de la sphincterotomie oddienne. *Rev. Int. Hepat.,* **16,** 487-496

Porsio, A. (1929). Contributo allo struttura della porzione intraparietale del dotto coledoco e del dotto pancreatico con special reguardo allo sfintere di Oddi. *Monitore Urol. Ital.,* **40,** 11-12, 265-268

Porsio, A. (1933). Studio sullo suiluppo della sfintere di Oddi dell' uomo. *Arch. Ital. Anat. Embriol.,* **30,** 603-625

Potter, J. C. and Mann, F. C. (1926). Pressure changes in the biliary tract. *Am. J. Med. Sci.,* **171,** 202-217

Reach, F. (1912). Untersuchungen zur physiologie und pharmakologie der gallenwege. *Zentr. Physiol.,* **26,** 1318-1325

Reynolds, B. M. (1966). Immediate effects of instrumental dilatation of the ampulla of Vater. Visual and histologic observations in man. *Am. Surg.,* **164,** 271-274

Ribiero, B. (1979). Personal communication

Ribiero, B. F., Cotton, P. B., Roberts, M. and Laurence, D. (1977). Duodenoscopic manometry of the bile duct and sphincter of Oddi. *Gut,* **18A,** 407

Rosch, W., Koch, H. and Demling, L. (1976). Manometric studies during ERCP and endoscopic papillotomy. *Endoscopy,* **8,** 30-33

Roux, M., Vayre, P. and Farah, A. (1965). Notre experience de la sphincterotomie oddienne. Indications et resultats. *Rev. Int. Hepat.,* **15,** 783-790

Salembier, Y. (1970). Etude critique de 207 observations de stenose oddiennes. *Ann. Chir.,* **24,** 1105-1110

Sandblom, P. (1933). Function of human gall bladder studies in connection with blood transfusions after stomach operations. *Acta Radiol.,* **14,** 249-258

Sandblom, P., Voegtlin, W. L. and Ivy, A. C. (1935). The effect of cholecystokinin on the choledochoduodenal mechanism (sphincter of Oddi). *Am. J. Physiol.,* **93,** 175-180

Sarles, J-C., Midejean, A. and Gayne, F. (1974). Etude electromyographique du sphincter d'Oddi. l. Technique et resultats chez le lapin 'in vivo' et 'in vitro'. *Biol. Gastroenterol.,* **7,** 19-27

Schein, C. J. and Beneventano, T. C. (1968). Choledochoduodenal junction stenosis in the post-cholecystectomy syndrome. *Surgery,* **64,** 1039-1046

Schreiber, H. (1944). Das Muskelapparat des duodenalen choledochusendes (papilla vateri) bein menschen. *Arch. Klin. Chir.,* **206,** 211-232

Schwegler, R. A. and Boyden, E. A. (1937a). The development of the pars intestinalis of the common bile duct in the human fetus with special reference to the origin of the ampulla of Vater and the sphincter of Oddi. I. The origin and involution of the ampulla. *Anat. Rec.,* **67,** 441-467

Schwegler, R. A. and Boyden, E. A. (1937b). The development of the pars intestinalis of the common bile duct in the human fetus with special reference to the origin of the ampulla of Vater and the sphincter of Oddi. II. The early development of the musculus proprius. *Anat. Rec.,* **68,** 17-42

Schwegler, R. A. and Boyden, E. A. (1937c). The development of the pars intestinalis of the common bile duct in the human fetus with special reference to the origin of the ampulla of Vater and the sphincter of Oddi. III. The composition of the musculus proprius. *Anat. Rec.,* **68,** 193-220

Sciacca, F. (1966). Anche per la sfinterotomia la verita' sta nel Giusto mezzo. *Rev. Int. Hepat.,* **16,** 479-486

Seifert, E. (1980). Complications of endoscopic sphincterotomy [Abstract], *International Biliary Association 2nd Annual Meeting*, 7

Shapiro, H. (1980). Endoscopic sphincterotomy—an American viewpoint [Abstract], *International Biliary Association 2nd Annual Meeting*, 6

Shennan, J. (1974). The value of operative post-exploratory T-tube cholangiography using an image intensifier with television monitoring. *J. R. Coll. Surg. Edin.*, **19**, 42-47

Shingleton, W. W. and Gamburg, D. (1970). Stenosis of the sphincter of Oddi. *Am. J. Surg.*, **119**, 35-37

Shore, J. M., Morgenstern, L. and Berci, G. (1971). An improved rigid choledochoscope. *Am. J. Surg.*, **122**, 567-578

Shore, J. M. and Shore, E. (1970). Operative biliary endoscopy: experience with the flexible choledochoscope in 100 consecutive choledocholithotomies. *Am. Surg.*, **171**, 269-278

Shore, J. M., Silverman, A., Siegel, M. and Bakal, M. (1971). Direct observations of the canine sphincter of Oddi. *Ann. Surg.*, **174**, 264-273

Stalport, J. (1964). A sensitive method for functional exploration of Oddi's sphincter. *Arch. Int. Pharmacodyn.*, **149**, 441-449

Stalport, J. (1965). Abord transoddien de la voie biliaire principale. *Rev. Int. Hepat.*, **15**, 791-801

Sterling, J. A. (1953). Significant facts concerning the papilla of Vater. *Am. J. Dig. Dis.*, **20**, 124-126

Tanaka, J. (1965). Electromyographic studies of the duodenum and choledochoduodenal junction. *Jap. J. Smooth Muscle Res.*, **1**, 50-71

Taniku, K. (1960). Study on the movement of the gall bladder and common bile duct with roentgenpneumatography and electromyography. *Mil Igaku*, **4**, 1838-1849

Terquen, J. (1969). Cent cas de sphincterotomie oddienne. *Bull. Soc. Chir. Paris*, **59**, 151-153

Thomas, C. G., Nicholson, C. P. and Owen, J. (1971). Effectiveness of choledocho-duodenostomy and transduodenal sphincterotomy in the treatment of benign obstruction of the common bile duct. *Am. Surg.*, **173**, 854-851

Toouli, J., Hogan, W. J., Glennen, J. E., Dodds, W. J., Arndorfer, R. A. and Stewart, E. J. (1980a). Variations in propagation of phasic pressure waves in the human sphincter of Oddi [Abstract], *International Biliary Association*, **41**

Toouli, J., Honda, R., Doods, W. J., Orlowski, J. M., Sarna, S. and Arndorfer, R. C. (1980b). Manometric and electromyographic features of the opossum sphincter of Oddi. *Gastroenterology*, **78**, 1279

Toouli, J. and Watts, J. M. (1972). Actions of cholecystokinin-pancreozymin, secretin and gastrin on extrahepatic biliary tract motility in vitro. *Ann. Surg.*, **175**, 439-447

Torsoli, A., Ramorino, M. L. and Carratu, R. (1973). On the use of cholecystokinin in the roentgenological examination of the extrahepatic biliary tract and intestines. In *Handbook of Experimental Pharmacology*, Vol. XXXIV, *Secretin, Cholecystokinin, Pancreozymin and Gastrin* (ed. J. E. Jorpes and V. Mutt), Springer-Verlag, Berlin, pp. 247-258

Torsoli, A., Ramorino, M. L., Colagrande, C. and Demaio, G. (1961). Experiments with cholecystokinin. *Acta Radiologica*, **55**, 193-206

Vassilakis, J. S., Chattopadhyay, D. K., Irvin, T. T. and Duthie, H. L. (1978). Primary closure of the common bile duct after elective choledochotomy. *J. R. Coll. Surg. Edin.*, **23**, 156-158

Vater, A. (1720). In Haller's *Disputationum Anatomicarum Selectarum*, Vol. 3, Gottingen, pp. 259-273

Vesalius, A. (1543). *De humani corporis fabrica lilri septum*, Basilea

Walters, W., Tama, L. and Magisano, J. (1961). Acute haemorrhagic pancreatitis and necrosis associated with choledochal sphincterotomy. *Surg. Clin. N. Am.*, **41**, 979-990

Warnes, T. W., Hine, P. and Kay, J. (1977). Intestinal alkaline phosphatase in the diagnosis of liver disease. *Gut*, **18**, 274-278

Warren, K. W. (1971). Chronic relapsing pancreatitis. In *The Craft of Surgery*, 2nd edn, Little Brown, New York, pp. 1289-1291

Watts, J. and Dunphy, J. E. (1966). The role of the common bile duct in biliary dynamics. *Surg., Gynec. Obstet.*, **122**, 1207-1218

Webb, W. R., e Guzman, V. C., Hoopes, J. E. and Doyle, R. A. (1964). Experimental evaluation of sphincteroplasty with and without long arm T-tubes. *Surg., Gynec. Obstet.*, **119**, 62-66

Whitaker, L. R. (1926). The mechanism of the gall bladder. *Am. J. Physiol.*, **78**, 411-436

White, T. T., Waisman, H., Hopton, D. and Kavlie, H. (1972). Radiomanometry, flow rates and cholangiography in the evaluation of common bile duct disease. *Am. J. Surg.*, **123**, 73-79

Wiechno, W. (1965). Sphincterotomy. *Rev. Int. Hepat.*, **15**, 999-1006

Wilkin, B. J. (1975). Primary closure of the common bile duct. *J. R. Coll. Surg. Edin.*, **20**, 115-119

Zinny, J. S. (1965). Choledoco-odditis retractil. *Pren. Med. Argent.*, **52**, 2403-2406

Zollinger, R., Branch, C. D. and Bailey, O. T. (1938). Instrumental dilatation of the papilla of Vater. *Surg., Gynec. Obstet.*, **66**, 100-104

7
The Pancreatic Sphincter

F. B. Keane and E. P. DiMagno

The pancreas was one of the last organs to receive the critical attention of early anatomists and physiologists; but since Langerhans described it histologically in 1869, its anatomy and physiology have been the subject of close scrutiny. The pancreatic sphincter mechanism, however, which normally should allow pancreatic secretion to flow into the duodenum and prevent reflux of bile or duodenal contents into the pancreatic ducts, has been difficult to study. Consequently, its physiological functions and the factors that control these functions are largely enigmatic.

The anatomy and physiology of the pancreatic sphincter mechanism in man cannot be understood without an appreciation of the anatomy and development of the pancreatic ductal system. Furthermore, since most physiological studies have been performed on laboratory animals, it is important to appreciate the comparative anatomy of these animals. Here we shall first review the pancreatic embryology and anatomy of man in detail and then the corresponding features of the most commonly used laboratory animals—namely the dog, baboon and cat. Next we shall review the physiology of the pancreatic sphincter mechanisms as interpreted from the data that have been collected by several investigators in studies of both animals and man.

ANATOMY

Human Anatomy

The pancreas first appears in the human embryo during the fourth week of gestation (Patten, 1968). Two outpouches, the ventral and the dorsal pancreas, develop from the endodermal lining of the duodenum (figure 7.1). The dorsal pancreas grows directly from the duodenum towards the

173

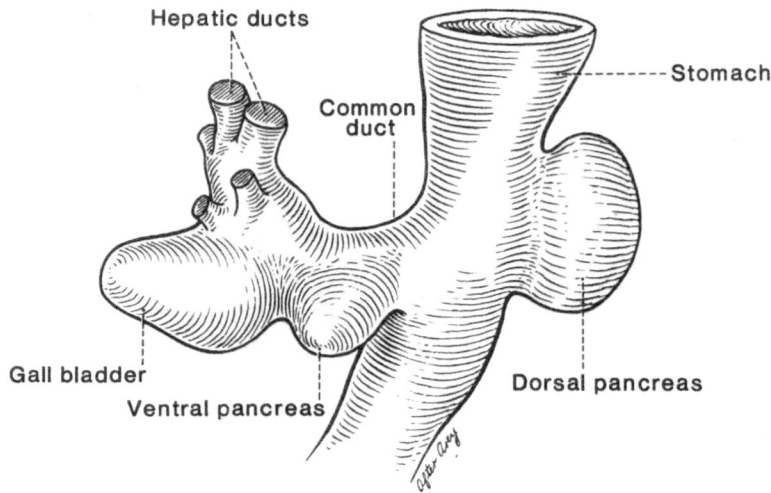

Figure 7.1   Pancreas at approximately 4 weeks of gestation (modified after Arey).

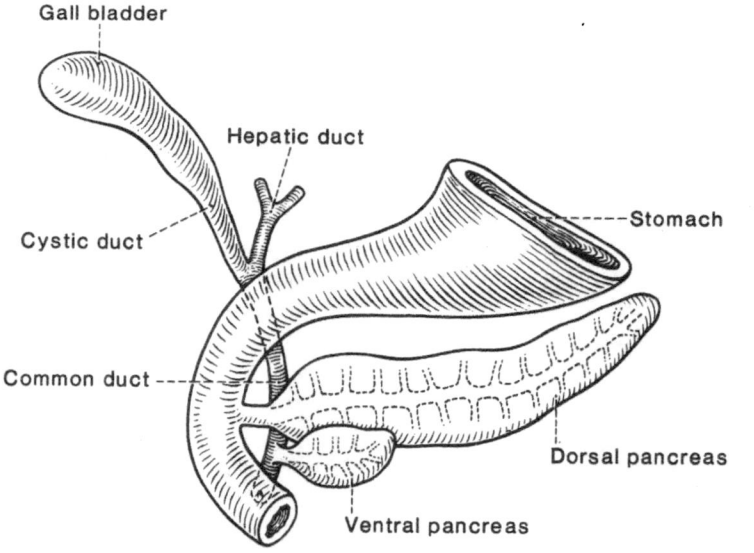

Figure 7.2   Pancreas at approximately 7 weeks. Fusion has occurred and ductular anastomosis is beginning (modified after Arey).

spleen and forms what later becomes part of the posterior wall of the lesser sac.

This portion of the gland empties into the duodenum via the accessory pancreatic duct (duct of Santorini). The ventral pancreatic bud is smaller and arises opposite the dorsal bud in conjunction with the bile duct. Later, owing to the uneven growth of the duodenum, the ventral bud rotates posteriorly; and eventually it is situated inferior to the dorsal pancreas. By the seventh week the ventral and dorsal buds fuse (figure 7.2). The dorsal component forms the tail, the body and part of the head of the pancreas; and the ventral pancreas forms the remainder of the head and the uncinate process.

Ducts

When the two pancreatic primordia fuse, their ductal systems also fuse, forming a main pancreatic duct. Most commonly the main pancreatic duct comprises parts of both the ventral and the dorsal ducts. Drainage of the main pancreatic duct into the duodenum is through the ventral pancreatic duct (duct of Wirsung), which unites with the common bile duct to form a common channel. In some cases the distal portion of this common channel dilates into an ampullary structure. Abraham Vater described this segment which now bears his name (the ampulla of Vater) as 'the place of mingling of bile and pancreatic juice' (Vater, 1748). The portion of the main pancreatic duct which drains the body and tail of the pancreas originates from the distal portion of the dorsal pancreatic duct. The more proximal portion of the dorsal pancreatic duct (Santorini) may open separately into the duodenum through the lesser papilla (figure 7.3) located proximal to the the major papilla, or end blindly, or be absent.

Indeed, anomalies in ductal fusion cause such diverse variations in the anatomy of the pancreatic ductal system that it is difficult to identify a normal pattern. Millbourn (1950) classified the most common ductal arrangements into three types. In type 1 (observed in 85.5 per cent of cases), the bile duct and the duct of Wirsung opened into the duodenum on the major papilla via a common channel, and the duct of Wirsung was the main avenue of drainage of pancreatic juice. The duct of Santorini could be absent or present and communicate or not communicate with the duct of Wirsung. In type II (5.5 per cent) the bile duct and the duct of the Wirsung had separate orifices on the major papilla. In type III (9 per cent) the duct of Santorini was the main route of drainage, and in some cases the duct of Wirsung was reduced to a fibrous cord.

Hand (1963), in a thorough review of 30 reports describing 3000 specimens, largely supported the findings of Millbourn, but further noted two important points. First, the minor papilla, though present in nearly all

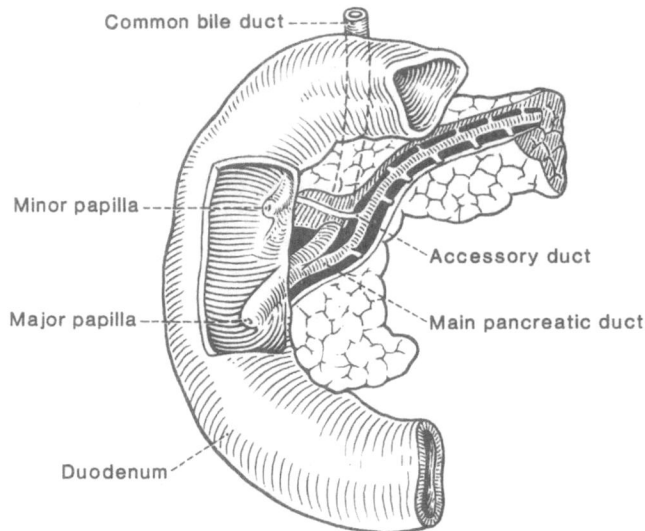

Common bile duct

Minor papilla

Accessory duct

Major papilla

Main pancreatic duct

Duodenum

Figure 7.3   Pancreas at birth (modified after Arey).

cases, was patent in only 60 per cent of cases. Second, in 75 per cent of cases the duct of Santorini communicated with the duct of Wirsung.

It has been suggested that the duct of Santorini may act as an important blow off or outflow valve (Berman *et al.,* 1960). Indeed, Mairose *et al.* (1978) found that a patent duct of Santorini significantly reduced the level of circulating pancreatic enzymes after endoscopic retrograde cholangio-pancreatography (ERCP). We therefore reviewed four studies in which a total of 375 specimens had been examined, and concluded that a patent duct of Santorini connected the duct of Wirsung with the duodenum in approximately 43 per cent of cases (Opie, 1903; Simkins, 1931; Schreiber, 1944; Rienhoff and Pickrell, 1945; Howard and Jones, 1947; Rösch *et al.,* 1976; Gregg, 1977; Cotton, 1979)

Recent preliminary data from the Mayo Clinic are in close agreement with these earlier works. In an autopsy study (Cubilla and Fitzgerald, 1975), 353 unfixed en bloc pancreaticoduodenal specimens were examined radiographically and anatomically. After injection of a 10 per cent formalin solution containing barium into the duodenal entrances of all ducts, stereoscopic X-rays were made. Specimens were studied anatomically by inserting a probe into the main pancreatic duct, filleting the pancreas and examining the relationships between ducts.

It was found that 74 per cent of the specimens had a common duct: 25 per cent with a *well-delineated ampulla* (defined as a common channel of the bile and pancreatic ducts which formed a bulbous, ampullary structure); 18 per cent with a *long common channel* (exceeding 3 mm in length, without an ampullary structure); and 31 per cent with a *short common channel* (less than 3 mm). The 26 per cent without a common channel comprised 7 per cent with an *interposed septum* (both ducts visualised as separate structures down to the duodenum, but entering it as a single opening) and 19 per cent with *separate openings* into the duodenum. The minor duct was identified in 38 per cent of the specimens. Similar to Hand's study (1963), when the minor duct was present, it emptied into the duodenum in 59 per cent and ended blindly in 41 per cent of the specimens.

Another variant of pancreatic duct anatomy is pancreas divisum, which has been observed during ERCP (Rösch *et al.*, 1976; Gregg, 1977). In pancreas divisum the two primordial pancreatic duct systems do not fuse but remain independent and drain separately into the duodenum (the ventral duct usually draining in conjunction with the common bile duct). It is said to be found in 2–3 per cent of post-mortem examinations. This anatomic variation may be important clinically, because chronic pancreatitis may develop in the portion of the gland drained by the dorsal duct (Cotton, 1979).

Sphincters

Whereas variation in pancreatic duct anatomy is extensive, pancreatic sphincter anatomy is no less complex. In most animals as well as in man, there is usually dual duct drainage into the duodenum, and therefore two sphincters might be expected. To demonstrate a true anatomical sphincter, the sphincter muscle should be shown to be separate from the surrounding duodenal muscle and, in the case of duct of Wirsung, to be independent of the common bile duct sphincter. Unfortunately, no anatomical study has clearly answered all questions about this difficult area.

Schreiber (1944) denied the existence of a separate muscle around the common bile and pancreatic ducts. He believed that the muscle of the ducts and duodenum was a single functional unit, 'the musculus complexus duodeni'. Boyden (1957a), however, after many years of study, concluded that there was a definite sphincter, independent of duodenal musculature. More specifically, in man he described two sphincteric muscle bands that might be capable of compressing the main pancreatic duct. One was a 'figure of 8' arrangement of muscle fibres that encircled both the bile and pancreatic ducts at their point of penetration through the gut wall, and the second was a common sphincter for both ducts, at the end of the papilla. Usually there was much less muscle around the pancreatic duct than the common bile duct. From a functional standpoint Boyden postulated that, in the presence of a common channel, contraction of the common sphincter might cause bile reflux into the pancreatic duct, whereas if the opening of each duct was separate, contraction of the distal sphincter would impede the flow from each duct. (Alternatively, from studies in the dog, we have suggested that separate openings of the bile duct and pancreatic duct could predispose to reflux of duodenal contents into the pancreatic duct, if duodenal pressure exceeds pancreatic duct pressure during relaxation of the pancreatic sphincter.)

Hand (1963) noted that the main pancreatic duct was free of surrounding muscle until it approached the duodenum. Thereafter it increased in amount until finally it surrounded the whole duct, producing a notch that can be seen macroscopically and radiologically. The pancreatic duct entered the duodenal wall with the common bile duct through the choledochal window, but their lumens never joined at this level. He found a common channel in 80 per cent of specimens, ranging between 2 and 17 mm in length and surrounded by muscular anatomy essentially similar to that found by Boyden. Hand further noted in all specimens that the major papilla projected into the duodenum to a variable extent. The orifice of the papilla was slit-like and frequently was filled by villus-like projections or valvules. Neither Boyden nor Hand reported whether the accessory (Santorini) duct of man possessed a separate sphincter muscle.

Animal Anatomy

Anatomical studies of the pancreatic sphincter have proven as difficult and complex in animals as in humans. One of the major criticisms of physiological studies on the pancreatic ducts of animals is that their anatomy and therefore their physiology are different from those of man. Further, the anatomical arrangements vary among species. However, there appear to be three generalisations that are true of both man and the animals that we have chosen to discuss. First, there usually are two ducts that drain pancreatic juice into the duodenum. Second, these ductal systems usually communicate within the gland itself. And third, one duct usually opens close by the opening of the common bile duct. In lower-order animals such as the hamster or rat the situation becomes more confusing, in that there are often several pancreatic ducts draining into the common bile duct, duodenum or both (Greene, 1935; Pour et al., 1977).

In regard to pancreatic anatomy, physiology and pathophysiology, the dog is the animal studied most extensively. The dog pancreas is C-shaped and lies across the dorsal wall of the abdominal cavity (figure 7.4). Its upper limb opposes the greater curvature of the stomach, and its lower limb is inside the curve of the duodenum (Miller, 1964). The upper limb or left lobe arises from the ventral primordial bud, while the lower or right lobe originates from the dorsal bud. There are two ductal systems but, in contrast to man, the dominant system or main duct is derived from the dorsal bud, which invariably drains both limbs of the pancreas through a separate opening into the duodenum about 8 cm below the pylorus. There

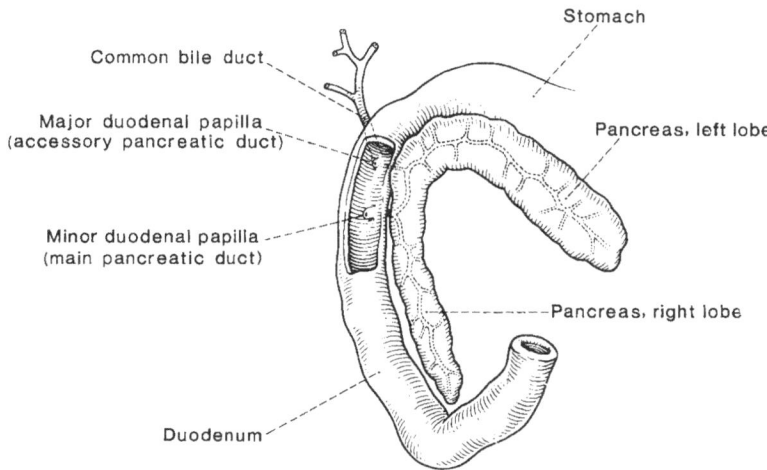

Figure 7.4   Normal ductular arrangement in the dog pancreas.

usually is a ventral or accessory duct that opens at the papilla with the common bile duct, some 4 cm proximal to the papilla of the main pancreatic duct.

Whereas the common bile duct of the dog passes obliquely through a tunnel of duodenal muscle, both the pancreatic ducts pass through the duodenal muscle directly (Eichhorn and Boyden, 1955). However, Keane *et al.* (unpublished) and Boyden (1957) have observed, around the submucosal portion of each of the pancreatic ducts, and especially the main duct, a substantial crescent of smooth muscle fibres and consider these crescents to be pancreatic sphincters.

Recently Tansy has studied the surface of the intramural portion of the major pancreatic ducts in the dog by light and electron microscopy and noted rounded mucosal surface convolutions that he interpreted as having a valve-like function in preventing reflux (Tansy *et al.*, 1977). We also have noted a constant specific mucosal structure around and within the pancreatic opening into the duodenum of the dog, which is different from the surrounding duodenal mucosa. Such arrangements might be analogous to the valvules at the opening of the common bile duct in man, described by Hand (1963).

The baboon has been suggested as a useful model for the study of pancreatic functions because the retroperitoneal position of the gland and the configuration of the ducts are similar to those in man (Bitter *et al.,* 1965). One anatomical study of five specimens revealed a common channel in two and a minor duct associated with interductal anastomosis in three. The baboon differs from man, however, in that the baboon minor duct enters the duodenum distal to the major papilla. Boyden (1966) described a definite bile duct sphincter in the baboon which is similar to that in man and consists of both superior and inferior portions. He also described superior and inferior sphincters around the accessory pancreatic duct within the minor papilla. However, the major pancreatic duct sphincters could not be separated as muscle groups distinct from the bile duct sphincter.

In the cat the common bile duct and the ventral pancreatic duct enter the duodenum through a window on the right lateral wall of the duodenum about 1.5 cm below the pylorus (Heuer, 1906; Boyden, 1957b). The ventral pancreatic duct (of Wirsung) is the main duct and is formed by the union of the ducts of the splenic and duodenal portions of the pancreas. The duct of the dorsal or accessory pancreas is smaller, and it anastomoses freely with branches of the main duct within the pancreas and opens into the duodenum 5–12 mm distal to the major papilla.

Because of the similarities in ductal anatomy between the cat and man, it has been suggested that the cat is a suitable model for study of pancreatic and biliary secretion and reflux. However, in the cat the common bile duct and pancreatic duct end in an 'ampulla' of Vater that differs from the human in that it is sacculated. Also, before the two ducts join, they lie adjacent separated by a specialised structure, the interductal septum, which is part of the duodenal muscle. The main pancreatic and bile duct sphincters of the cat are not clearly separate, and no accessory pancreatic duct sphincter has been described.

Despite variation of pancreatic sphincter anatomy in different species (particularly dogs and cats) and also within species, it appears that the innervation is similar in these animals. Kyösala and Rechardt (1974) studied the anatomy and innervation of the sphincter of Oddi in the cat and the dog and found dense innervation of this structure by cholinergic fibres. The anatomical structure of the sphincter indicates that, in contrast to the gut, it may have complex motor and possibly sensory functions (Kyösola and Rechardt, 1974, 1975). In addition, adrenergic transmission and adrenoreceptor function have been demonstrated in the cat sphincter of Oddi. This suggests that there is a neuroanatomical basis for the integration of finely graded motor activity which may play a part in secretory control and in prevention of reflux by the sphincter mechanisms (Persson, 1971).

PHYSIOLOGY

By definition, since the pancreas has a ductal system that delivers water, electrolytes and enzymes into the duodenum, it is classified as an exocrine gland. The pancreatic duct sphincter has two functions: first, to control the release of exocrine secretions into the duodenum, and second, to prevent duodenal contents or bile from refluxing into the pancreatic duct. However simple the idea may seem, investigation of these functions remains difficult because of anatomical size, variation and species difference. The pancreatic sphincter or sphincters have therefore remained elusive to direct examination, and what knowledge we have comes largely from the measurement of pancreatic duct pressures. Intrapancreatic ductal pressure is thought to reflect sphincteric activity, but other factors also have a part in intraductal pressure, as shown in figure 7.5. Here we shall review the experience of several investigators who have measured intrapancreatic ductal pressure in dogs and man, and then consider the part played by each of the factors listed in figure 7.5 in the modulation of this pressure.

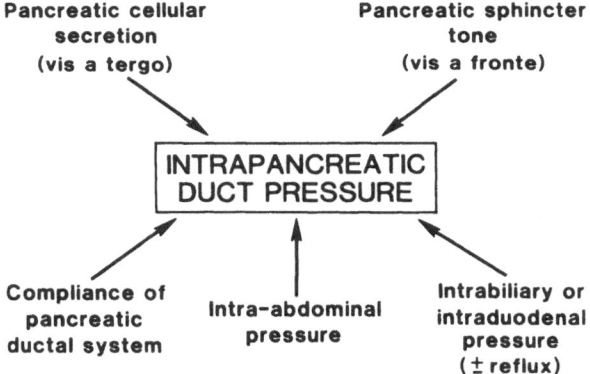

Figure 7.5   Factors influencing intrapancreatic duct pressures.

Intrapancreatic Duct Pressure

In early studies Jordan and Hallenbeck (1952) found the maximum secretory pressures of the pancreas in the dog after stimulation by histamine and beeswax to be about 44 cm of water. However, their experiments required occlusion of the ducts and creation of a pancreatic fistula, thereby excluding the pancreatic sphincter. Parry *et al.* (1955) were the first investigators to develop a method of recording pancreatic duct pressures in the chronic dog model without interfering with the sphincter mechanism, and they found the resting pancreatic duct pressure to be variable (mean of 9.1 cmH$_2$O) but consistently greater than the pressures in the common bile duct. It should be noted that they studied dogs resting on their sides and took their arbitrary zero as half the dogs' body thickness at the 11th rib. Subsequent studies have been performed with dogs standing in a Pavlov sling, and differences in the mean resting pressures can be accounted for by differences in the zero reference points.

Menguy *et al.* (1958) found that the pancreatic duct pressure varied from day to day and from dog to dog but averaged 14 cmH$_2$O. Again this pressure was consistently greater than the common bile duct pressure. Meals, alcohol and especially morphine increased the pancreatic duct pressure; atropine and epinephrine appeared to lower it. Intraduodenal acid or intravenous secretin produced no change in pressure, and the investigators concluded that a mere increase in the rate of external secretion of the pancreas did not alter intrapancreatic duct pressure.

Later, Owyang and co-workers (1977) found the mean fasting pancreatic duct pressures in the dog to be 28.9 cmH$_2$O, which was consistently higher than the mean duodenal pressure of 22.9. However, after a meal the mean pancreatic duct pressure rose to a peak of 45 cmH$_2$O at 75 min; and the duodenal pressure rose more quickly to a peak of about 48 cmH$_2$O at 45 min. They concluded that this postprandial pressure relationship might favour duodenopancreatic reflux.

Human pancreatic duct pressures were first recorded by Duval (1958), who measured pressures in nine patients with chronic pancreatitis after distal pancreatectomy and in four patients with cutaneous pancreatic fistulas due to trauma. The mean was 28.3 cmH$_2$O in the chronic pancreatitis group and 13.3 in the fistula group. Anderson and Hagstrom (1962), in a patient with a pancreatic fistula and a T-tube in the common bile duct, found the mean pancreatic duct pressure to be 24.4 cmH$_2$O and the mean common bile duct pressure 17. In this patient the mean pancreatic duct pressure diminished after meals to 22.9 cmH$_2$O, although there was an increase in the number of spike elevations of pressure. Both morphine and acid, when introduced into the duodenum, increased the pancreatic duct pressure; but alcohol had no effect. As in the dog, stimulation or depression of exocrine secretion did not have a pronounced influence on pressures in the pancreatic duct.

Endoscopic measurements of human pancratic duct pressures have now been reported by a number of authors; but these recordings, like those of Jordan and Hallenbeck (1952) in the dog, exclude the influence of pancreatic sphincter action. Gregg and Sharma (1978) measured the maximum secretory pressures in the pancreatic ducts after giving a bolus of secretin intravenously. The mean maximum secretory pressure was 40.3 cmH$_2$O in controls, 40.2 in patients with acute relapsing pancreatitis and 75 in patients with pancreatic carcinoma.

Bar-Meir *et al.* (1979) have studied biliary and pancreatic duct pressures in cases of suspected papillary stenosis from which other causes of biliary obstruction were excluded. Groups of three kinds were compared: control, suspected common bile duct obstruction, and idiopathic recurrent pancreatitis. In most cases the basal and phasic pressures of the sphincter of Oddi were measured, as well as the gradients between duodenum and common bile duct and between duodenum and pancreatic duct. In all these measurements data from the idiopathic recurrent pancreatitis group were similar to those from the control group; but in the group with suspected common bile duct obstruction the pressure at the sphincter of Oddi and the gradient between duodenum and common bile duct were increased. In this group of cases no attempt was made to obtain the gradient between duodenum and pancreatic duct or the pressure at the pancreatic sphincter. The authors concluded that endoscopic manometry was a useful procedure for identifying patients with papillary stenosis who might benefit from sphincterotomy.

Pancreatic Cellular Secretion

The *vis a tergo* contribution to intrapancreatic duct pressure is accounted for by pancreatic cellular secretion (figure 7.5). Pancreatic juice has two major components, an alkaline fluid and enzymes. The two components are secreted in variable proportions, depending on the stimulus. The alkaline fluid, rich in bicarbonate, arises from the centroacinar, intralobular and immediately extralobular ductular cells; the enzymes originate from the acinar cells. The control of exocrine secretion is both neural and hormonal, and only a brief description of these factors can be given in this review. Both vagus and splanchnic nerves play a part in the modulation of pancreatic secretion, although recently, with the advent of radioimmunoassay, hormonal control has received more attention. Gastrin, secretin and cholecystokinin-pancreozymin are the three primary gut hormones that regulate pancreatic secretion, but other hormones such as glucagon, vasoactive intestinal peptide, chymodenin, somatostatin, pancreatic polypeptide, motilin and bombesin may play a part. Other humoral agents such as serotonin, dopamine and prostaglandin may be implicated also. A complex relationship exists between the autonomic nervous system and the release of hormones and their effect on pancreatic acinar and ductal cells (Singh and Webster, 1978).

In essence, food intake stimulates pancreatic cellular secretion and pancreatic flow into the duodenum. Fasting has been presumed to bring about suspension or irregularity of pancreatic secretion. However, Keane *et al.* (1980) recently measured pancreatic secretion in the dog and related it to periodic duodenal interdigestive motor activity (figure 7.6). During phase I motor activity there was minimal secretion of pancreatic enzyme and bicarbonate; but secretory rate increased during phase II activity, and reached a peak immediately before the beginning of phase III. Peak enzyme outputs occurred earlier than peak bicarbonate outputs. From this study we concluded that fasting pancreatic secretion occurs regularly and is linked closely with the different phases of upper gastrointestinal motility. The factors that control fasting pancreatic secretion are probably different from

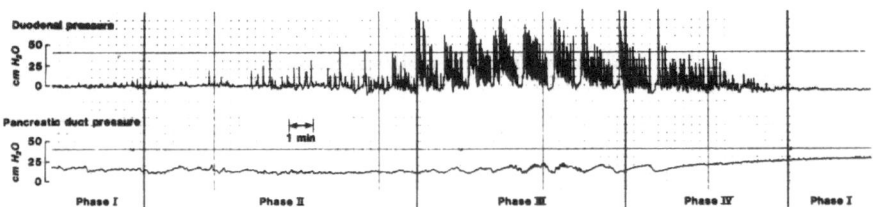

Figure 7.6   Simultaneous recording of duodenal and pancreatic duct pressures in the dog. The phases refer to periods of motor activity in the duodenum. Normally, during fasting, phase I activity lasts about 70 min, phase II 20 min, phase III 10 min and phase IV 5 min.

those that govern postprandial secretion. Disturbance of fasting intestinal motility (as by division of the bowel in creation of a pancreatic fistula) may disturb fasting pancreatic secretion. Finally, despite a tenfold increase of pancreatic secretory rate during phases II and III motor activity, there is only a small increase of intrapancreatic duct pressure during this time (DiMagno *et al.*, 1979; figure 7.6). This further suggests that increase of the pancreatic secretory rate does not appreciably alter intrapancreatic duct pressure, and it implies sphincteric relaxation.

Pancreatic Sphincter Tone

The *vis a fronte* component of intrapancreatic duct pressure is accounted for by pancreatic sphincter tone. The degree to which the duodenal muscle surrounding the pancreatic sphincter contributes to sphincter tone is unknown. Gilsdorf *et al.* (1967) infused saline into the pancreatic ducts of chronic dog preparations at a rate of 0.764 ml min^{-1} and found that the mean pressure at this rate was 18.3 cmH$_2$O. It increased with central sympathetic nervous stimulation, indicating an increase of sphincter tone, and decreased with central parasympathetic nervous stimulation, reflecting a decrease of sphincter tone.

Tansy *et al.* (1977) assessed sphincter tone in anaesthetised dogs by measuring opening pressure with a hydraulic ramp generator. He found the mean opening pressure to be 20–25 cm of saline. Vagotomy in these preparations gave no consistent results; but central vagal stimulation increased the opening pressure and increased the blood pressure, whereas peripheral vagal stimulation decreased both the opening pressure and blood pressure. Also, locally applied bethanechol increased the opening pressure and locally applied norepinephrine decreased it. From these observations, together with morphologic findings, the investigators concluded that the competence of the orifice of the canine pancreatic duct was accounted for by a mucosal flutter valve. The egress of pancreatic secretions, they suggested, depends on the state of mucosal congestion, which in turn is controlled by the local blood supply. It seems that the organised mucosal arrangement must certainly possess antireflux properties; but in contrast to Tansy and co-workers, we further believe that the consistent muscle sphincter arrangement surrounding the pancreatic orifice in the dog also is likely to have functional antireflux capability.

Indeed, Sankaran et al. (1978) have studied an isolated dog pancreatic sphincter preparation with use of a perfusion system and a drop counter. Their findings suggested that local application of acetylcholine and adrenalin caused contraction, whereas saline and atropine had no effect and caerulin produced relaxation.

Compliance of the Pancreatic Ducts and Intra-abdominal Pressures

Compliance of the pancreatic ductal system and its contribution to intrapancreatic duct pressure has not been studied, and the effects of changes in intra-abdominal pressure also need to be clearly documented. Anderson and Hagstrom (1962) confirmed the findings of Drye (1948) that changes in intraperitoneal pressures definitely influenced both biliary and pancreatic pressures in man. Since intra-abdominal pressure probably affects intraduodenal, biliary and pancreatic systems equally, the resultant pressures should be dependent on the respective volume and resistance to flow in each system.

Intrabiliary and Intraduodenal Pressures

Under most circumstances intrapancreatic duct pressure exceeds biliary pressure in both man and dog (Parry et al., 1955; Menguy et al., 1958; Anderson and Hagstrom, 1962). In man the main pancreatic duct usually joins the common bile duct, and therefore it is unlikely that biliary pressures influence intrapancreatic duct pressures. In the dog the main pancreatic duct opens into the duodenum apart from the bile duct, and it is known that the mean duodenal pressure can exceed mean pancreatic duct pressure, both during phase III fasting duodenal motor activity (figure 7.6) and in the postprandial period (Owyang et al., 1977; DiMagno et al., 1979). Mean intrapancreatic duct pressure does not rise proportionally with intraduodenal pressure. This lack of relationship between duodenal and pancreatic duct pressure suggests the action of a competent valve mechanism, which may be the mucosal valve mechanism, the pancreatic sphincter muscle or the sphincteric action of the duodenal muscle arranged around the duct orifice, or a combination of these possibilites. And yet, despite this competent valve mechanism, the pancreas is known to secrete both during the postprandial period and during phase III interdigestive activity (Keane *et al.*, 1980). As pancreatic pressures usually are above baseline duodenal pressures (figure 7.6), the pancreas must secrete during periods of duodenal relaxation.

An incompetent valve or sphincter mechanism would predispose to reflux of either bile or duodenal contents into the pancreatic duct, if the pressure relationships were suitable. Whether reflux of bile occurs in man under normal circumstances has long been a controversial issue. During operative cholangiography some reflux from the biliary tract occurs in 40 per cent of cases (Ivy and Gibbs,1952). However, in a review of over 2034 intravenous cholangiograms, Wise (1962) could find no evidence of reflux of contrast into the pancreatic duct. And we have been able to find reports of only three instances of reflux occurring during intravenous cholangiography (Yvergneaux, 1969; Ominsky, 1974).

In the dog, Rosato *et al.* (1971) were unable to induce consistent reflux, despite high pressures in a Pfeffer loop. Similarly, Rosenbaum *et al.* (1971) were unable to produce consistent reflux of contrast medium from the duodenum of cats with closed duodenal loops. However, more recent experiments have demonstrated reflux of small amounts of radioactive markers from the duodenum in dogs postprandially and from the biliary tree of rhesus monkeys (Becker *et al.*, 1979; Hendricks *et al.*, to be published). Even so, most of the data suggest that the pancreatic sphincteric mechanism is, under normal circumstances, essentially competent.

MEDICAL AND SURGICAL THERAPEUTIC IMPLICATIONS IN HEALTH AND DISEASE

The functional integrity of the pancreatic sphincter is of obvious importance in clarifying the aetiological factors in diseases of the pancreas and in deciding upon their treatment or prevention.

The concept that bile reflux into the pancreatic duct is secondary to blockage of its common channel by gallstones and could cause acute pancreatitis was first introduced by Opie (1901). Although impaction of stones in the common channel can be demonstrated in only about 5 per cent of patients with acute pancreatitis found at post mortem (Maingot, 1974), it is known that patients with acute pancreatitis and associated gallstones frequently pass gallstones in the faeces. This event usually is preceded by a relief of symptoms and rapid decrease of serum amylase and bilirubin concentrations (Acosta and Ledesma, 1974). Therefore, it is well accepted that gallstones and common duct stones are associated with acute pancreatitis.

However, much of the evidence incriminating bile reflux as a cause of acute pancreatitis is not convincing. In humans it has been noted that reflux of contrast medium from the bile duct into the pancreatic duct is possible at the time of operative cholangiography in patients who have no evidence of pancreatitis (Ivy and Gibbs, 1952). Experimental pancreatitis induced by injection of bile into the pancreatic duct is probably a non-specific effect—merely a manifestation of the destruction of the pancreas by marked raising of the intrapancreatic duct pressure. Furthermore, it is probable that the secretory pressure of the pancreas is sufficient to protect against bile reflux.

An alternative explanation for acute pancreatitis secondary to gallstones is that impaction or passage of a gallstone at the terminal end of the bile duct or through the ampulla might damage the sphincteric mechanism guarding against reflux of duodenal contents into the pancreatic duct. Then reflux of duodenal contents (which contain enterokinase) and the activation of trypsinogen might induce acute pancreatitis. Several clinical situations have been described wherein reflux of duodenal contents into the pancreatic duct seems to cause acute pancreatitis. Examples include afferent loop distension after Billroth II partial gastrectomy (Perman, 1935), intestinal obstruction (Byrne et al., 1964) and duodenal distension (Dreiling et al., 1960; Keane et al., 1978). McCutcheon and Race (1962) were able to produce acute pancreatitis in dogs with a Pfeffer loop and an open pancreatic duct. They also showed that the presence of bile was not necessary to induce pancreatitis and that it could be prevented by ligating the pancreatic duct, a finding which has been confirmed by others (Wisniewski et al., 1963). Johnson and Doppman (1967) produced haemorrhagic pancreatitis in the rhesus monkey by administration of cholecystokinin and secretin together with duodenal distension. This suggests that a hormonal imbalance might also be contributory.

The aetiology of pancreatic cancer is unknown. However, good evidence suggests that environmental factors and cigarette smoking may be predisposing factors (Go and DiMagno, 1977). Reflux may be implicated by location of the majority of carcinomas in the head of the gland and by the 75 per cent preponderance of ductal carcinoma among histologic types (Cubilla and Fitzgerald, 1975). In an autopsy study at the Mayo Clinic, abnormal pancreatic duct histology has tended to be more frequent among cases wherein the duodenal orifices of the pancreatic and common bile ducts were separate (Cubilla and Fitzgerald, 1975).

Wynder (1975) has suggested that a link between cigarette smoking and pancreatic cancer could be accounted for by hepatic conversion of inactive precursors to carcinogens, which then reflux from the biliary tree into the pancreas. This concept is supported by Pour et al. (1974), who administered di-isopropanolnitrosamine, a potent carcinogen chemically related to nitrosamines present in tobacco smoke, to hamsters and produced ductal carcinomas very similar histologically to pancreatic ductal carcinomas in humans.

Much has been written on the value of sphincteroplasty in biliary and pancreatic surgery for the unclear pathologic entities variously described as papillary stenosis (Bar-Meir *et al.*, 1979), ampullary stenosis (Jones *et al.*, 1969), stenosis of the sphincter of Oddi (Shingleton and Gamburg, 1970; Vassilakis *et al.*, 1979), postcholecystectomy syndrome (Rothwell-Jackson, 1968), biliary dyskinesia (Cotton, 1977), papillitis (Acosta and Nardi, 1966), and non-calculous obstruction (Haff and Tormua, 1975). However, the place of sphincteroplasty for pancreatic disease remains uncertain.

White (1973) reported that stricture of the pancreatic duct sphincter can occur alone or in combination with a stricture of the sphincter of Oddi. For these lesions he recommended additional pancreatic duct sphincteroplasty and pancreatography. Bartlett and Nardi (1960) reported three cases in which pancreatitis continued to recur after Oddi sphincterotomy. Re-exploration in two of them disclosed inadequacy of the exposure of the duct of Wirsung, which required further division of the muscle sling around the lower ends of the common bile and pancreatic ducts. In the third case the duct of Santorini was the main pancreatic duct and its orifice was tightly stenosed, so a plastic correction of the orifice was done. None of the three patients had further episodes of pancreatitis.

Endoscopic sphincterotomy has little place in the treatment of pancreatic disease at the present time. Cremer has used this technique to remove stones from the duct of Wirsung, but others are more cautious about its use in pancreatic disease and it is specifically contraindicated in active acute pancreatitis (Third International Symposium, 1977; Ligoury and Loriga, 1978). Pancreas divisum may be associated with recurrent pancreatitis, and Cotton (1979) has reported successful treatment of two patients with this condition by endoscopic sphincterotomy.

Sphincteroplasty for the treatment of chronic relapsing pancreatitis has few advocates. The operations in common use are either some form of pancreatic duct drainage or resection of a variable amount of the gland (Editorial, 1977). However, Adson (1979) has pointed out that sphincteroplasty might provide satisfactory results in patients with only mild or moderate gross pancreatic parenchymal changes and no segmental ductal obstruction. Occasionally, in these cases, he performs a plastic repair of the pancreatic duct opening together with sphincteroplasty—the 'double' sphincteroplasty.

INVESTIGATIVE TECHNIQUES IN MAN AND POSSIBLE FUTURE ADVANCES

Pancreatic sphincter pressures in man have not been documented as have those at the sphincter of Oddi. Endoscopic cannulation of the pancreatic duct with the low-compliance, water-perfused, side-hole catheter, described by Andorfer, is likely to reveal a high-pressure zone at the pancreatic duct orifice (Arndorfer *et al.,* 1977). But a high-pressure zone may be intermittent, and isolated readings may be of little relevance to a patient's symptoms. However, accumulating knowledge of intestinal motility and the now-established link between pancreatic secretion and phases of fasting duodenal motility should provide an ideal background for study of pancreatic sphincter activity during and in the absence of predictable physiological secretion, both in animals and in man (Vantrappen *et al.,* 1979; Keane *et al.,* 1980).

REFERENCES

Acosta, J. M. and Ledesma, C. L. (1974). Gallstone migration as a cause of acute pancreatitis. *New Engl J. Med.,* **290,** 484-487

Acosta, J. M. and Nardi, G. L. (1966). Papillitis: inflammatory disease of the ampulla of Vater. *Arch. Surg.,* **92,** 354-361

Adson, M. A. (1979). Surgical treatment of pancreatitis: review of a series. *Mayo Clin. Proc.,* **54,** 443-448

Anderson, M. C. and Hagstrom, W. J. Jr. (1962). A comparison of pancreatic and biliary pressures recorded simultaneously in man. *Can. J. Surg.,* **5,** 461-470

Arndorfer, R. C., Stef, J. J., Dodds, W. J., Linehan, J. H. and Hogan, W. J. (1977). Improved infusion system for intraluminal esophageal manometry. *Gastroenterology,* **73,** 23-27

Bar-Meir, S., Geenen, J. E., Hogan, W. J., Dodds, W. J., Stewart, E. T. and Arndorfer, R. C. (1979). Biliary and pancreatic duct pressures measured by ERCP manometry in patients with suspected papillary stenosis. *Dig. Dis. Sci.,* **24,** 209-213

Bartlett, M. K. and Nardi, G. L. (1960). Treatment of recurrent pancreatitis by transduodenal sphincterotomy and exploration of the pancreatic duct. *New Engl J. Med.,* **262,** 643-648

Becker, J. M. Ti, T. K., Moody, F. G., McGreevy, J. M. and Nelson, J. A. (1979). A model of biliary pancreatic reflux. *Surgery,* **85,** 147-153

Berman, L. G., Prior, J. T., Abramow, S. M. and Ziegler, D. D. (1960). A study of the pancreatic duct system in man by the use of vinyl acetate casts of postmortem preparations. *Surg. Gynec. Obstet.,* **110,** 391-403

Bitter, J. M., Telander, R. L. and Hitchcock, C. R. (1965). A comparison of the pancreas of the baboon, dog and man using vinyl resin techniques. In *The Baboon in Medical Research,* Vol. 1 (ed. H. Vagtborg), University of Texas Press, Austin

Boyden, E. A. (1957a). The anatomy of the choledochoduodenal junction in man. *Surg. Gynec. Obstet.,* **104,** 641-652

Boyden, E. A. (1957b). The choledochoduodenal junction in the cat. *Surgery,* **41,** 773-786

Boyden, E. A. (1966). The pancreatic sphincters of the baboon as revealed by serial sections of the choledochoduodenal junction. *Surgery,* **60,** 1187-1194

Byrne, J. J., Reilly, P. S. and Toutounghi, F. M. (1964). Regurgitation in experimental pancreatitis. *Ann. Surg.,* **159,** 27-31

Cotton, P. B. (1977). ERCP: progress report. *Gut,* **18,** 316-341

Cotton, P. B. (1979). Pancreas divisum: a new cause for pancreatic pain and recurrent pancreatitis [Abstract]. *Gastroenterology,* **76,** 1116

Cubilla, A. L. and Fitzgerald, P. J. (1975). Morphological patterns of primary nonendocrine human pancreas carcinoma. *Cancer Res.,* **35,** 2234-2246

DiMagno, E. P., Hendricks, J. C., Go, V. L. W. and Dozois, R. R. (1979). Relationships among canine fasting pancreatic and biliary secretions, pancreatic duct pressure and duodenal type III motor activity—Boldyreff revisited. *Dig. Dis. Sci.,* **24,** 684-693

Dreiling, D. A., Kirschner, P. A. and Nemser, H. (1960). Chronic duodenal obstruction: a mechano-vascular etiology of pancreatitis. I. Report of 6 cases illustrating this clinical variety. *Am. J. Dig. Dis.,* **5,** 991-1005

Drye, J. C. (1948). Intraperitoneal pressure in the human. *Surg. Gynec. Obstet.*, **87**, 472-475

Duval, M. K. Jr (1958). The effect of chronic pancreatitis on pressure tolerance in the human pancreatic duct. *Surgery*, **43**, 798-801

Editorial (1977). Surgical treatment of chronic relapsing pancreatitis. *Lancet*, **i**, 460-462

Eichhorn, E. P. Jr and Boyden, E. A. (1955). The choledochoduodenal junction in the dog: a restudy of Oddi's sphincter. *Am. J. Anat.*, **97**, 431-459

Gilsdorf, R. B., Urdaneta, L. F., Delaney, J. P. and Leonard, A. S. (1967). Central nervous system influences on pancreatic secretion, sphincteric mechanisms, and blood flow and their role in the course of pancreatitis. *Surgery*, **62**, 581-588

Go, V. L. W. and DiMagno, E. P. (1977). The pancreas: pancreatic exocrine adenocarcinoma. *Br. J. Hosp. Med.*, **18**, 567-576

Greene, E. C. (1935). Anatomy of the rat. *Trans. Am. Phil. Soc.*, **27**, 1-370

Gregg, J. A. (1977). Pancreas divisum: its association with pancreatitis. *Am. J. Surg.*, **134**, 539-543

Gregg, J. A. and Sharma, M. M. (1978). Endoscopic measurement of pancreatic juice secretory flow rates and pancreatic secretory pressures after secretin administration in human controls and in patients with acute relapsing pancreatitis, chronic pancreatitis, and pancreatic cancer. *Am. J. Surg.*, **136**, 569-574

Haff, R. C. and Torma, M. J. (1975). Oddi sphincteroplasty in the management of complicated biliary and pancreatic disease. *Am. J. Surg.*, **129**, 509-512

Hand, B. H. (1963). An anatomical study of the choledochoduodenal area. *Br. J. Surg.*, **50**, 486-494

Hendricks, J. C., DiMagno, E. P., Go, V. L. W. and Dozois, R. R. (to be published). Reflux of duodenal contents into the pancreatic duct of dogs. Submitted to *Surgery*

Heuer, G. J. (1906). The pancreatic ducts in the cat. *Johns Hopkins Hosp. Bull.*, **17**, 106-111

Howard, J. and Jones, R. (1947). The anatomy of the pancreatic ducts: the etiology of acute pancreatitis. *Am. J. Med. Sci.*, **214**, 617-622

Ivy, A. C. and Gibbs, G. E. (1952). Pancreatitis: a review. *Surgery*, **31**, 614-642

Johnson, R. H. and Doppman, J. (1967). Duodenal reflux and the etiology of pancreatitis. *Surgery*, **62**, 462–467

Jones, S. A., Steedman, R. A., Keller, T. B. and Smith, L. L. (1969). Transduodenal sphincteroplasty (not sphincterotomy) for biliary and pancreatic disease: indications, contraindications, and results. *Am. J. Surg.*, **118**, 292-304

Jordan, G. L. Jr. and Hallenbeck, G. A. (1952). Effect of increased secretory pressure on canine pancreatic secretion. *Am. J. Physiol.*, **170**, 211-216

Keane, F. B., DiMagno, E. P., Dozois, R. R. and Go, V. L. W. Unpublished data

Keane, F. B., DiMagno, E. P., Dozois, R. R. and Go, V. L. W. (1980). The relationships among canine interdigestive exocrine pancreatic and biliary flow, duodenal motor activity, plasma pancreatic polypeptide, and motilin. *Gastroenterology*, **78**, 310–316

Keane, F. B. V., Fennell, J. S. and Tomkin, G. H. (1978). Acute pancreatitis, acute gastric dilation and duodenal ileus following refeeding in anorexia nervosa. *Irish J. Med. Sci.*, **147**, 191-192

Kyösola, K. and Rechardt, L. (1974). The anatomy and innervation of the sphincter of Oddi in the dog and cat. *Am. J. Anat.*, **140**, 497-521

Kyösola, K. and Rechardt, L. (1975). Electron microscopic observations on the innervation of the sphincter of Oddi in the dog. *Cell Tissue Res.*, **161**, 167-176

Liguory, Cl. and Loriga, P. (1978). Endoscopic sphincteromy: analysis of 155 cases. *Am. J. Surg.*, **136**, 609-613

McCutcheon, A. D. and Race, D. (1962). Experimental pancreatitis: a possible etiology of postoperative pancreatitis. *Ann. Surg.*, **155**, 523-531

Maingot, R. (1974). *Abdominal Operations*, 6th edn, Appleton-Century-Crofts, New York, p. 768

Mairose, U. B., Wurbs, D. and Classen, M. (1978). Santorini's duct: an insignificant variant from normal or an important outflow valve. *Endoscopy*, **10**, 24-29

Menguy, R. B., Hallenbeck, G. A., Bollman, J. L. and Grindlay, J. H. (1958). Intraductal pressures and sphincteric resistance in canine pancreatic and biliary ducts after various stimuli. *Surg., Gynec. Obstet.*, **106**, 306-320

Millbourn, E. (1950). On the excretory ducts of the pancreas in man, with special reference to their relationships to each other, the common bile duct and to the duodenum: a radiological and anatomical study. *Acta Anat.*, **9**, 1-34

Miller, M. E. (1964). *Anatomy of the Dog*, Saunders, Philadelphia

Ominsky, S. H. (1974). Intravenous cholangiogram contrast medium reflux into pancreatic duct in a patient with acute pancreatitis. *Radiology*, **111**, 97-98

Opie, E. L. (1901). The etiology of acute haemorrhagic pancreatitis. *Johns Hopkins Hosp. Bull.*, **12**, 182-188

Opie, E. L. (1903). *Disease of the Pancreas: its Cause and Nature*, Lippincott, Philadelphia

Owyang, C., Dozois, R. R., DiMagno, E. P. and Go, V. L. W. (1977). Relationships between fasting and postprandial pancreaticoduodenal pressures, pancreatic secretion, and duodenal volume flow in the dog. *Gastroenterology*, **73**, 1046-1049

Parry, E. W., Hallenbeck, G. A. and Grindlay, J. H. (1955). Pressures in the pancreatic and common ducts: values during fasting after various meals, and after sphincterotomy; an experimental study. *Arch. Surg.*, **70**, 757-765

Patten, B. M. (1968). *Human Embryology*, 3rd edn, Blakiston Division, McGraw-Hill, New York

Perman, E. (1935). Surgical treatment of gastric and duodenal ulcer. *Acta Chir. Scand.*, **77**, 142

Persson, C. G. A. (1971). Adrenoreceptor functions in the cat choledochoduodenal junction in vitro. *Br. J. Pharmacol.*, **42**, 447-461

Pour, P., Althoff, J. and Takahashi, M. (1977). Early lesions of pancreatic ductal carcinoma in the hamster model. *Am. J. Pathol.*, **88**, 291-308

Pour, P., Kruger, F. W. Chem, D., Althoff, J., Cardesa, A., and Mohr, U. (1974). Cancer of the pancreas induced in the Syrian golden hamster. *Am. J. Path.*, **76**, 349-358

Rienhoff, W. F. Jr and Pickrell, K. L. (1945). Pancreatitis: an anatomic study of the pancreatic and extrahepatic biliary systems. *Arch. Surg.*, **51**, 205-219

Rosato, E. F., Oram-Smith, J. C., Reber, H. A., Czernobilsky, B. and Rosato, F. E. (1971). Papillary integrity as a factor in pancreatic reflux. *Am. J. Surg.*, **121**, 13-15

Rösch, W., Koch, H., Schaffner, O. and Demling, L. (1976). The clinical significance of the pancreas divisum. *Gastrointest. Endosc.*, **22**, 206-207

Rosenbaum, H. D., Barker, E. G. Jr, Gibson, D. E. and Griffen, W. O. Jr. (1971). Reflux pancreatography: experimental observations in the cat. *Invest. Radiol.*, **6**, 321-325

Rothwell-Jackson, R. L. (1968). Sphincteroplasty in the treatment of biliary and pancreatic disease. *Br. J. Surg.*, **55**, 616-622

Sankaran, H. Fitzgerald, O. and McGeeney, K. F. (1978). Sphincteric mechanism of the main pancreatic duct in the dog: an experimental model of the isolated sphincteric preparation. *Digestion*, **72**, 221-228

Schreiber, H. (1944). Der muskelapparat des duodenalen choledochusendes (Papilla Vateri) beim Menschen. *Arch. klin. Chir.*, **206**, 211-232

Shingleton, W. W. and Gambourg, D. (1970). Stenosis of the sphincter of Oddi. *Am. J. Surg.*, **119**, 35-37

Simkins, S. (1931). Variations in the pancreatic ducts and the minor duodenal papilla. *Am. J. Med. Sci.*, **182**, 629-639

Singh, M. and Webster. P. D. III (1978). Neurohormonal control of pancreatic secretion: a review. *Gastroenterology*, **74**, 294-309

Tansy, M. F., Salkin, L. M., Innes, D. L., Martin, J. S., Landin, W. E. and Kendall, F. M. (1977). The occlusive competence of the duodenal orifice of the canine pancreatic duct. *Surg., Gynec. Obstet.*, **144**, 865-868

Third International Symposium of Digestive Endoscopy, Brussels, February 1977

Vantrappen, G., Peeters, T. L. and Janssens, J. (1979). The interdigestive complexes of man have both secretory and motor components [Abstract]. *Gastroenterology*, **76**, 1264

Vassilakis, J. S., Manolas, K. and Boundouris, J. (1979). Transduodenal sphincteroplasty. *Arch. Surg.*, **114**, 181-184

Vater, A. (1748). Dissertatio anatomica, qua novum bilis diverticulum circa orificum ductus cholidochi ut et valvulosam colli vesicae felleae constructionem ad disceptandum proponit, atque singularis utriusque structurae eximiam utilitatem in via bilis determinanda exponit. In Albrecht von Haller's *Disputationum Anatomicarum Selectarium*, Vol. 3, A. Vandenhoeck, Gottingen, pp. 259-273

White, T. T. (1973). Indications for sphincteroplasty as opposed to choledochoduodenostomy. *Am. J. Surg.,* **126,** 165-168
Wise, R. E. (1962). *Intravenous Cholangiography,* Thomas, Springfield, Ill., pp. 105-115
Wisniewski, C. Williams, H. T. G. and MacKenzie, W. C. (1963). An experimental study of pancreatitis following Pólya gastrectomy. *Can. J. Surg.,* **6,** 210-217
Wynder, E. L. (1975). An epidemiological evaluation of the causes of cancer of the pancreas. *Cancer Res.,* **35,** 2228-2232
Yvergneaux, J. P. (1969). Le reflux wirsungien à la lumière du cliché dentaire intra-abdominal, complément de la radiomanométrie. *Acta Gastroent. Belg.,* **32,** 225-263

8
The Ileocaecal Junction

T. W. Balfour

'The cause, perhaps, of a valve at the termination of the ileum is that the putrid contents might not regurgitate. If we understand the use of a valve we shall understand the use of a caecum.'

John Hunter (1728–1793)

Unfortunately, this mysterious valve has not yielded its secrets as easily as John Hunter predicted. Two hundred years later the standard textbooks of anatomy and physiology (whether pure, applied or surgical) still cannot tell us how the valve functions, other than to claim that it regulates flow from the ileum to colon. There is much specialised knowledge about the motility of the small intestine in man; somewhat less is known about colonic motility; and almost nothing about the junctional zone between the ileum and colon.

ANATOMY

The gross anatomical features of the ileocaecal junction in man and other animals are well described by Didio and Anderson (1968). Many of the minor variations described can be attributed to the state of the tissues at the time of fixation, and these are of little clinical significance.

Since the original description by Macewen (1904), there have been many isolated reports of direct observation of the ileocaecal junction in patients with the area surgically exteriorised. Such studies suffer from the disadvantage of surgical distortion and the effects of the underlying disease process or trauma for which the surgery was undertaken. The best observations of the dynamic appearance of the ileocaecal junction can now be obtained at colonoscopy, where it is routine practice to pass the endoscope as far as the caecum and even into the distal ileum. Under the

193

conditions of normal endoscopy the ileocaecal papilla appears as a smooth reddish projection, elliptical or hemispherical in shape, from 1.5 to 2.0 cm in diameter and projecting 1 cm above the pink folded mucosa of the caecum.

Studies of comparative anatomy are largely unrewarding, since the ileocaecal region varies so greatly in different animals—for example, the large convoluted caecum dominates the area in herbivores such as the rabbit and the opossum; the caecum becomes short and convoluted (almost appendix-like) in the dog; while in man the true caecum is simply the blind-ending pouch distal to the point of entry of the ileum. Embryologically, the ileocaecal junction appears to be primarily a sphincter, and the valve-like appearance is a secondary development (Beattie, 1924; Jit, 1956).

PHYSIOLOGY

The latest edition of a standard textbook of physiology (Guyton, 1971) states that the ileocaecal valve is controlled by 'various viscerosympathetic reflexes', including the ill-understood gastroileocolic reflex. The vague statement is probably a fair summary of present-day knowledge about the control mechanisms. Controversy has long raged as to whether the junctional zone between the ileum and the colon was a simple valve (Buirge, 1943), a sphincter (White *et al.*, 1934), or both (Ulin *et al.*, 1956). The physiological sphincter was demonstrated in dogs by Hinrichsen and Ivy (1931), who produced consistent contraction of the sphincter by stimulation of the sympathetic nerves or by distension of other viscera. However, the most detailed experiments, both *in vivo* and *in vitro*, were conducted by Gazet (1964a). He concluded that there was a definite anatomical sphincter in man with a mean length of 1.0 cm. There was a demonstrable physiological sphincter, confined to the anatomically defined area in man but extending beyond it into the terminal ileum in the dog. The sphincter contracted in response to sympathetic nerve stimulation, to adrenaline and noradrenaline, and to parasympathomimetic drugs; it relaxed with isoprenaline; and produced variable results after stimulation of the vagal nerves. Certain of these control mechanisms have subsequently been challenged, but there is little more to be gained clinically from such detailed study of the nervous control of the ileocaecal sphincter. Certainly the classical 'sympathetic' and 'parasympathetic' concepts serve only to confuse. There is some measure of agreement that *in vitro* the sphincteric muscle always contracts with acetylcholine and alpha-adrenergic stimulation, but relaxes to beta-adrenergic stimulation (Farrar and Zfass, 1967). The pharmacological basis of this sphincteric action and the exact neurotransmitters involved remain obscure. The effect of the gastrointestinal hormones on the physiological sphincter in man is not confidently known, although there is a suggestion that it is contracted by secretin but relaxed by gastrin. If proved, these latter observations will be most interesting, since they are diametrically opposed to the responses of the lower oesophageal sphincter.

Attempts have been made to study ileocaecal function in the dog by recording myoelectrical activity of the region from surgically implanted electrodes, both in intact animals and in isolated perfused preparations (Balfour and Hardcastle, 1978). These preliminary studies indicate that the ileal part of the sphincter complex shows uncomplicated small intestinal electrical activity; the colonic component is more difficult to record, but appears to have an intermittent slow wave; the anatomical junction between ileum and colon presents a narrow band of electrical silence. The significance of this is not clear, but McCoy and Bass (1963) recorded the same phenomenon at the pylorus. This band of electrical silence may simply represent recording artefact due to neutralisation of two electrical potentials or may add weight to the observations made by others in the cat (Weinbeck and Janssen, 1973), which suggest that the ileocaecal junction exhibits the electrical characteristics of a semi-permeable and selective electrical insulator. It is not known whether this applies to man.

TECHNIQUES OF INVESTIGATION

The ileocaecal junction is probably the most inaccessible portion of the gastrointestinal tract, which makes direct observation difficult. Until recently direct studies were limited to appropriately situated surgical (or traumatic) stomata. Such work is difficult to interpret, because of the artificial presence of the stoma, which may actually produce abnormal results. In addition, the adjacent intestine is usually abnormal from associated inflammatory bowel disease or mechanical trauma, and this may interfere greatly with myoelectrical and pressure records. Acute human studies under anaesthesia are rarely practicable, and their value under the depressant effect of general anaesthesia is debatable. The only significant advance in direct observation of the area has been the recent widespread introduction of colonoscopy. It is now possible to pass a colonoscope with comparative ease under minimal sedation into the caecum and inspect directly the ileocaecal valve of man. The gross anatomical features and ever-changing shape of the ileocaecal valve have been well recorded by this technique (Nagasako and Takemoto, 1973), but as yet no detailed information is available about its control mechanisms or the effects of the gastrointestinal hormones on sphincter function.

There have been a few good surveys of the radiographic appearance of the ileocaecal junction in man (Samuel, 1962; Berk and Lasser, 1975). Cineradiography, after barium enema, follow-through or small bowel enema, has demonstrated the variable appearances of the ileocaecal junction in man. For instance, there is a posterior insertion of the ileum into the caecum in 7 per cent of contrast examination. Ileal reflux occurs with a variable degree of caecal distension. During routine barium enema examination a hydrostatic pressure of 45 cm of barium will produce ready reflux in some patients, and yet in others the entire colon can fill with overflow from the anus before the ileocaecal sphincter becomes incompetent. During barium follow-through examinations the peristaltic waves in the ileum seem to stop short of the terminal narrowed intracolonic segment of ileum. The barium enters the colon as an intermittent flow rather than as the sharp spurts which are seen in the duodenal cap distal to the pyloric sphincter. The terminal ileum never seems to distend against the apparently closed sphincter, such as can be seen at the lower end of the oesophagus above the gastro-oesophageal sphincter. Unfortunately, the disadvantage of all such radiological studies is that the barium suspensions interfere with normal motility. In addition, the nature of the examination is such that the radiographic screening must be done with the patient non-ambulant, and usually lying supine. This is important, since normal walking movements are undoubtedly involved in 'normal' ileocaecal function. Many characteristic morphological appearances of the ileocaecal region have been reported during barium studies in man—including lipomas, Crohn's disease, intussusception and prolapse, and a bewildering variety of rare tumours, the commonest being carcinoid.

Other important radiological observations can be made in patients with colonic obstruction. It is a common clinical experience to see an abdominal radiograph showing a massively distended caecum which may go on to perforate before the ileocaecal valve allows of reflux into the ileum; and yet in others the degree of reflux is so great that the small bowel distension completely dominates the clinical picture. The reasons for this difference are unclear.

There have been a few enthusiastic reports of surface recordings of intestinal electrical activity, the so-called electroenterogram (Bertrand and Thillier, 1975; Fleckenstein, 1978). However, it is difficult to obtain reproducible myoelectrical records from the small intestine or the colon, and it seems highly unlikely that the more confusing electrical events of the ileocaecal junction will be revealed by this technique. As has been mentioned above, now that colonoscopy is a routine procedure in unanaesthetised patients, it should be possible to record motility and myoelectrical activity by introducing fine recording devices through the biopsy channel of the colonoscope or by attaching recorders to the instrument itself. Any results obtained by this method could be influenced by the presence of a large foreign body (the colonoscope) in the intestinal lumen and also by the effects of any patient sedation. If the colonoscope were removed, leaving the intraluminal recorders *in situ,* then the value of direct vision is lost and there is then uncertainty about the exact location of the sensors. It has been possible at surgical operation to introduce a fine needle electrode under the serosa of the intestine and to leave it *in situ* for several days afterwards (Taylor *et al.,* 1975). The electrode can then be safely withdrawn at the same time as the surgical drain. However, this technique has not been used to study the ileocaecal region.

The methods of obtaining chronic recordings in unanaesthetised experimental animals with surgically implanted electrodes (Balfour and Hardcastle, 1978) are, unfortunately, not applicable to man. Similarly, strain gauge transducers sewn on the serosal surface of the intestine show great promise for recording muscular activity (at least in experimental animals), but these have not yet produced reliable results from the ileocaecal region.

In general, therefore, the direct intraluminal recording techniques which can be used successfully to investigate the oesophagus and anal sphincters are difficult to use in the investigation of the ileocaecal region, because of its remoteness.

THERAPEUTIC IMPLICATIONS

The classical operation of a right hemicolectomy for carcinoma of the caecum or ascending colon may be followed by some degree of diarrhoea, but it is fair to say that the vast majority of patients adapt extremely well. It might be thought that the loss of a sophisticated flow-controlling mechanism such as the ileocaecal sphincter would produce much greater dysfunction. That this is not so is supported by experimental work in the dog (Singleton *et al.,* 1964), which showed that the ileocaecal valve resection itself had little effect unless combined with ileal resection. This is well known in clinical practice, although the analogy is not quite fair, as most patients who have ileal resections also have underlying inflammatory disease of the bowel. Gazet (1964b) postulated that the diarrhoea of the 'ileo-caecal syndrome' was due not so much to the removal of the ileocaecal valve as to the cathartic effect of bile passing directly into the large bowel.

Because of its assumed sphincteric function the ileocaecal segment has been used as a surgical replacement in situations where reflux is thought undesirable—both in urological surgery, where it was said to be 'an ideal substitute for ureter and bladder' (Gil-Vernet, 1965), and as a replacement for the stomach following total gastrectomy, where 'the ileo-caecal valve can function as effectively as the oesophago-gastric cardia' (Lee, 1951). Despite such early optimism, neither of the procedures has been generally adopted in surgical practice.

CONCLUSION

We can add little to John Hunter's opening remark. The ileocaecal sphincter appears to modify the entry of the ileal contents into the colon and seems to prevent free reflux from the colon into the ileum. Despite advances in modern investigative and recording techniques, we can say little more about its control or about the changes (if any) which take place in motility disorders, particularly those leading to diarrhoea. It is possible that detailed investigations into the control mechanisms and the effect of gastrointestinal polypeptides will be totally unrewarding; the ileocaecal junction, like the adjacent appendix, may be largely vestigial and totally lacking in physiological sophistication.

REFERENCES

Balfour, T. W. and Hardcastle, J. D. (1978). The identification of an electrically silent zone at the ileo-caeco-colic junction. In *Gastrointestinal Motility in Health and Disease* (ed. H. L. Duthie), MTP Press, Lancaster, pp. 407-409

Beattie, J. (1924). The early stages of the development of the ileo-colic sphincter. *J. Anat.,* **59,** 56-59

Berk, R. N. and Lasser, E. C. (1975). *Radiology of the Ileo-caecal Area,* Saunders, Philadelphia

Bertrand, J. and Thiller, J. L. (1975). L'electromyographic digestive externe. *Med. Chir. Dig.,* **4,** 327-331

Buirge, R. E. (1943). Gross variations in ileo-caecal valve; study of factors underlying incompetency. *Anat. Rec.,* **86,** 373-385

Didio, L. J. A. and Anderson, M. C. (1968). *The 'Sphincters' of the Digestive System,* Williams and Wilkins, Baltimore

Farrar, J. F. and Zfass, A. M. (1967). Small intestinal motility. *Gastroenterology,* **52,** 1019-37

Fleckenstein, P. (1978). Migrating electrical spike activity in the fasting human small intestine. *Am. J. Dig. Dis.,* **23,** 769-775

Gazet, J. C. (1964a). 'A study of the ileo-caecal regions; its surgical significance in man'. M.S. Thesis, University of London

Gazet, J. C. (1964b). The ileo-caecal valve syndrome. *Br. J. Surg.,* **61,** 371-374

Gil-Vernet, J. M. Jr (1965). The ileo-colic segment in urologic surgery. *J. Urol.,* **94,** 418-426

Guyton, A. C. (1971). *Textbook of Medical Physiology,* 4th edn, Saunders, Philadelphia, p. 749

Hinrichsen, J. and Ivy, A. C. (1931). Studies on ileo-caecal sphincter of dog. *Am. J. Physiol.,* **96,** 494-507

Jit, I. (1956). Structure and development of ileo-colic valve and its frenula. *Indian J. Med. Res.,* **44,** 361-373

Lee, C. M. Jr (1951) Transposition of colon segment as gastric reservoir after total gastrectomy. *Surg., Gynec. Obstet.,* **92,** 456-465

McCoy, E. J. and Bass, P. (1963). Chronic electrical activity of gastroduodenal area: effects of food and certain catecholamines. *Am. J. Physiol.,* **205,** 439-445

Macewen, W. (1904). The Huxley Lecture on the function of the caecum and appendix. *Lancet,* **ii,** 995-1000

Nagasako, K. and Takemoto, T. (1973). Endoscopy of the ileo-caecal area. *Gastroenterology,* **65,** 403-411

Samuel, E. (1962). In *Surgical Physiology of the Gastrointestinal Tract* (ed. A. N. Smith), The Royal College of Surgeons of Edinburgh, pp. 135-140

Singleton, A. O. Jr, Redmond, D. C. and McMurray, J. E. (1964). Ileo-caecal resection and small bowel transit and absorption. *Ann. Surg.,* **159**, 690-694

Taylor, I., Duthie, H. L., Smallwood, R. and Linkens, D. (1975). Large bowel myoelectrical activity in man. *Gut,* **16**, 808-814

Ulin, A. W., Shoemaker, W. G. and Deutsch, J. (1956). Ileo-caecal valve and papilla; observations relating to pathophysiology of acute colon obstruction. *Arch. Int. Med.,* **97**, 409-420

Weinbeck, M. and Janssen, H. (1973). Electrical control mechanisms at the ileo-colic junction. *Rend. Gastro-enterol.,* **5**, 128-129

White, H. L., Rainey, W. R., Monaghan, B. and Harris, A. S. (1934). Observations on nervous control of ileo-caecal sphincter and on intestinal movements in unanaesthetised human subject. *Am. J. Physiol.,* **108**, 449-457

9
The Rectosigmoid Junction Zone: Another Sphincter?

W. N. W. Baker and C. V. Mann

EVIDENCE FOR A RECTOSIGMOID SPHINCTER MECHANISM

The junctional areas between the different parts of the gastrointestinal tract are usually defined by valves or sphincters. This rule is almost universal, in so far as there is the cardiac sphincter between the oesophagus and the stomach, the pyloric sphincter between the stomach and the duodenum, and the ileocaecal 'valve' between the terminal portion of the small intestine and the commencement of the large bowel.

However, between the pelvic colon and the rectum no such sphincteric arrangement has ever been defined, although it is clearly recognised that colonic functions are profoundly different from those of the rectum. There would be every reason to suspect that a valvular or sphincteric mechanism ought to exist, even if proof were lacking. The reasons to support this statement may be summarised broadly under the following headings: anatomical, physiological, pharmacological, radiographic, clinical and histopathological.

Anatomical

Gray's Anatomy does not describe an anatomical arrangement that is specific for the rectosigmoid junction zone, although surgeons recognise that there is a narrowed area lying between the termination of the sigmoid (pelvic) colon and the top of the more ballooned rectal ampulla: this area is commonly described as the rectosigmoid junction, and malignant growths of the region are referred to as 'rectosigmoid carcinomas'. In broad terms, it lies opposite the brim of the pelvis, in front of the lumbosacral

201

promontory. This junctional zone is higher than the anatomists would recognise: they describe the rectum as starting opposite the third sacral vertebra, but they also agree that it is difficult to be sure where the sigmoid colon ends and the rectum begins. Detailed studies of the junction zone were carried out by Mayo (1917) and Prata (1955). Prata failed to establish that a specific anatomical arrangement existed in the area, and repudiated the idea that an anatomical sphincter was present at this site, although Mayo had reached the opposite conclusion.

Nevertheless, it is appropriate at this point to recall that no sphincter apparatus of a specific structural type appears to be present at the gastro-oesophageal junction, but since the pioneering work of Code (Fyke *et al.*, 1956) it is now commonly accepted that a physiological sphincter mechanism is present between the lower end of the oesophagus and the entrance into the stomach.

It is apparent from such studies that the functions of an area can be sphincteric in type without the necessity for a specialised anatomical structure to support the activity that is present in the area.

Physiological

It would not be a correct statement to say that the physiological activity of the rectosigmoid junction zone has been as sharply defined as for the gastro-oesophageal sphincter. Indeed, quite the reverse is the case. Early efforts to define a sphincteric zone by manometric methods proved unrewarding (Hill *et al.*, 1960; Ritchie *et al.*, 1962; Painter, 1964). Although Ritchie and Tuckey (1969) subsequently showed a high-pressure zone 17 cm from the anus (a figure which would agree with the 'surgical' point at which the rectum merges into the sigmoid colon), most observers have been more convinced of the lack of good data provided by manometric investigations of the region.

Nevertheless, it is now realised that the absence of such manometric data does not mean that a zone of functional sphincter-like activity cannot be present in this area. Manometric testing of the human pyloroduodenal function has also failed to provide evidence of a functioning 'sphincter' in the sense of a closed zone of high pressure that will open or shut less or more tightly according to the stimulus that it receives. In response to this difficulty posed by the lack of supporting manometric evidence from the pyloric zone when it was so clearly capable of regulating the emptying of the stomach contents, the sophisticated idea of an 'open sphincter' was propounded. By this concept, an area (such as the pylorus) that did not constantly exhibit such a high degree of tonus that its lumen was normally obliterated could on appropriate occasions shut tightly to oppose onward movement of contents, and subsequently relax again to allow progress of fluids and/or solids to be resumed. If such a 'sphincter' were tested by standard manometric methods involving fine perfused tubes or small balloons during its normal 'open' state, no discernible outline of a high-pressure sphincteric zone would be elicited.

By this reasoning the absence of convincing manometric data to define the presence of a sphincter at the rectosigmoid junction does not deny the possibility that a mechanism similar to the open-sphincter type could be active in this region. What little evidence there is would support the view that such a physiological apparatus does exist.

Pharmacological

In studies of the paediatric rectosigmoid muscle Trounce and Nightingale (1960) demonstrated that nicotine caused relaxation of the muscle of this area. Baker (1975) showed that circular muscle strips taken from this zone frequently relaxed when exposed to acetylcholine, but similar strips from the sigmoid colon showed consistently a contractile response.

When a clinician experiences difficulty in traversing the rectosigmoid junction zone with a sigmoidoscope, the manoeuvre can be facilitated by the administration of an anticholinergic drug (e.g. IV Buscopan) which will induce relaxation of the muscle of the junction.

This evidence is highly suggestive for the presence of a short zone possessing high intrinsic tone situated at the region of the junction between the sigmoid colon above and the rectum below. The work of Trounce and Nightingale (1960) would be compatible with the belief that the high intrinsic tone of the area was maintained through the ganglion cell network. Baker's work, which strongly supports this concept, will be considered in greater detail later in this chapter (see under 'Experimental observations').

Radiographic

Radiological 'sphincters' were described for this area by Templeton and Lawson (1931), by Bailli (1939) and by Templeton (1960). This area is well known to radiologists as one where resistance to barium inflow is encountered frequently, which on many occasions has to be reduced by the administration of an anticholinergic drug. Hughes (1970) has demonstrated a persistently constricted zone in the rectosigmoid junctional area by a plastic foam enema technique. On barium studies of the lower intestine, a constricted portion of bowel 1–2 cm long can be seen frequently between the sigmoid colon above and the rectum below.

Clinical

It has been remarked already that surgeons and endoscopists are aware that the area of the rectosigmoid junction can be very difficult to traverse with instruments. Frequently the difficulty seems to be caused by the presence of spasm in the junctional area, although it is apparent in many cases that the lumen has not been completely closed: this impression of a segment of high resistance is reinforced by those patients to whom an anticholinergic drug is given, when the area can be seen to actively relax to allow of easy progress of the instrument where beforehand it had been impossible.

O'Bierne (1883) described a sphincter at the rectosigmoid junction and related its presence to various disorders, especially constipation. More recently, evidence has accrued from the treatment of diverticular disease by myotomy (Reilly, 1966, 1969) that the muscle of the rectosigmoid junction is an important factor to take into account in relation to surgical management. Unless the muscle of this area is divided, the condition fails to remit: the parallel with the operative technique of myotomy at the gastro-oesophageal junction (Heller's procedure) for the treatment of achalasia is very striking. In both situations an area of resistance, caused by deranged neuromuscular activity, has to be overcome by a surgical technique designed to facilitate passage through the segment by reducing or abolishing segmental muscular resistance.

Histopathological

Morson (1963) has drawn attention to the muscular hypertrophy present in the walls of colectomy specimens removed for diverticular disease (or its complications). Diverticular disease affects the lower left colon more often than any other site, and the changes stop at the rectosigmoid junction and never involve the rectum itself.

Painter has done a great deal to investigate the physiological defects underlying the pathological changes (Painter, 1964, 1968, 1969, 1973; Painter and Truelove, 1964). Further studies have been carried out by other authors (Ritchie et al., 1962; Smith, 1970). All are in agreement that in diverticular disease the sigmoid colon exhibits increased muscular activity with higher than normal intraluminal pressures being recorded both at rest and in response to stimulation. The increased pressure responses are linked with the histological evidence of hypertrophic muscle in this disease, but do not tell us whether they are the cause of or result from the increased muscle mass. However, in 5 per cent of cases the muscle hypertrophy is the first and only abnormality present, and this is strongly suggestive that the muscle hypertrophy is the factor that is responsible for the increased contractile power, rather than vice versa.

Radiologists also agree that the colons of patients afflicted by diverticular changes show increased irritability to barium instillation, with excessive spasms and segmental contractile activity being observed. They describe 'pre-diverticular' changes with a corrugated appearance of the colon wall by barium enema examination. These changes are thought to be caused by the irritable hypertrophied muscle of the bowel wall, and precede the development of the mucosal out-pouchings which are characteristic of the established condition.

But if muscle hypertrophy is the first and universal accompaniment of acquired diverticular disease, this immediately raises the question 'what is the cause of the muscular hypertrophy?' Could it be that it is the normal response to an extra work-load which is being performed to overcome increased resistance at the rectosigmoid junction.

Because cumulative evidence from so many widely different sources seemed to point to the conclusion that the rectosigmoid junction zone was an area of change from propulsive (colonic) activity to storage (rectal) function, and that such a change could be explained most easily by postulating a mechanism of the 'open-sphincter' type at the rectosigmoid junction, it was decided to carry out a specific programme of investigations at St Mark's Hospital to study this possibility.

EXPERIMENTAL OBSERVATIONS

Since many competent observers had previously carried out numerous manometric studies of the rectosigmoid junction with largely inconclusive or ill-defined results, it was decided not to repeat such studies on intact human volunteers. Instead it was decided to make use of the many lower sigmoid colons and rectums that were removed substantially intact by the operation of abdominoperineal resection for carcinoma of the lower third of the rectum. It was found that by mounting these specimens in a perfusion circuit they could be kept in an excellent state for physiological experiments, often for many hours. Bucknell and Clarke (1967) had previously reported a preparation of isolated perfused colon segments, and this provided an impetus for establishing the basis of the perfusion technique with the assistance of Mr C. Cabré-Martinez, FRCS. The technique was subsequently developed and refined by one of the authors (WNWB), and the experiments carried out with this preparation were the foundation for his M.S. thesis (1975). The details of importance in the perfusion technique were as follows.

Perfusion was carried out through the intact inferior mesenteric artery attached to each specimen. Free venous drainage was allowed from the cut edges of the specimen: such free venous drainage prevented any rapid accumulation of oedema fluid in the specimen. The perfusate was

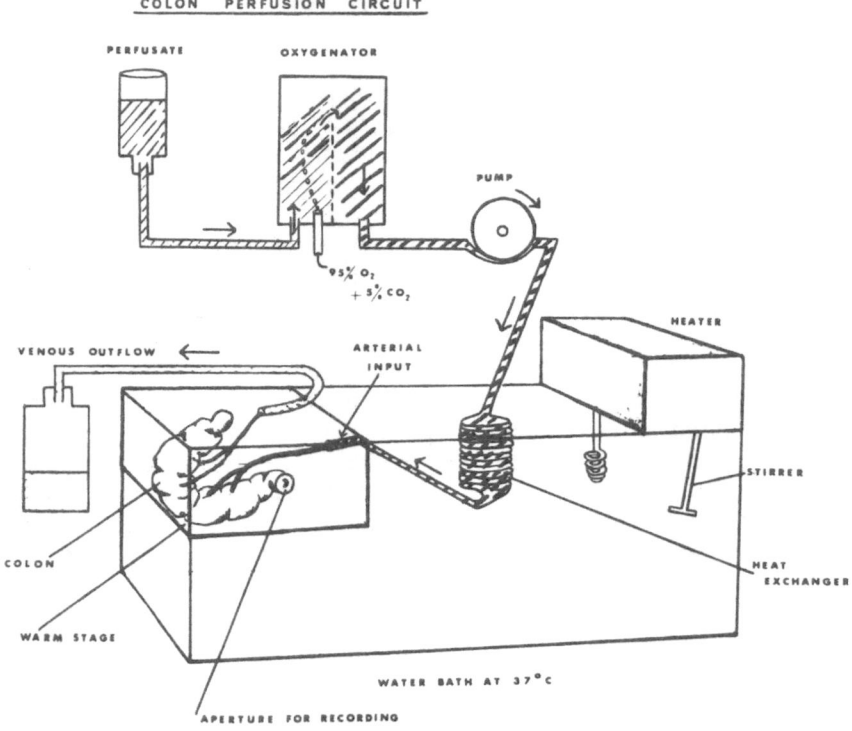

Figure 9.1   A labelled diagram of the various parts of the perfusion circuit (the thermistor probe for recording the temperature of the specimen is omitted).

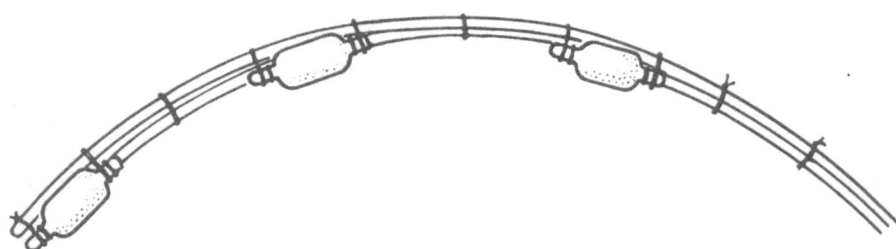

TRIPLE BALLOON SYSTEM

EACH BALLOON = 1·0 cm X 0·5 cm

Figure 9.2   The triple balloon system for recording intraluminal pressures (circular muscle contractions).

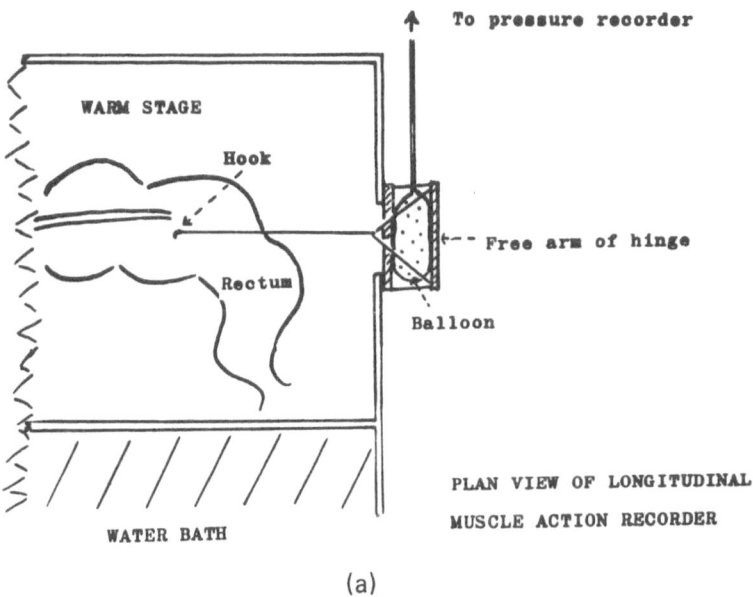

(a)

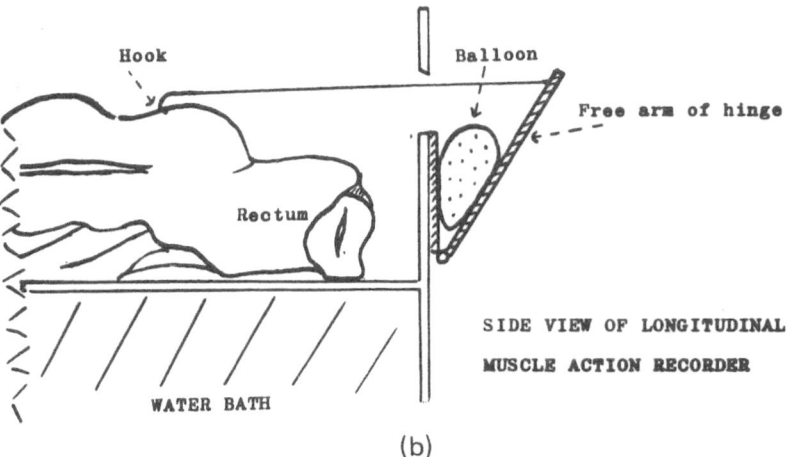

(b)

Figure 9.3   The hook-and-lever system for recording longitudinal (taenia) muscle shortening: (a) plan view; (b) side view. The degree of shortening was reflected by the magnitude of the squeeze on the balloon placed between the jaws of the hinge.

oxygenated Tyrode's solution with added 6 per cent Dextran (to preserve osmotic equilibrium), infused at a rate of between 10 and 18 cm³ min⁻¹. The solution was pre-warmed to 37.5°C and the whole specimen was mounted in a warm perfusion chamber (figure 9.1). Intraluminal pressures were monitored by three small (0.5 × 1.0 cm) air-filled balloons placed in tandem 5 cm apart and attached to an amplifying–recording apparatus (Schwartzer): each of these balloons delivered an individual pressure tracing and was considered to reflect mainly the contractile 'squeeze' response of the circular muscle (figure 9.2). Shortening was measured by a lever system attached by a hook and pulley to a taenia muscle: this system was considered to reflect the activity of the longitudinal (taenia) muscle (figure 9.3).

With this preparation, it was possible to demonstrate the following unique features of the rectosigmoid junction zone, which are best explained by the 'open-sphincter' postulate:

(1) The zone possessed intrinsic tone (higher than the sigmoid colon above or rectum below) which could be reduced by both nicotine and atropine.

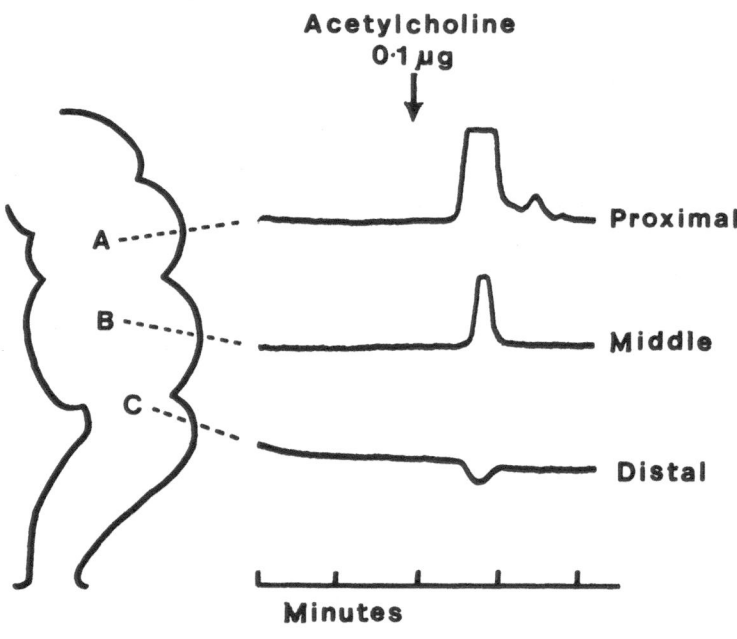

Figure 9.4   Relaxation response at the rectosigmoid junction of acetylcholine (0.1 μg). Note the simultaneous strong contraction of the muscle of the sigmoid colon.

(2) The zone was able to exhibit the ability to relax—both spontaneously as well as to physical stimulation (stroking or pinching/pricking the surface of the colon at this point (figure 9.4).

(3) The zone would relax to bolus injections of acetylcholine delivered through the inferior mesenteric arterial line. While the rectosigmoid junction zone relaxed, the muscle of the sigmoid colon above reacted conventionally by a contractile response (figure 9.5). This would be the expected response in a sphincter-like zone of resistance when a peristaltic propulsive wave descended down the left colon, driving a faecal bolus in front of it, and is directly analogous to the relaxation of the gastro-oesophageal sphincter in front of a typical oesophageal (swallow) peristaltic wave.

(4) The presence of regular slow rhythmic contraction waves in this zone plus the regular observance of waves of retrograde peristaltic activity starting at the rectosigmoid junction and progressing in a cephalad direction up the sigmoid colon.

The ability of the smooth muscle of the rectosigmoid junction to relax was verified by subjecting strips of circular muscle from the junction zone

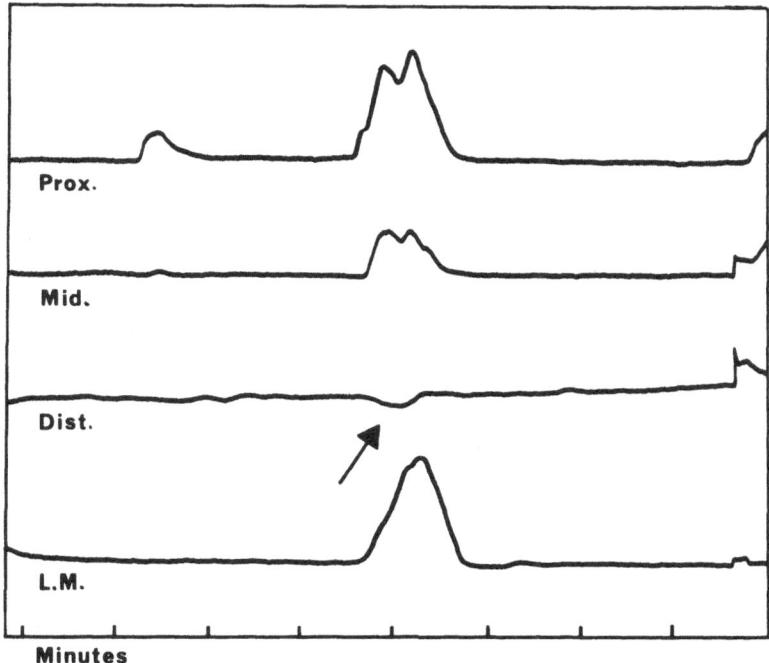

Figure 9.5   Spontaneous relaxation at the rectosigmoid zone (arrow). Note the simultaneous strong contractions in both the circular and the longitudinal muscles of the sigmoid colon.

to *in vitro* (water-bath) pharmacological testing by the technique devised by Fishlock (1966). The reaction of the strips to pharmacological agents was compared with similar strips taken from the sigmoid colon proper and tested simultaneously. In 25 separate paired experiments the circular muscle from the rectosigmoid junction zone relaxed in response to acetylcholine on 21 occasions, while the muscle from the sigmoid colon never relaxed on any occasion.

DISCUSSION

There is little doubt in the minds of most clinical observers familiar with the distal bowel that the area of the rectosigmoid junction zone is a recognisably distinct zone with its own behaviour patterns. It is not, however, an area that has anatomical definition.

The quite separate observations from widely different fields can be explained best on the postulate of an open sphincter, and there is experimental evidence to back up this concept.

In addition to conferring credibility on the observations of the 'normal' rectosigmoid junction zone, the concept of sphincter-like activity at the junction provides a more convincing background to the explanations currently held for the development of diverticular disease. If, through processes of ageing or neuromuscular degeneration, the rectosigmoid junction zone became unable to relax sufficiently to allow of unobstructed faecal pasage, a partial resistance would develop in the area: the sigmoid colon muscle would hypertrophy as a work response to this obstruction and all the histopathological processes would follow inexorably in their turn. Painter and Burkitt (1971) have drawn attention to the effects of faulty diet in inducing the changes of diverticulosis, and provide a good case for the hypothesis that this disease may be due to neuromuscular abnormality at the rectosigmoid 'sphincter'.

REFERENCES

Bailli, R. (1939). The sphincter of the colon. *Radiology*, 33, 372-376
Baker, W. N. W. (1975). Mural mechanisms controlling the motor activity of the human sigmoid colon and recto-sigmoid junctional zone. M.S. Thesis, University of London, pp. 126-131
Bucknell, A. and Clarke, C. (1967). An experimental method for recording the behaviour of human isolated colonic segments. *Gut*, 8, 569-537
Fishlock, D. J. (1966). The action of nicotine, histamine and 5-hydroxytryptamine on the circular muscle of the human ileum and colon in vitro. Ph.D. Thesis, University of London
Fyke, F. E., Code, C. F. and Schlegel, J. F. (1956). The gastro-oesophageal sphincter in healthy human beings. *Gastroenterologia*, 86, 135-150
Hill, J. R., Kelley, M. L., Schegel, J. F. and Code, C. F. (1960). Pressure profile of the rectum and anus of healthy persons. *Dis. Colon Rectum*, 3, 203-209

Hughes, L. E. (1970). A study of abnormal muscular patterns in diverticular disease of the colon using the polysiloxane foam enema. *Gut*, **11**, 111-117

Mayo, W. J. (1917). A study of the recto-sigmoid. *Surg., Gynec. Obstet.*, **25**, 616-621

Morson, B. C. (1963). The muscle abnormality in diverticular disease of the sigmoid colon. *Br. J. Radiol.*, **36**, 385-392

O'Bierne J. (1883). *New Views on the Process of Defaecation and their Application to the Pathology and Treatment of Diseases of the Stomach, Bowels and Other Organs*, Hedges and Smith, Dublin

Painter, N. S. (1964). The aetiology of diverticulosis of the colon with special reference to the action of certain drugs on the behaviour of the colon. *Ann. R. Coll. Surg. Engl.*, **34**, 98 – 119

Painter, N. S. (1968). The correlation of the pressures in the human colon with the shape of the colonic lumen as shown by cineradiography combined with simultaneous pressure recording. *Am. J. Dig. Dis.*, **13**, 468-479

Painter, N. S. (1969). Diverticular disease of the colon, a disease of this century. *Lancet*, **ii**, 586-588

Painter, N. S. (1973). In *Topics in Gastroenterology*, No. 1, *Diverticular Disease* (ed. Truelove and Sewell)

Painter, N. S. and Burkitt, D. P. (1971). Diverticular disease of the colon, a deficiency disease of Western civilisation. *Br. Med. J.*, **2**, 450

Painter, N. S. and Truelove, S. C. (1964). The intraluminal pressure patterns in diverticulosis of the colon. *Gut*, **5**, 201-365

Prata, P. (1955). Anatomical study of the transition between the sigmoid colon and the rectum with discussion of the so-called recto-sigmoid sphincter. *Arch. Chir. Klin. Exp.*, **18**, 39-86

Reilly, M. (1966). Sigmoid myotomy. *Br. J. Surg.*, **53**, 859-863

Reilly, M. (1969). Sigmoid myotomy; interim report. *Proc. R. Soc. Med.*, **62**, 715-717

Ritchie, J. A., Ardran, G. M. and Truelove, S. C. (1962). Motor activity of the sigmoid colon of humans. A combined study by intraluminal pressure recording and cineradiography. *Gastroenterology*, **43**, 642-668

Ritchie, J. A. and Tuckey, M. S. (1969). Intraluminal pressure studies at different distances from the anus in normal subjects and in patients with the irritable colon syndrome. *Am. J. Dig. Dis.*, **14**, 96-106

Smith, B. (1970). Disorders of the myenteric plexus. *Gut*, **11**, 271-274

Templeton, A. W. (1960). Colon sphincter simulating organic disease. *Radiology*, **75**, 237-241

Templeton, R. D. and Lawson, H. (1931). Studies in the motor activity of the large intestine. 1. Normal motility in the dog recorded by the tandem balloon method. *Am. J. Physiol.*, **96**, 667-676

Trounce, J. R. and Nightingale, A. (1960). Studies in Hirschsprung's disease. *Arch. Dis. Childhood*, **35**, 373-377

10
The Anal Sphincters

H. L. Duthie

STRUCTURE

External Anal Sphincters

The classical description of the external sphincter has been of a group of muscle fibres surrounding the anal canal and continuing with the pelvic floor at the edge, puborectalis portion, of the levator ani muscle. Studies have been made of this region by histological sections and by various methods of direct dissection. There has been considerable debate about the sub-divisions comprising the external sphincter. Initially it was described as being in three separate parts—subcutaneous, superficial and deep. Many authors supported this arrangement, which found its way into standard anatomy textbooks. The sphincter has also been described as consisting only of two parts—subcutaneous and deep (Goligher *et al.,* 1955). This dispute has been largely resolved by two studies using careful dissection together with meticulous histological examination of the structures in this region (Oh and Kark, 1972: Shafik, 1975). They show that part of the reason for the discrepancy in the previous findings is that the relationships of the various parts of the sphincter muscles are not the same around the circumference of the anus. Thus, while in the mid-line posteriorly three layers are not difficult to distinguish, in the lateral aspects of the anus the deep and superficial parts may quite well be fused, and unless they are traced either anteriorly or posteriorly, they could not clearly be separated. Even these studies do differ in some detail and this, again, may be due to different interpretations of the structures dissected out. Oh and Kark (1972) have clearly defined three layers of muscle in the external anal sphincter, as in the classical description. The subcutaneous part is below and outside the end of the internal anal sphincter and in their description is an annular muscle which is penetrated by longitudinal bands of conjoined smooth

213

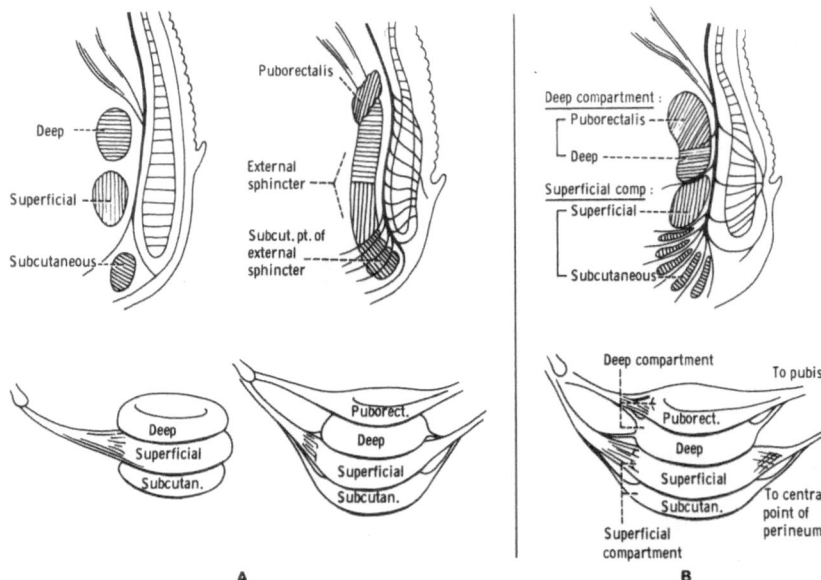

Figure 10.1 Coronal sections and diagrams of anteroposterior attachments of external anal sphincter. A: Above, showing bilaminar and trilaminar arrangements. Below, two suggested patterns of posterior attachments. B: Oh and Kark's concepts of three layers in deep and superficial compartments and both anterior and posterior connections for the components of the external anal sphincter. (Redrawn from Oh and Kark, 1972.)

muscle (figure 10.1). The superficial portion is elliptical in form, and above and slightly inside the subcutaneous part. Some fibres of the longitudinal muscle also penetrate the superficial portion, which has a major attachment posteriorly on the dorsal surface of the coccyx. The deep portion of the sphincter is fused with the puborectalis part of the levator ani and is mainly an annular muscle. Although describing three portions, these authors prefer to allow for the variation round the lateral aspect of the anal canal and describe the external anal sphincter as consisting of a part in the deep compartment (that is, the puborectalis and the deep muscle) and a superficial compartment which contains the superficial and subcutaneous. Their particular contribution has been to emphasise the difference in the anterior part of the anal sphincters between male and female, and their findings are clearly set out in figure 10.2. The other study (Shafik, 1975) also emphasises the presence of three layers in the sphincter. However, Shafik does not think that these three layers fuse posteriorly to become two layers. In addition, he has found that the subcutaneous layer is attached mainly anteriorly to the perineal body. Both groups are in agreement that the superficial layer of the sphincter, which Shafik calls the middle loop, is

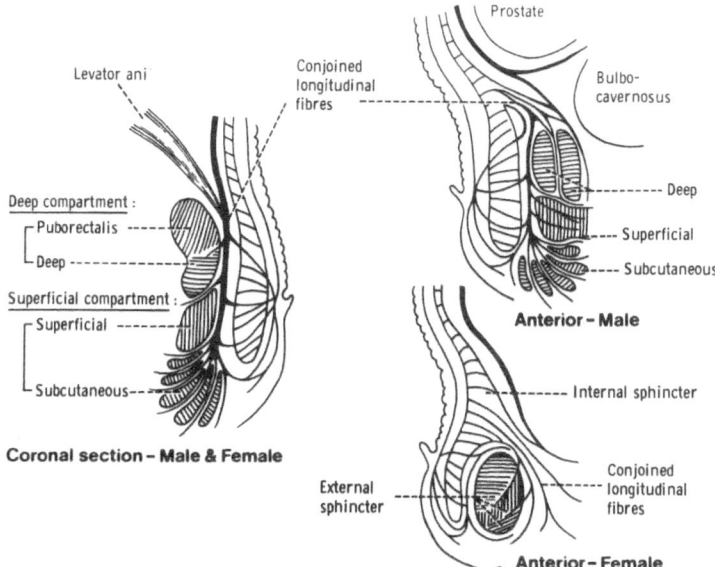

Figure 10.2   Diagrams of anterior parasagittal and coronal sections of the sphincter in the male and female. Anteriorly, the longitudinal fibres extensively encapsulate and ramify through the deep sphincter, as compared with the sparseness of longitudinal fibres laterally. In the male the conjoined long fibres envelop the deep external sphincter with occasional bisection of its muscle. However, the laminar pattern is well maintained. In the female all the external sphincters are encapsulated by conjoined longitudinal fibres. In both the male and female the longitudinal fibres join with sprouting fibres of the internal sphincter which firmly fasten the anal wall to the adjacent structures. (Redrawn from Oh and Kark, 1972.)

attached to the posterior aspect of the coccyx (figure 10.3). The deep portion of the sphincter or top loop is intimately blended with puborectalis in this study also but it does not show many circular fibres. In summary, the disputes concerning the number of anatomical divisions in the external anal sphincter have been largely resolved by the finding that there are variations around the anal canal. For ease of description and from the fact that these classical divisions have been used for so long, I think it would still be wise to consider that there are three layers which tend to be fused laterally into two layers.

Two types of striated muscle fibres have been identified in the external anal sphincter: a tonic type and a kinetic type. This has been done by analysis of responses in using electromyograms of the muscle (Kawakami, 1954) and also by differential histological staining techniques (Parks *et al.*, 1977).

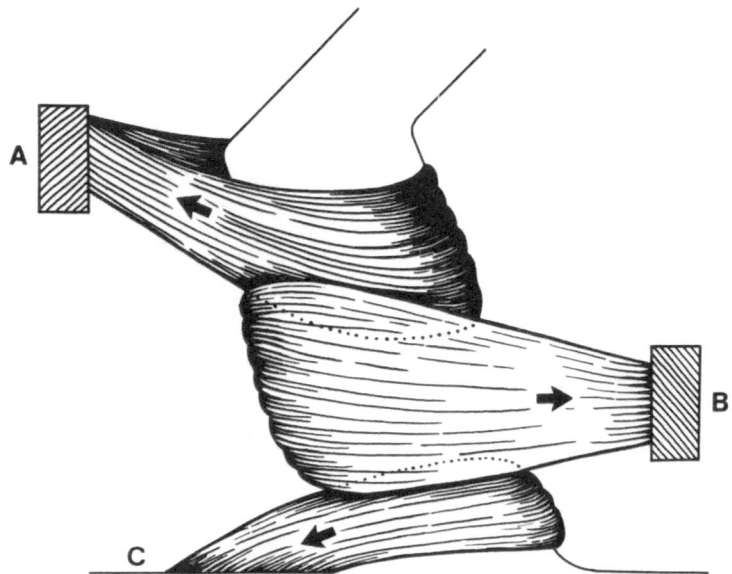

Figure 10.3   Diagram illustrating the triple-loop system of the external anal sphincter. A, top loop attached to pubis; B, intermediate loop attached to coccyx; C, base loop attached to perianal skin. (Redrawn from Shafik, 1975.)

Longitudinal Fibres

It has been generally agreed that a prolongation of the longitudinal smooth muscle coat of the rectum splits up in a fan-like manner and penetrates the fibres of the external anal sphincter to gain attachment to the skin around the anus. All agree that the subcutaneous portion of the external sphincter is split up into bundles by these processes, and most authors include part of the superficial sphincter in this. A much more complicated arrangement has been suggested on the basis of histological findings (Shafik, 1976), and three well-formed layers of longitudinal muscle were identified, each with a different origin and separated from the others by fascial septa (figure 10.4). The medial longitudinal muscle is innermost and related to the internal sphincter, and is the true prolongation of the longitudinal muscle coat of the rectum. The intermediate longitudinal muscle is apparently a direct prolongation of pubococcygeus and is only related to the lateral and posterior aspects of the anal canal. The third layer of the lateral longitudinal muscle is said to be a prolongation of the deep external anal sphincter. It is claimed that these longitudinal muscle layers have a role to play in the defaecation reflex.

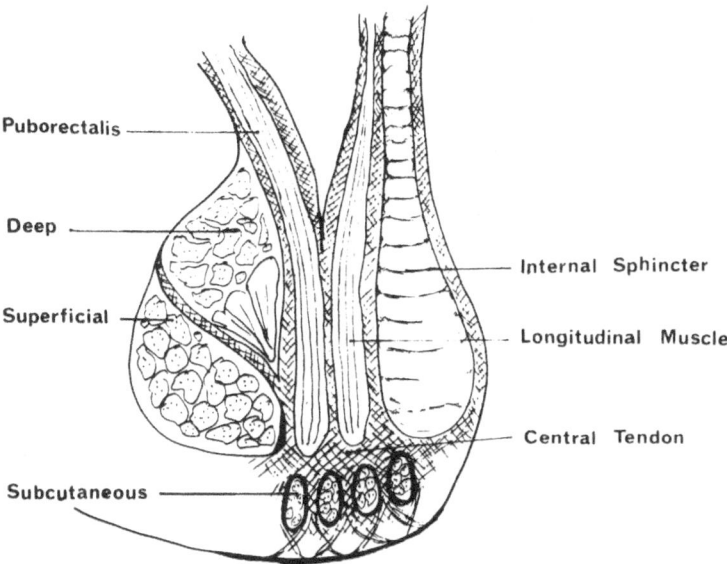

Figure 10.4   Diagram illustrates the structure of the longitudinal muscle and the related fascial septa. The fascial layers (indicated by cross-hatching) fuse into the central tendon and slips from this traverse the subcutaneous part of the external anal sphincter. (Redrawn from Shafik, 1976.)

Internal Anal Sphincter

This consists of a thickening of the circular muscle of the rectal coat. It lies within the external anal sphincter and extends from the puborectalis ring to the anal verge. It is penetrated by fibrous septa which are said to arise either from the longitudinal muscle itself or from the fibrous sheath surrounding it.

Nerve Supply

The external anal sphincter receives its innervation from the pelvic nerves—the subcutaneous portion from the inferior haemorrhoidal nerve, the superficial portion by the perineal branch of the fourth sacral nerve and the deep portion from branches of the pudendal nerve. Somatic sensation in the anal canal is found to just above the level of the anal valve, and this is subserved by a rich plexus of organised nerve endings (Duthie and Gairns, 1960; figure 10.5).

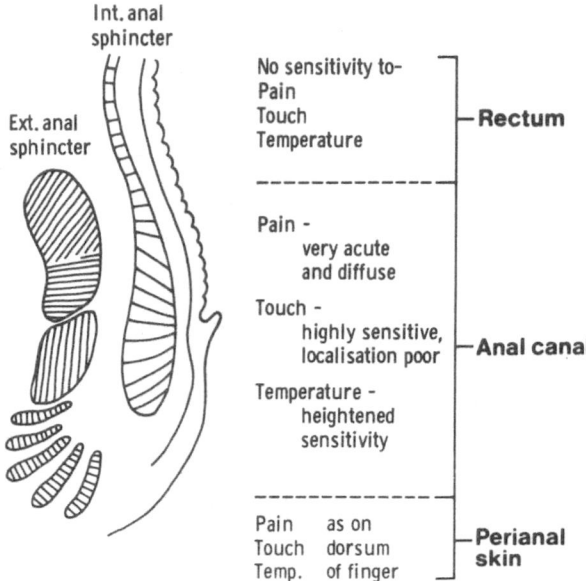

Figure 10.5 Diagrammatic representation of the distribution of appreciation of different sensory modalities (redrawn from Duthie and Gairns, 1960).

Anal Canal

As a result of the muscle distribution round it, the anal canal at rest is an anteroposterior slit rather than a fine line, with a rosette of mucosal folds (Phillips and Edwards, 1965). In addition, it is important to note that it makes with the axis of the rectum an anorectal deflexion angle, which averages about 80° in the patient standing, although it is reduced to 60° by full flexion of the hip-joint (Tagart, 1966). The anal canal is lined in its caudal part by stratified squamous epithelium to the level of the anal valves, which lie from 1.5 to 2 cm from the anal verge. At this level it changes to stratified columnar epithelium and about 1.5 cm further proximal becomes columnar epithelium. The line separating these latter two epithelia is rather wavy round the upper part of the anal canal, and it has been emphasised that the somatic sensation is present up to this line—that is, proximal to the anal valves.

FUNCTION

Extensive studies of the function of the anal sphincter have depended largely on measurement of pressure responses within the anal canal and as such are the result of the effects of both external and internal sphincters.

Pressure measurements have been made with fine tubes connected to transducers (Hill *et al.*, 1960), with balloons (Schuster *et al.*, 1963) and with obturators (Yanchev, 1963), and strain gauges have been used to measure force directly (Collins *et al.*, 1969). Attempts have been made by placing balloons in different parts of the canal to differentiate actions that are mainly due to the internal anal sphincter in the proximal part of the canal from those that are mainly external sphincter in the distal part. However, these muscles overlap to such a great extent that this distinction is hardly valid. The action of the external sphincter and the pelvic floor muscles can be measured by introducing electromyographic electrodes into them, usually by concentric needle electrodes (Kawakami, 1954; Parks *et al.*, 1962), but this can only give a qualitative assessment, as the actual force engendered may not necessarily reflect the activity of the muscle fibres adjacent to the electrodes. Similarly, with the internal anal sphincter, electrical measurements can be made of its activity (Kerremans, 1968; Wankling *et al.*, 1968). In many instances combinations of these techniques are used (Ihre, 1974).

In the Resting Subject

External Anal Sphincter

All the workers in this field have noted that the external anal sphincter, in contradistinction to striated voluntary muscle elsewhere, exhibits continual activity when the patient is at rest. This activity increases in time with respiration and when abdominal pressure is increased—for example, by a Valsalva manoeuvre. The response to distension of the rectum is initially a transiently increased activity when the balloon is inflated and again a short burst of spike activity when the balloon is deflated. Over a certain volume, usually about 150 ml of air, the activity in the external sphincter becomes inhibited, and this is felt to be the sequence of events in defaecation (Porter, 1962). Inhibition can also be elicited by moving a solid object in the anal canal (Kawakami, 1954).

Internal Anal Sphincter

Differential studies of pressure within the anal canal in patients before and after neuromuscular block of the external anal sphincter have shown that the internal anal sphincter contributes the major part of the pressure within the anal canal measured by fine tubes, but that when a small bolus such as a balloon is introduced, the external sphincter makes a contribution (Duthie and Watts, 1965). The tonic activity of the internal anal sphincter is reduced in the upper part of the anal canal in response to distension of the rectum. It is known as the internal sphincter or rectoanal reflex, and has been the subject of a large number of studies. It is present in almost all conditions in this area, including denervation, apart from patients with Hirschsprung's disease (Lawson and Nixon, 1967). It is shown to be intact in patients with spinal injuries (Frenckner, 1975), with sacral root resections (Gunterberg *et al.*, 1976), with sacral meningocoele (Meunier and Mollard, 1977) and even in some patients after resection of the rectum (Lane and Parks, 1977). Various theories concerning possible pathways for this reflex have each successively had to be modified as further study has shown the reflex still to be present even after resection of the rectum and substitution of the descending colon. It has been suggested that the distension acts through the 'rectal' wall and affects receptors in the puborectalis muscle and that by a local nerve net this then reflexly affects the internal sphincter itself.

Response to Rectal Distension

The three phases of response to distension of the rectum are found (figure 10.6). Initially a small distension mimicking some material entering the rectum from above results in a transient increase in the activity of the

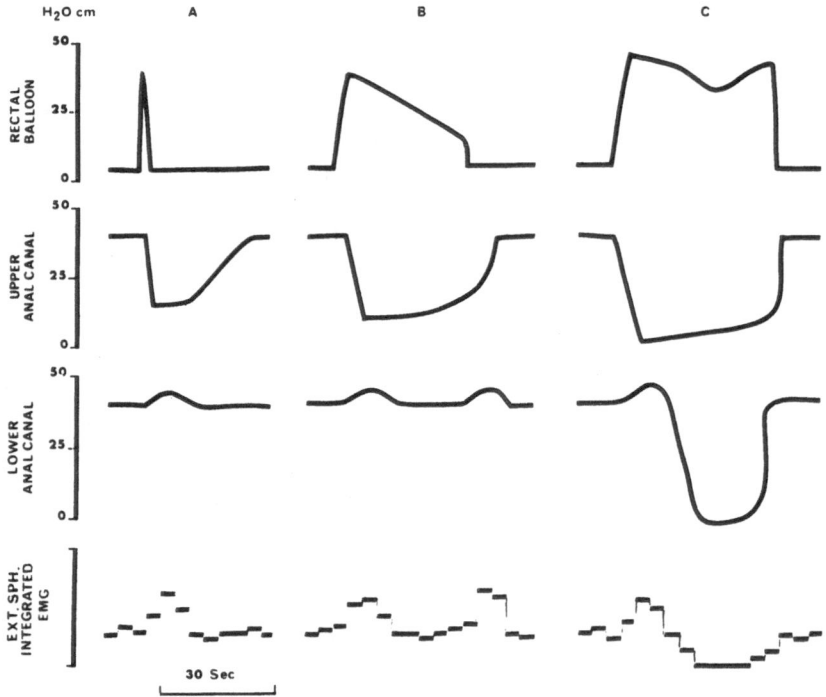

Figure 10.6 Diagram showing pressure recordings from rectal balloon and small balloons in the anal canal together with electromyography of the external anal sphincter complex. The responses of A (sampling), B (accommodation) and C (defaecation) are illustrated. (Redrawn from Duthie, 1975.)

external anal sphincter and a rise in intrarectal pressure. The rectum itselt accommodates to this and the pressure tends to return towards the resting pressure. When the balloon is deflated, there is again a transient increase in pressure and activity in the external sphincter. During the inflation period the internal anal sphincter itself is relaxed slightly. This reflex occurs even when the patient is not aware of any rectal sensation, and because rectal contents could contact the somatic sensory area of the anal canal, is known as the *sampling reflex.*

Next a slightly higher volume in the balloon is appreciated initially as an urge to defaecate, which passes off with relaxation of the rectum. The sphincteric responses are as above. This reflex is known as the *accommodation reflex* (Duthie, 1975).

Thirdly, a *defaecation response* occurs when a balloon in the rectum is blown up to sufficient level to reach the maximum tolerable volume (Ihre, 1974), when the rectum accommodation ceases and, in addition to the inhibition of the upper part of the anal canal, the external anal sphincter is inhibited and the bolus passed.

PATHOPHYSIOLOGY

Minor Anorectal Conditions

Haemorrhoids

When pressure in the anal canal is studied in patients with internal haemorrhoids, an increased incidence of ultra-slow pressure waves has been observed (Hancock, 1977a). These ultra-slow pressure waves occur just over once per minute, in distinction to the usual wave activity found at 16 cycles per minute. These waveforms have also been detected in the electrical recordings from this region. Ultra-slow waves are present in from 5 per cent (Hancock, 1977a) to 30 per cent (Wankling *et al.,* 1968) of normal subjects. However, both of these are much below the incidence found in patients with haemorrhoids, ranging from 44 per cent to 80 per cent. An increase in the resting pressure within the anal canal is also found in patients with haemorrhoids. Both the increase in ultra-slow waves and the increase in basal pressure are relieved in patients submitted to forcible anal canal distension in the treatment of haemorrhoids (Lord's procedure; Hancock and Smith, 1975). The significant decrease in pressure after this procedure was not found in a more recent study (Ortiz *et al.,* 1978), where standard Milligan Morgan haemorrhoidectomy gave a significant decrease, confirming previous work showing that patients after standard haemorrhoidectomy show no significant difference in the anal canal pressure characteristics from those of normal subjects (Bennett and Duthie, 1965).

Anal Fissure

The clinical finding of spasm of the anal sphincters on digital examination in the presence of an acute fissure in ano is in contrast with measurements of the resting pressure in the anal canal made with a fine polythene tube in patients with spasm. The anal canal pressure was not significantly higher than in normal subjects (Duthie and Bennett, 1964), and it was concluded that the spasm of the sphincter was only important when the anal canal was distended by the passage of faeces and that the effect of sphincter stretching, which was shown to be transient over 8 days, was in abolishing this spasm rather than reducing a high resting pressure. When anal sphincter pressure in patients with fissure in ano were studied by use of balloons, a higher resting pressure was found, to some extent explicable by the larger diameter of the recording apparatus (Nothman and Schuster, 1974; Hancock, 1977b). Other abnormalities were also discovered which were held to point to disturbance of internal sphincter function. Nothman and Schuster found that the normal relaxation of the upper part of the anal sphincters to rectal distension was accompanied by an overshoot in patients

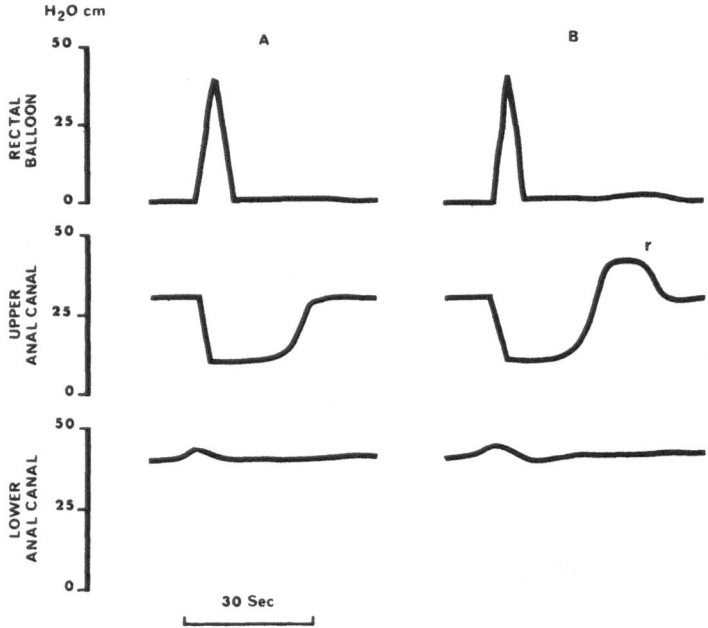

Figure 10.7 A: Normal internal sphincter inhibition (upper anal canal pressure) response to rectal distension with transient external sphincter contraction (lower anal canal pressure) B: In a patient with fissure in ano a rebound (r) occurs in internal sphincter pressure following the relaxation. (Redrawn from Nothman and Schuster, 1974.)

with fissure (figure 10.7). In another study using a balloon, Hancock (1977b) found a high incidence of ultra-slow waves (as mentioned above under 'Haemorrhoids') in patients with anal fissure. Thus, there is manometric evidence of internal sphincter dysfunction which may help to explain the clinical results of lateral sphincterotomy, classical internal sphincterotomy or sphincter stretching, which are all efficacious ways of treating fissure in ano.

Hirschsprung's Disease

It is well established that the reflex inhibition of the internal anal sphincter produced by distension of the rectum is absent in cases of Hirschsprung's disease (Lawson and Nixon, 1967). This provides a useful diagnostic test to distinguish it from megarectum when the reflex is present (Meunier *et al.*, 1976). However, these latter patients have a grossly impaired rectal sensation which allows of accumulation of faeces in the rectum and encopresis. The use of manometric tests to diagnose Hirschsprung's disease must be qualified by the finding that it takes some days after birth for the majority of infants to develop the reflex, reaching 100 per cent of cases after 12 days (Holschneider *et al.*, 1976).

Restorative Resection of the Rectum

With the increasing popularity of sphincter-preserving operations for low rectal growths, opportunity has arisen to assess postoperative sphincteric function both symptomatically and manometrically. In the classical low anterior resection completed from the abdominal approach, it has been shown that distension of the colon which is brought down to provide the anastomosis in the pelvis can give rise to reflex inhibition of the internal anal sphincter (Goligher *et al.*, 1965). On the other hand, the abdominoanal pull-through technique seems to disturb the function of the sphincters, because eversion of the anal canal is required in this operative procedure and the reflex response of the sphincters is impaired considerably. By use of the transanal technique to provide a very low anastomosis, continence can be preserved in the majority of patients, and while sphincteric function is impaired a month following operation, on testing at a year or more normal response of sphincteric inhibition to distension in the colon was found in the majority of patients (Lane and Parks, 1977). As observed before, the previous concept that normal rectal sensation is essential for this reflex has to be modified to include the suggestion that endings in the pelvic floor itself will provide the afferent sensory part for the reflex.

Incontinence

In addition to the above studies in patients after rectal resection, information concerning the basic mechanism of anal continence has been derived from subjects with various neurological lesions and after local regional block (Ihre, 1974). Comparison of groups of patients who are continent with those who have deficient function has been done using several methods of measurement. In patients with intussusception of the rectum who were incontinent internal anal sphincter function was held to be deficient (Frenckner and Ihre, 1976). When lesions involving the sacral nerves were considered, it was found that the external sphincter complex could be maintained if at least one root at the second sacral segmental level was left intact, whereas the internal sphincter reflex was unaffected (Gunterberg et al., 1976). Similarly, in men with spinal injuries it was found that the internal sphincter reflex was intact and the external sphincter electromyogram was more easily stimulated and inhibited by balloon distension than when the spinal cord was intact. In patients with operative treatment of congenital defects in this area—in particular, imperforate anus—the degree of the continence correlates with the number of abnormalities detected with manometric studies (Taylor et al., 1973; Ahran et al., 1976). When histological studies are made of the striated muscle in the external anal sphincteric complex in patients with incontinence, a pattern of partial denervation is observed which in patients with rectal prolapse has been suggested to be secondary to straining with an effect on the pudendal or perineal nerves (Parks et al., 1977).

SUMMARY

The function of the anal sphincters is dependent on their intimate anatomical relationship with one another and with the muscles of the pelvic floor, and the change in direction of the rectal axis making an angle of 80° with the anal canal axis. These relationships, combined with the sensory information derived from the anal canal, the pelvic floor and the rectal ampulla, provide the basis for the maintenance of continence. It is generally agreed that at rest the internal anal sphincter has a larger role in maintaining the pressure within the anal canal and that in periods of stress the external anal sphincter can provide voluntary support which can be maintained for up to a minute.

Pathological changes in the area, notably those secondary to minor surgical procedures, fortunately only provide a slight disruption to the sphincteric mechanism, and most patients are completely continent. When larger operations are undertaken (in particular, rectal resections), the effects can be minimised if the operative technique does not disrupt the connections of the internal and external anal sphincters.

REFERENCES

Ahran, P., Faverdin, C., Devroede, G., Dubois, F., Coupris, L. and Pellerin, D. (1976). Manometric assessment of continence after surgery for imperforate anus. *J. Pediat. Surg.,* **11,** 157-166

Bennett, R. C. and Duthie, H. L. (1965). Pressure and sensation in the anal canal after minor anorectal procedures. *Dis. Colon Rectum,* **8,** 131-136

Collins, C. D., Brown, B. H., Whittaker, G. E. and Duthie, H. L. (1969). New method of measuring forces in the anal canal. *Gut,* **10,** 160-163

Duthie, H. L. (1975). Dynamics of the rectum and anus. *Clin. Gastroenterol.,* **3,** 467-477

Duthie, H. L. and Bennett, R. C. (1964). Anal sphincter pressure in fissure in ano. *Surg., Gynec. Obstet.,* **119,** 19-21

Duthie, H. L. and Gairns, F. W. (1960). Sensory nerve-endings and sensation in the anal region of man. *Br. J. Surg.,* **47,** 585-595

Duthie, H. L. and Watts, J. M. (1965). Contribution of the external anal sphincter to the pressure zone in the anal canal. *Gut,* **6,** 64-68

Frenckner, B. (1975). Function of the anal sphincters in spinal man. *Gut,* **16,** 638-644

Frenckner, B. and Ihre, T. (1976). Function of the anal sphincters in patients with intussusception of the rectum. *Gut,* **17,** 147-151

Goligher, J. C., Duthie, H. L., DeDombal, F. T. and Watts, J. M. (1965). Abdomino-anal pull-through excision for tumours of the mid-third of the rectum. A comparison with low anterior resection. *Br. J. Surg.,* **52,** 323-335

Goligher, J. C., Leacock, A. G. and Brossy, J-J (1955). The surgical anatomy of the anal canal. *Br. J. Surg.,* **43,** 51-61

Gunterberg, B., Kewenter, J., Petersen, I. and Stener, B. (1976). Anorectal function after major resections of the sacrum with bilateral or unilateral sacrifice of sacral nerves. *Br. J. Surg.,* **63,** 546-554

Hancock, B. D. (1977a). Internal sphincter and the nature of haemorrhoids. *Gut,* **18,** 651-655

Hancock, B. D. (1977b). The internal anal sphincter and anal fissure. *Br. J. Surg.,* **64,** 92-95

Hancock, B. D. and Smith, K. (1975). The internal sphincter and Lord's procedure for haemorrhoids. *Br. J. Surg.,* **62,** 833-836

Hill, J. R., Kelley, M. L. Jr, Schlegel, J. F. and Code, C. F. (1960). Pressure profile of the rectum and anus of healthy persons. *Dis. Colon Rectum,* **2,** 203-209

Holschneider, A. M., Kellner, E., Streibl, P. and Sippell, W. G. (1976). The development of anorectal continence and its significance in the diagnosis of Hirschsprung's disease. *J. Pediat. Surg.,* **11,** 151-156

Ihre, T. (1974). Studies on anal function in continent and incontinent patients. *Scand. J. Gastroenterol.,* **9,** Suppl. 25

Kawakami, M. (1954). Electromyographic investigation on the human external sphincter muscle of the anus. *Jap. J. Physiol.,* **4,** 196-204

Kerremans, R. (1968). Electrical activity and motility of the internal anal sphincter. *Acta Gastroenterol. Belg.,* **31,** 465-482

Lane, R. H. S. and Parks, A. G. (1977). Function of the anal sphincters following coloanal anastomosis. *Br. J. Surg.,* **64,** 596-599

Lawson, J. O. N. and Nixon, H. H. (1967). Anal canal pressures in the diagnosis of Hirschsprung's disease. *J. Pediat. Surg.,* **2,** 544-552

Meunier, P. and Mollard, P. (1977). Control of the internal anal sphincter: manometric study with human subjects. *Pflugers Arch.,* **370,** 233-239

Meunier, P., Mollard, P. and Marechal, J. M. (1976). Physiopathology of megarectum: the association of megarectum with encopresis. *Gut,* **17,** 224-227

Nothman, B. J. and Schuster, M. M. (1974). Internal anal sphincter derangement with anal fissures. *Gastroenterology,* **67,** 216-220

Oh, C. and Kark, A. E. (1972). Anatomy of the external anal sphincter. *Br. J. Surg.,* **59,** 717–723

Ortiz, H., Marti, J., Jaurrieta, E., Masdevall, C., Ferrer, J. and Sitges, A. (1978). Lord's procedure: a critical study of its basic principle. *Br. J. Surg.,* **65,** 281-284

Parks, A. G., Porter, N. H. and Melzak, J. (1962). Experimental study of the reflex mechanism controlling the muscles of the pelvic floor. *Dis. Colon Rectum,* **5,** 407-414

Parks, A. G., Swash, M. and Urich, H. (1977). Sphincter denervation in anorectal prolapse. *Gut,* **18,** 656-665

Phillips, S. F. and Edwards, D. A. W. (1965). Some aspects of anal continence and defaecation. *Gut,* **6,** 396-406

Porter, N. H. (1962). A physiological study of the pelvic floor in rectal prolapse. *Ann. R. Coll. Surg. Engl.,* **31,** 379-404

Schuster, M., Hendrix, T. R. and Mendeloff, A. I. (1963). The internal anal sphincter response: manometric studies on its normal physiology, neural pathways and alterations in bowel disorders. *J. Clin. Invest.,* **42,** 196-207

Shafik, A. (1975). A new concept of the anatomy of the anal sphincter mechanism and the physiology of defecation. The external anal sphincter: a triple loop system. *Invest. Urol.,* **12,** 412-419

Shafik, A. (1976). A new concept of the anatomy of the anal sphincter mechanism and the physiology of defecation. III. The longitudinal anal muscle: anatomy and role in anal sphincter mechanism. *Invest. Urol.,* **13,** 271-277

Tagart, R. E. B. (1966). The anal canal and rectum. Their varying relationship and its effect on anal continence. *Dis. Colon Rectum,* **9,** 449-452

Taylor, I., Duthie, H. L. and Zachary, R. B. (1973). Anal continence following surgery for imperforate anus. *J. Pediat. Surg.,* **8,** 497-503

Wankling, W. J., Brown, B. H., Collins, C. D. and Duthie, H. L. (1968). Basal electrical activity in the anal canal in man. *Gut,* **9,** 459-460

Yanchev, V. G. (1963). Anal tonometry. *Fed. Proc.* (Translation supplement), **22,** T110-T113

11
Editorial Summation

While the term 'sphincter' has been generally used in this book for junction areas between different organs of the gastrointestinal tract, it is accepted that alternative terms such as 'pylorus' and 'valve' have also been used to describe some of these specialised areas. None of these terms, however, seems totally applicable. In so far as flow through these regions is usually unidirectional, the concept of a valve is sound, but it has the disadvantage that it conceals the fact that some movement of content can occur normally in an orad direction. In addition, the mechanistic concept of a valve underestimates the innate variability of activity that some of these areas demonstrate. The term 'pylorus' literally means a door-keeper. While it can be employed broadly to describe the function of all these specialised areas, because it is used specifically to describe the gastric outlet its application to any of the other areas is precluded. This therefore appears to limit these areas to being grouped together as 'sphincters'.

What is a sphincter? It can be defined 'physiologically' as an area of the gastrointestinal tract which is tonically closed and has the ability to relax and contract. The best examples of this type of sphincter are the cricopharyngeal, gastro-oesophageal and anal sphincters. The biliary and pancreatic sphincters probably also fall into this category. However, the pylorus and the rectosigmoid junction, while they have the ability to relax and contract, are not always closed—and this has given rise to the concept of the physiological 'open' sphincter mechanism.

Alternatively, sphincters can be defined 'anatomically' as 'a thickening of circular muscle fibres in a hollow viscus'. This describes collectively all of the specialised areas apart from the gastro-oesophageal junction in man (although recent reports suggest such a thickening does exist) and the rectosigmoid junction.

Finally, in pharmacological terms the sphincter region can be identified by the so-called theory of 'reciprocal innervation' whereby sympathetic activity produces sphincteric contraction and parasympathetic activity induces relaxation—effects which are opposite to those observed on neighbouring gastrointestinal smooth muscle. This definition is sound for all smooth muscle sphincters but is not applicable to the cricopharyngeal and external anal sphincters—both of which contain striated muscle. It has to be accepted, therefore, that none of the definitions which are used at present is ideal but in the absence of a more unifying description a 'physiological sphincter mechanism'—most of which are of a closed variety (table 11.1)—seems the best compromise.

Table 11.1   Definition of sphincter mechanism

Sphincter	Physiological	Anatomical	Pharmacological
Cricopharyngeal	Closed	Yes	No
Gastro-oesophageal	Closed	No	Yes
Pyloric	Open	Yes	Yes
Choledochal	Closed	Yes	Yes
Pancreatic	Closed	Yes	Not known
Ileocaecal	Closed	Yes	Yes
Rectosigmoid	Open	No	Not known
Anal	Closed	Yes	Internal anal—yes
			External anal—no

In general, the gastrointestinal sphincters have two functions—they control the rate of transit of material through the alimentary tract and they limit retrograde flow or reflux. At first glance it seems probable that all of the sphincter regions offer resistance to forward movement of content, but on closer examination it is plain that normal transit patterns depend on some sphincters being open. For example, both of the oesophageal sphincters relax on swallowing, and the movement of food from mouth to stomach is dependent on the co-ordinated peristalsis of the pharyngeal and oesophageal muscles. In this respect, little is known about the function of the ileocaecal or rectosigmoid regions, although it seems likely that the patterns of flow through them will also reflect the pattern of more proximal activity. Relaxation of the pancreatic sphincter is unlikely to be linked to pancreatic duct contraction, as the latter has no smooth muscle. It probably reflects, in part, changes in pancreatic duct pressure, and this is dependent on the duct's compliance and the rate of pancreatic secretion.

The pylorus is perhaps the best example of an open sphincter which controls forward movement. Its sieve-like function allows only small particles and fluids to pass into the duodenum and forms part of an intricate mechanism controlling the rate of emptying of a solid meal by the stomach. It also protects the small intestine from larger, non-digestible solids during the digestive period, although these materials are subsequently emptied during the interdigestive phase of gastric motility. This differential emptying pattern of digestible and non-digestible solids is also a good example of the possible different roles that sphincters may play during the fed and fasting phases of gastrointestinal activity. The anal sphincter, on the other hand, is an example of a closed sphincter whose sole function is to prevent forward movement and thereby maintain continence.

The biliary sphincter appears to play both roles. First, in most species its tonic closure diverts bile into the gall bladder and allows concentration of the bile to occur. Second, in response to a meal-induced gall bladder contraction the sphincter behaves like the oesophageal sphincters by relaxing to permit of uninterrupted flow of concentrated bile into the duodenum.

It is generally accepted that sphincters of the upper gastrointestinal tract play an important role as anti-reflux devices. The best example is at the gastro-oesophageal junction, where the physiological sphincter (together with other anatomical components of the junction) is of vital importance because the abdominothoracic pressure gradient across the oesophageal hiatus favours acid reflux. It also seems important to stress that the anti-reflux function of any sphincter should not be regarded in isolation. The motor activity of the tract on either side of a sphincter seems, at least in some areas, to be well adapted to deal with any reflux that may escape sphincter control. For example, instillation of fluid into the distal oesophagus induces a secondary peristaltic wave which then clears the oesophagus. The rate at which the oesophagus clears instillate may be an important aspect of the pathogenesis of oesophagitis. Similarly, the rate at which the distal stomach returns duodenal content to the duodenum may represent an important mechanism preventing prolonged contact of duodenal juice with the gastric mucosa.

Apart from the external anal sphincter, all of the alimentary sphincters are controlled involuntarily. It is evident from the preceding chapters that detailed pharmacological maps of the various neurohumoral receptor sites at each of the sphincter areas are now available and they demonstrate that all of the smooth muscle sphincters contain autonomic and hormonal receptors. What is not clear is the exact role that these effector mechanisms play in the control of sphincter function. It is still not clear whether hormones have a direct physiological effect on sphincter smooth muscle—the critical experiments of cross-perfusion or transplantation of sphincteric regions are yet to be performed. It does seem likely that hormones will have a physiological role, probably as paracrine agents, because pharmacological experiments demonstrate that the muscle itself is more sensitive to the effect of these substances when compared with adjacent smooth muscle. Until it is possible to measure local tissue concentration of hormones, further advances seem unlikely. Correlating changes in circulating hormone levels with alteration in sphincter function looks now to be unrewarding.

It is the editors' view that further experimentation on sphincters may be helped by regarding flow through sphincters in terms of basic physical principles (figure 11.1). Flow in either direction will depend on the pressure differentials between two cavities ($P_1 >$ or $< P_2$) and the resistance offered to flow by both the consistency of the luminal content (D) and the closure tone of the sphincter (R). While applicable to all sphincters, the relative importance of each of these factors will vary according to the site.

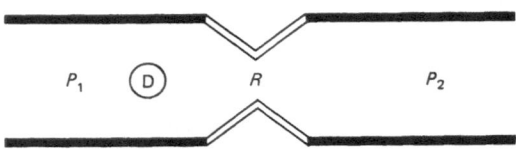

Figure 11.1   Flow through a sphincter will depend on the pressure differential ($P_1 - P_2$ or $P_2 - P_1$) across it, the sphincteric resistance to flow (R) and the physical form of luminal content (D)

With the exception of the anal sphincters, the pressures (P_1 and P_2) on either side of any of the other alimentary sphincters are continually changing. The hollow viscera adjacent to sphincters have contractible patterns which vary not only with site, but also with the digestive state of the gastrointestinal tract. It follows that the pressure differential across a sphincter at any one moment in time will be dependent on a temporal integration of intraluminal contractile activity on either side of it. Apart from the gastro-oesophageal and anal sphincters, changes in intra-abdominal pressure should affect the pressure on either side of the sphincter equally.

Simultaneous measurement of P_1 and P_2 over long periods will need to be made if profiles of the net motive force are to be obtained, and the volume of data so collected will probably make computer analysis mandatory. The chief practical problem at present is one of access, as it is at only the oesophageal sphincters, pylorus and anal sphincter that both P_1 and P_2 can be measured simultaneously with any ease. There is no way of measuring P_1 in studies on the pancreatic and biliary sphincters unless one resorts to post-surgical states or animal models. Similarly, in the lower alimentary tract both pressures at the rectosigmoid and ileocaecal junctions are difficult to measure under normal conditions.

The only available tool for measuring sphincter closure tone is an intraluminal pressure recorder. Strain gauge or myoelectrical recordings are alternative techniques but have yet to prove of quantitative use. Pressure recordings have been of great use in defining the relaxation and contractile activity in the oesophageal and anal sphincters, but their value as measurers of 'tone' is questionable. The accurate measurement of resting pressure (or tone) in a closed sphincter is impossible. The difficulties are expressed by the 'Heisenberg uncertainty principle', which states that one cannot make a measurement without at the same time altering that which one wishes to measure. The presence within a closed sphincter of a recording device distorts the sphincter muscle and thereby alters the pressure recorded—this explains the variable pressures that occur with probes of different diameters and different rates of infusion. It has to be accepted that at present no adequate means of quantifying sphincter tone exists. Intraluminal pressure recorders will continue to be used, but it seems important that standardisation of the diameter of the probes and the rates of infusion should occur.

For a given level of resistance to flow through any of the sphincters, the force required to propel intraluminal content through it will be determined by the physical nature of content. For example, solid particles will only pass if their diameter is smaller than that of the sphincteric lumen or if the force is large enough to dilate the sphincter ring. Solid intraluminal content is a feature of the upper and the lower alimentary tract, and it is perhaps no accident that the oesophageal and the anal sphincters all relax in anticipation of passage of a solid bolus, lowering the resistance to flow and obviating the need for a proximal contraction of even larger amplitude. It may be anticipated that the rectosigmoid junction will behave similarly. The pylorus is the only other sphincter which is normally in contact with solid particles, and has been shown to behave differently postprandially and during fasting in the way it handles such material. Only very small particles (< 1 mm) empty during the digestive phase, while larger non-digestible particles remain in the stomach. However, when cyclical interdigestive motor activity begins, these particles empty rapidly. The distal gastric contractions during fasting are of large amplitude and probably overcome pyloric resistance by forcibly distending the pyloric ring. Liquids, on the other hand, will pass more easily as long as the force exerted on either side of the sphincter is sufficient to overcome sphincteric resistance. The direction of flow will be determined by the direction of the pressure gradient.

When flow across sphincters is studied, the 'markers' used need to reflect accurately the nature of the materials which are known to normally flow through the area of study. In this respect, lessons have been learnt from gastric emptying studies. It is now recognised that in an organ which empties the varying components of intraluminal content at different rates, the markers of flow need to form an integral part of the content under study. The use of liver labelled *in vivo* with radioactive B_{12} as a test meal of emptying of solids is probably the only way of accurately measuring solid emptying. Any other markers mixed with the content probably empty in the liquid phase.

While there is no shortage of ideas on further experimentation, further advances are greatly dependent on technological improvements. The availability of radiotelemetry as a relatively non-invasive technique of recording motility patterns over long periods, scintiscanning as a measure of flow and endoscopy as a means of gaining access to the more distant sphincters would seem to provide possible ways of advancing knowledge of sphincteric function.

Index